ANNUAL REVIEW OF NURSING RESEARCH

Volume 15, 1997

ANNUAL REVIEW OF NURSING RESEARCH

Volume 15, 1997

Joyce J. Fitzpatrick, Ph.D.
Jane Norbeck, D.N.Sc.

Editors

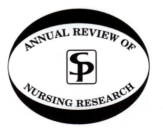

SPRINGER PUBLISHING COMPANY
New York

Order ANNUAL REVIEW OF NURSING RESEARCH, Volume 16, 1998, prior to publication and receive a 10% discount. An order coupon can be found at the back of this volume.

Springer Publishing Company, Inc.
536 Broadway
New York, NY 10012

97 98 99 00 01 / 5 4 3 2 1

ISBN-0-8261-8234-8
ISSN-0739-6686

ANNUAL REVIEW OF NURSING RESEARCH is indexed in *Cumulative Index to Nursing and Allied Health Literature* and *Index Medicus.*

Printed in the United States of America

Contents

Preface

We have reached another landmark in the *Annual Review of Nursing Research (ARNR)* series: This is the fifteenth volume. During the past decade and a half we have witnessed the remarkable development of the discipline of nursing and a considerable expansion of nursing research.

Volume 15 includes several chapters in the area of nursing practice. Diane Holditch-Davis and Margaret Miles have critiqued the research on parenting the prematurely born child. Diane Cronin-Stubbs reviewed research on interventions for cognitive impairment and neurobehavioral disturbances of older adults. Research on uncertainty in acute illness is reviewed by Merle Mishel and violence in the workplace is reviewed by Jeanne Hewitt and Pamela Levin. Jean Goeppinger and Kate Lorig have critiqued the research on interventions to reduce the impact of chronic disease, with attention to community-based arthritis patient education. Susan Riesch reviewed the area of parent–adolescent communication in nondistressed families and Felissa Cohen analyzed nursing research on tuberculosis.

One chapter is included in the section on nursing care delivery. Sally Lusk critiqued research on health promotion and disease prevention in the worksite. Two general chapters and one international chapter are included in the other research section. Quincealea Brunk reviewed historical research on nursing during wars and Janet Fulton critiqued research on long-term vascular access devices. We are pleased to have an international chapter included in this volume. Shyang-Yun Pamela Koong Shiao and Yu-Mei Yu Chao have reviewed nursing research in Taiwan.

This volume marks the conclusion of the current Advisory Board Members' terms. We are indebted to all of them for the expert direction and leadership they have demonstrated during the past several volumes. Volume 15 also marks the end of Jane Norbeck's term as coeditor. I have very much appreciated her colleagueship and her outstanding contributions to not only the editing process, but most especially to the scholarly pursuits for nursing.

One other important transition occurs with this volume: After 12 years of work on *ARNR*, Nikki Polis is stepping down as Associate Editor. Nikki worked with me on the *ARNR* series even before I assumed the role of senior editor. Many of you are well aware of her behind-the-scenes orchestration of the multiple levels of work related to the series. I cannot thank her enough.

Plans for Volume 16 are well under way; it will have a special focus on nursing research in health promotion. We look forward to continuing to highlight significant areas for nursing research. Please let us know your thoughts and suggestions for topics for review.

Joyce J. Fitzpatrick
Senior Editor

Contributors

Quincealea Brunk, PhD
School of Nursing
The Pennsylvania State
  University
University Park, PA

Yu-Mei Yu Chao, PhD
Bureau of National Health
  Insurance
Department of Health
The Executive Yuan
and
School of Nursing
National Taiwan University
Taipei, Taiwan, R.O.C.

Felissa L. Cohen, PhD
School of Nursing
Southern Illinois University at
  Edwardsville
Edwardsville, IL

Diane Cronin-Stubbs, PhD
College of Nursing
Rush University
Chicago, IL

Janet S. Fulton, PhD
College of Nursing and Health
Wright State University
Dayton, OH

Jean Goeppinger, PhD
School of Nursing
University of North Carolina
  at Chapel Hill
Chapel Hill, NC

Jeanne Beauchamp Hewitt, PhD
School of Nursing
University of Wisconsin-
  Milwaukee
Milwaukee, WI

Diane Holditch-Davis, PhD
School of Nursing
The University of North Carolina
  at Chapel Hill
Chapel Hill, NC

Pamela F. Levin, PhD
College of Nursing
University of Illinois at Chicago
Chicago, IL

Kate Lorig, DPH
Stanford Patient Education
  Research Center
Stanford University
Palo Alto, CA

Sally Lechlitner Lusk, PhD
School of Nursing
The University of Michigan
Ann Arbor, MI

Margaret Shandor Miles, PhD
School of Nursing
The University of North Carolina
  at Chapel Hill
Chapel Hill, NC

Merle H. Mishel, PhD
School of Nursing
The University of North Carolina
  at Chapel Hill
Chapel Hill, NC

Susan K. Riesch, DNSc
School of Nursing
University of Wisconsin-Madison
Madison, WI

**Shyang-Yun Pamela Koong
  Shiao, PhD**
Frances Payne Bolton School of
  Nursing
Case Western Reserve University
Cleveland, OH

Forthcoming

ANNUAL REVIEW OF
NURSING RESEARCH, Volume 16

Tentative Contents

PART I

Research on Nursing Practice

Chapter 1

Parenting the Prematurely Born Child

DIANE HOLDITCH-DAVIS
SCHOOL OF NURSING
UNIVERSITY OF NORTH CAROLINA AT CHAPEL HILL

MARGARET SHANDOR MILES
SCHOOL OF NURSING
UNIVERSITY OF NORTH CAROLINA AT CHAPEL HILL

ABSTRACT

The purpose of this chapter is to summarize the findings of the nursing research on parenting the prematurely born child. This research focused on eight general areas: impact of the home environment on infant development status, the relationship between premature infants and their mothers during the first 2 years, parenting during hospitalization, maternal concerns about infant discharge, fathering, subpopulations of premature infants, parenting after the first 2 years, and interventions to improve parenting. There is a need to strengthen the design and conceptualization of these studies, to move toward more intervention research, and to do research that is more culturally sensitive, especially toward fathers, ethnic and cultural minority groups, and the poor.

Keywords: Preterm Infants, Premature Infants, Parenting, Mothers, Fathers

Premature infants and their parents have long been of major interest to nurse researchers. Reviews of maternal–child and pediatric nursing research have found that studies of premature infants and their parents made up a significant proportion of the literature (Barnard, 1984; Beck, 1988, 1989; Walker, 1992). However, this interest in parenting is rather recent. McBride's 1984 review of parenting published in *Annual Review of Nursing Research* did not include any information on parenting premature infants.

The purpose of this review is to summarize the findings of nursing research on parenting the prematurely born child and to identify directions for further study. A literature search of MEDLINE was conducted to identify all studies written in English published in nursing journals since 1985 on parenting prematurely born children. Articles dealing exclusively with the infant or child, those in which parental report was used only to describe the child, or those that were focused exclusively on the emotional responses or stresses of parents were excluded. Articles focused on aspects of parenting not specific to prematurity also were excluded, even if some or all of the parents had premature infants, unless there were findings directly related to prematurity. In addition, nonnursing literature was reviewed to obtain additional articles written by major nurse authors. Nursing research articles written by major nursing authors prior to 1985 also are included in this review. Studies were considered to be nursing research if they were published in the nursing literature, if a nurse was one of the first two listed authors, or if a nurse coauthor had an ongoing body of research in this area. A total of 65 articles met these criteria.

As a result of this review, it was apparent that the earliest nursing studies of parenting the premature infant examined two areas: the impact of the quality of the home environment provided by parents on the developmental status of premature infants, and the relationship between relatively healthy premature infants and their mothers during the first 2 years after hospital discharge. Other areas of nursing research on the parent-premature infant relationship developed as extensions of these two areas of study.

EFFECT OF HOME ENVIRONMENT ON PREMATURE INFANT OUTCOMES

The association between the quality of the home environment provided by parents and the developmental status of premature infants was the earliest area of nursing research interest. Medoff-Cooper and Schraeder (1982) found that 42% of 26 premature infants between 4 and 14 months were at risk for developmental problems, but there was no correlation between developmental status and quality of parenting as measured by the home observation measurement of the environment (HOME) Inventory, an observational and interview tool that rates parental involvement, parental emotional availability, and characteristics of the home environment. However, there were correlations between HOME score and infant distractibility and mood. When these infants were 16 and 26 months of age, Schraeder and Medoff-Cooper (1983) again found no association between HOME scores and developmental outcome, but found that HOME scores were related to infant temperament.

In a series of reports, Schraeder explored the relation between development and home environment in a group of 41 preterm infants, about half of whom were White and half minority (Schraeder, 1986; Schraeder, Heverly, O'Brien, & McEvoy-Shields, 1992; Schraeder et al., 1990; Schraeder, Rappaport, & Courtwright, 1987; Tobey & Schraeder, 1990). During the first year, the quality of the home environment—as measured by the HOME Inventory— accounted for 67% of the variance in the mother's report of the child's developmental status with biological variables having only a minor impact (Schraeder, 1986). However, the percentage accounted for is unclear, because length of hospitalization was included as an environmental variable, though this variable is better operationalized as an indicator of the severity of the infant's illness. At 36 months, the quality of the home environment remained the most important predictor of the mother's report of development, followed by length of hospitalization and degree of intraventricular hemorrhage (Schraeder et al., 1987). Language stimulation and stimulation of academic behavior were the aspects of the home environment most directly related to developmental status. The quality of the home environment at 6 months was more strongly related to the mother's report of development at 48 months than demographic and medical variables, and equally predictive of 48-month learning abilities determined by an examiner (Schraeder et al., 1990). At 5 years, children who were more immature and hyperactive had caretakers who experienced higher levels of daily stress and less positive home environments (Tobey & Schraeder, 1990). Partial correlations indicated that daily stress affected child behavior through its effect on the quality of the home environment. At 7 years of age, the sample was compared to a matched group of children of normal birth weight (Schraeder et al., 1992). Again, environmental variables—age of mother at first birth and quality of the social environment— had the largest impact on academic achievement and global cognitive abilities. Birth weight, which differentiated between the full-term and premature children, did not significantly affect academic achievement and had only minor effects on cognitive abilities.

Feingold (1994) also studied the quality of the home environment, as measured by the HOME Inventory, for 30 prematurely born toddlers from low-income families (63% of whom were White). The HOME was the only variable correlated with the Bayley Mental Development Index (MDI). Maternal education was positively correlated with the HOME score, and maternal depression scores and infant birth weight were negatively correlated with the HOME score.

Censullo (1994) studied 47 premature infants and their mothers and 47 full-terms and their mothers. Mothers were married, middle-class, and primarily White. At 2 years, the prematurely born children scored lower on the Bayley MDI than did the full-terms, but they did not differ on the Psychomotor Developmental Index. The quality of the home environment, as measured by the HOME Inventory, was related to the MDI scores, and accounted for more of the variance in MDI scores than either infant characteristics or distal environmental factors (such as paternal employment and SES). These associations were stronger for the prematurely born children than for the full-terms.

Thompson et al. (1994) studied 102 premature infants with birth weights less than 1500 gm, and their mothers. Slightly more than half the infants were non-White. Multiple regression indicated that neonatal neurological insults and maternal stress were related to Bayley mental scores at each age; whereas SES and race, more general measures of parenting risk, were only related at 24 months. Psychomotor scores were related to neonatal neurological insults, gender, and maternal stress at 6 months, and to neurological insults, gender, and maternal education at 24 months.

Brandt, Magyary, Hammond, and Barnard (1992) followed 68 premature infants from initial hospitalization to second grade. The 35 children with learning problems displayed less positive behavior during a teaching situation at 8 months, had lower scores on the HOME inventory at 24 months, and lived in families with more stresses—particularly financial problems and maternal job loss—at 8 years than did the children without learning problems. The 17 children with behavioral/emotional problems (14 of whom also had learning problems) displayed less positive behavior during a teaching situation at 8 months and lived in a family with more stress—problematic marriages, death of a close family member, problems with maternal job, financial problems, and problems finding time for family recreation—at 8 years.

Thus, there is evidence from a variety of nursing studies that the quality of parenting and the home environment, as measured by the HOME Inventory, is related to the cognitive development and the occurrence of behavioral problems in prematurely born children. These findings are consistent with that of an extensive literature from other disciplines (see for example, Aylward, 1992; Aylward, Pfeiffer, Wright, & Verhurst, 1989; Hack et al., 1992). However, the HOME Inventory, the primary measure of the social environment for all studies except Brandt et al. (1992) and Thompson et al. (1994), is essentially a screening tool that is designed to differentiate adequate home environments from inadequate ones. It provides little information about specific aspects of the home environment that might be modified to improve the outcome of prematures. In order to provide guidance for intervention studies, there is a need for research that utilizes sensitive instruments to examine specific aspects of the home environment and relates this information to the long-term outcome of prematurely born children.

Intervention efforts also need to be based in research that examines potentially changeable aspects of parents' experiences that impact on the quality of the social environment, thus on the infant's outcome. The relatively recent studies of Thompson et al. (1994) and Brandt et al. (1992), by examining the effects of maternal psychological distress and family stresses, provide a good beginning, but more investigation of this topic is needed.

To date, researchers studying the effect of parenting on premature infant outcomes have either used predominantly White samples, or have used samples of mixed racial groups without examining the effects of ethnic background. The social environment is known to have different effects on the outcomes of premature and full-term infants (Censullo, 1994). It would not be surprising if the social environments of premature infants from different ethnic groups had different effects on outcomes. Thus, studies with diverse samples are needed. In addition, all of these studies were limited to the mother. Although an initial concentration on the mother was probably justified, based on mothers' greater accessibility to researchers and their greater involvement in the caretaking of infants, the father and other family members also affect the outcomes of infants, and their impact needs to be studied.

MOTHERING DURING THE FIRST 2 YEARS AFTER HOSPITAL DISCHARGE

The mothering of premature infants during the first 2 years after hospital discharge was another early area of nursing research interest. The earliest nursing study in this area was conducted by Magyary (1983). Videotapes of mothers interacting with their premature infants of unspecified racial backgrounds were divided into four interactional patterns: both mother and infant interacting, mother only interacting, infant only interacting, and neither interacting. At 4 and 8 months past term, these dyads spent the majority of time engaged in an asynchronous social exchange, with an attentive mother and inattentive infant, or in disengagement, in which neither mother nor infant was attentive to the other. When both mother and infant were disengaged, the mother was much more likely to initiate interaction. It is impossible to determine whether these patterns were similar or differed from those of full-term infants and their mothers since no full-term comparison group was included in this study.

Barnard, Bee, and Hammond (1984) rated the behavior of mothers and infants of unspecified racial backgrounds during brief play and teaching situations at 4 months, 8 months, and 24 months past term. These researchers found that mothers of prematures provided fewer positive and negative messages, used fewer techniques, and used less facilitation in a teaching situation than did mothers of full-term infants. Mother behaviors did not differ in the feeding situation. The differences between mothers of premature and full-term infants decreased over the first 2 years, but mothers of premature infants continued to be somewhat less involved with them.

Censullo, Lester, and Hoffman (1985) studied 15 White premature and 15 White full-term infants and their mothers during 3-minute videotaped interactions at term. The videotapes were scored for levels of interactive involvement, and spectral analysis was conducted on the scored data. Reliable rhythmic patterns were found for all mother–infant dyads, and there were no significant differences in the rhythmic patterns between premature and full-term infants.

Holditch-Davis and Thoman (1988) conducted 7-hour observations in the home during the first 4 weeks after term, during which they scored maternal and infant behaviors every 10 seconds. Ten White mothers of premature infants moved, talked to, looked at, and held their infants less often than did 28 White mothers of full-terms. The mothers of prematures did not differ from mothers of full-terms in the amount of stimulation they provided when with their infants, but they provided less total stimulation because they left the infant alone more.

Zahr (1991) studied the interactions between 49 premature infants and their low-income mothers over the first year; 88% of the infants were Black. Maternal caretaking skills, maternal affective behaviors, and infant behaviors were rated during play and feeding situations at 4 and 8 months. Multiple regression indicated that infant temperament was the most important predictor of interaction quality at both ages. At 4 months, mothers interacted more favorably with infants who were less dull, were more adaptable, and had higher birth weights. At 8 months, mothers interacted more favorably with more difficult infants than with infants with easier temperaments. It is impossible to determine whether these patterns differed from those of full-term infants and their mothers because no full-term comparison group was studied.

Maternal characteristics have also been found to affect the quality of caregiving provided for premature infants. Engelke and Engelke (1992) found that for 109 premature infants treated in an NICU (65% of whom were African American), the quality of the home environment at 6 months, as measured by the HOME Inventory, was positively related to an internal locus of control for parenting and to higher socioeconomic status. Specific subscales of the HOME had different predictors. For example, maternal responsivity was related to maternal age, parity, parenting locus of control, and infant gender; provision of play material and maternal involvement were related only to SES and parenting locus of control.

Gross, Rocissano, and Roncoli (1989) found that 62 mothers of prematurely born toddlers (mean age 20 months; 77% White) did not differ from 70 mothers of toddlers born at term (96% White) in their perception of the effectiveness of their parenting. For the mothers of prematures, parenting confidence was positively related to child-care experience and child age, and negatively related to cerebral palsy; for mothers of full-terms, it was positively related to child-care experience, birth weight, maternal age, maternal education, and ethnic group.

Vasquez (1995) conducted a qualitative study of the perceptions of 10 married couples and 4 single mothers of unspecified ethnic backgrounds about the first 5 months at home with a very low-birth-weight infant. Although this study included fathers, their data was combined with their wives', so it was impossible to determine whether fathers had any unique views of this time period. Immediately after discharge, parents were focused on gathering the resources they need to care for the infant, and particularly on gathering information and finding ways to protect the infant. By about 3 months after discharge, parents gradually became less protective of the infant and became more involved in reciprocal interaction with the infant. Finally at 5 months, parents saw themselves as a family with the infant, became more comfortable taking the infant out in public, and began to worry about possible long-term sequelae. The degree to which these perceived changes reflected actual changes in interactions was not studied.

Thus, these studies demonstrated that the interaction patterns for mothers and their premature infants differ from those of full-terms and their mothers, although a number of similarities also were found (Barnard et al., 1984; Censullo et al., 1985; Holditch-Davis & Thoman, 1988). However, the extent to which these differences are beneficial or detrimental to the development of the premature infants is unknown. The behaviors of premature infants are known to differ from those of full-terms (e.g., Holditch-Davis, 1990; Holditch-Davis & Thoman, 1987) so there is no reason to believe that their interactive needs would be the same. This is an area that needs additional study.

In addition, the impact of infant and mother characteristics on mothering is unclear. Some researchers found that differences between mothers of full-term and premature infants in parenting could not be explained by either parity or maternal education (Barnard et al., 1984; Holditch-Davis & Thoman, 1988), but others found that quality of mothering was related to characteristics of the mother and infant, including maternal age, parity, child-care experience, locus of control, infant temperament, and infant health status (Engelke & Engelke, 1992; Gross et al., 1989; Zahr, 1991). In addition, influence of mothers' and infants' characteristics on mothering was different for premature and full-term infants (Gross et al., 1989). This topic needs to be studied more extensively, as does the impact of maternal emotional responses to the premature birth (e.g., Miles, Funk, & Kasper, 1992; Gennaro, 1986; Gennaro, York, & Brooten, 1990); attitudes about parenting (such as were studied by Gross et al., 1989); and perceptions of parenting on the mother–premature infant relationship (Vasquez, 1995).

PARENTING DURING THE INITIAL HOSPITALIZATION

The findings of differences in mothers' relationships with premature and full-term infants, and an association between the quality of parenting and premature infant outcomes, have increased interest in studying other aspects of the parent–premature infant relationship. Nurse researchers have explored the nature of the interactions between parents and premature infants during the neonatal hospitalization in order to identify the origins of the interactive patterns that differ from those of full-terms and parents. Several nurse researchers have investigated the visiting patterns of parents of preterm infants. Brown, York, Jacobsen, Gennaro, and Brooten (1989) studied parental visits and phone calls recorded in the medical records of 65 premature infants (79% of whom were African American). Giacoia, Rutledge, and West (1985) also used nurse-recorded parental visiting patterns of 167 infants of unspecified racial backgrounds, although they did not state whether they utilized chart review or had special parental contact logs. Both studies found that mothers visited and telephoned much more often than fathers. Only in the first week did the number of paternal visits approach the number of maternal visits (Brown et al., 1989). After the first week, fathers usually visited with the mother, but mothers also continued to visit by themselves. Parents of lower socioeconomic class, unmarried parents, those who lived greater distances from the hospital, those with higher financial costs per visit, and those who did not own a car visited less frequently (Brown et al., 1989; Giacoia et al., 1985). These two studies need to be replicated because it is unclear how accurately nurses record visits and telephone calls. Also, the visiting patterns of married fathers might be expected to differ markedly from those of single fathers, but neither study compared these two groups. Instead, they only compared mothers with fathers.

Other nurse researchers have studied parent–infant interactions during hospital visits. Yu, Jamieson, and Astbury (1981) had 38 Australian parents complete a questionnaire about their experiences during visits. More than 75% of mothers and fathers reported that they had touched, talked to, and cuddled the infant during visits. The only significant difference between mothers and fathers was that mothers were more likely to have changed the infant's diaper. However, self-reports were the only measure used to determine parental activities during visits, and thus, the estimates of parental activities may not have been accurate.

In a series of reports, L. L. Harrison videotaped mothers, fathers, and grandmothers of 36 preterm infants (2/3 of whom were African American) touching their infants during the first 2 weeks. Oxygen saturation was lower during parental touch, but only rarely was the decreased oxygenation clinically significant (L. L. Harrison, Leeper, & Yoon, 1990). Heart rate was not affected. Regression analyses indicated that infant gestational age had the greatest effect on oxygen saturation; birth weight and prior handling had the greatest effect on heart rate (L. L. Harrison, Leeper, & Yoon, 1991). L. L. Harrison and Woods (1991) found that parents used 14 different types of touches, with holding, stroking, and contact being most common. Mothers spent the most time touching the infant, and fathers the least. There were relatively few differences in the touch addressed to male and female infants, though male infants were held more. Infants younger than 28 weeks experienced shorter durations of touch and fewer touch episodes than older infants.

The interactions of nurses and parents with preterm infants were compared by Miller and Holditch-Davis (1992). Twenty-nine high-risk preterm infants (59% of whom were White) were observed once weekly. A single observation for each infant that contained a minimum of 2 minutes of parental care and 2 minutes of nursing care was selected for analysis. Results showed that nurses and parents provided different types of stimulation, with nurses more likely to engage in procedural care and parents more likely to hold, talk to, move, and touch the infants affectionately. Infants showed more sleep–wake transition, large body movements, and jitters when with nurses, and more active sleep and more smiles when with parents. Infants older than 33 weeks postconceptional age showed greater differences in their responses to parents and nurses than did younger infants. The different infant behavioral responses appeared to result primarily from the different stimulation provided by parents and nurses.

Oehler (Eckerman & Oehler, 1992) interviewed 12 mothers (10 of whom were White) about their interactions with their infants twice during the preterm hospitalization, at 2 weeks after discharge, and at 6 months corrected age, and videotaped them interacting with their infants. During the preterm period, all mothers reported attempting to get their infant to respond to them, and most believed that their infant did respond. The behaviors mothers perceived as responsive included eye-opening, reaching for or touching mother's clothes or hand, smiling, general body movements, and calming down when fussing. The most salient infant behaviors for the mothers were eyes—opening, looking, or closing—and sleep–wake states. Most mothers felt that the major benefit of the early interactions in the hospital was helping the infant get to know the parent. The mothers' knowledge of infant cues continued to increase after hospital discharge (Oehler, 1995). The mothers' behaviors during the interaction were fairly consistent over the weeks: at all infant ages, they primarily looked at the infant continuously, had pleasant or smiling facial expressions, and talked for 5–10 seconds of every 15-second period of interaction, but as the infant got older they spent more time in mutual engagement (Oehler, 1995).

In a related study, Oehler, Hannan, and Catlett (1993) interviewed 47 mothers (60% of whom were African American) of preterm infants weighing less than 1500 gm twice during the first 6 weeks after the infant's birth. Mothers reported significantly more positive emotions, confidence in their parenting, and knowledge of the infant's behavior at the second interview. More than half the mothers reported feeling angry, happy, sad, and scared at each interview. Mothers reported talking to and touching their infants to get them to respond to them. Eighty percent of the mothers felt that their infant responded to them at the first interview, usually by eye-opening, eye-orienting, and/or body movements. This percentage increased to 96% at the second interview. The mothers tended to attribute meaning to the infants' behaviors. At the first interview, less than a quarter of the mothers made no attributions of meaning, and almost half found that two or more behaviors had meaning. By the second interview, only 9% did not attribute any meaning to their infants' behaviors, and 70% found two or more behaviors to have meaning.

One of the most natural and unique ways for mothers to relate to their premature infants during hospitalization is through breast-feeding. In a series of studies, Meier demonstrated that premature infants can safely breast-feed at earlier ages than they can bottle-feed, with fewer decreases in oxygenation and no decrease in body temperature (Meier, 1988; Meier & Anderson, 1987; Meier & Pugh, 1985). Most mothers (79%) can express breast milk without contamination by pathogenic organisms and with only low to moderate level of colonization with nonpathogenic organisms (Meier & Wilks, 1987). However, ongoing culturing of expressed breast milk is recommended, as a small percentage of mothers developed at least one contaminated culture after exhibiting acceptable expressed breast milk (Meier & Wilks, 1987).

Mead, Chuffo, Lawlor-Klean, and Meier (1992) used these findings as a basis for providing support for a mother breast-feeding premature quadruplets. The infants were born at 34 weeks gestational age. Two began breast-feeding on the second day of life and the other two, who required ventilatory support, began at 1 week of age. In the hospital, all infants received both breast- and bottle-feedings, and all consumed as much or more milk while breast-feeding than when bottle-feeding. The mother identified the intensive, individualized assistance received from the research team as a major support during the in-hospital feedings; staff concerns that she would not be able to breast-feed all four infants was seen as the major barrier. The mother continued to both breast- and bottle-feed until the infants were older than a year.

Kaufman and Hall (1989) studied 125 English-speaking, Canadian mothers of preterm infants (98% White); 88 of these mothers chose to breast-feed and provided expressed breast milk and/or breast-fed their infants. These mothers perceived their social network, and particularly their husbands, as being significantly more positive about breast-feeding than did mothers who never breast-fed. Over the 9 months of the study, 62 mothers stopped breast-feeding; 43 of these never established effective infant suckling. The most common sources of support for breast-feeding were husbands and nurses. There was a direct relationship between the number of breast-feeding supports reported and the duration of breast-feeding.

Stainton conducted a series of case studies on the experiences of mothers of preterm infants. Hayes, Stainton, and McNeil (1993) analyzed a single 2-hour interview of a mother of a surviving twin who had been hospitalized for 6 months. During this interview, the mother disclosed that she was mentally rehearsing for discharge. She saw her experiences as shrouded in uncertainty, her infant as actively working to come to know her and to accept her, and her role as a mother as unclear. She envisioned discharge as cutting her off from the NICU and leaving her alone and vulnerable. Lasby, Newton, Sherrow, Stainton, and McNeil (1994) conducted nine interviews with a mother about her experiences with her third premature infant during the 113 days of the infant's hospitalization. They found that the mother engaged in a number of forms of maternal work, including being present to fulfill the infant's need for comfort and love, trying to find meaningful ways to think of the infant's birth and accomplishments, using downward comparisons, and accepting setbacks. Accomplishing this work while maintaining other roles required extensive commitment that allowed little time for herself. The nursing staff and other health care providers both supported and hindered this work.

Scharer and Brooks (1994) used a grounded theory methodology to examine the growing relationship between nine White, primary nurses and 10 mothers of infants with prolonged NICU hospitalizations (60% of whom were White). They found that there was a gradual shift of responsibility from the nurse to the mother. This process had four stages—nurse providing all care;

sharing of normal infant care; sharing normal and technical care; and parent providing most care—and was influenced by the medical status of the infant, family support, the nurse's expectations of the mother, and the relationship between the mother and nurse.

Miles and Frauman (1993) studied mothers of medically fragile infants, most of whom were premature, and the staff nurses caring for them. They noted that mothers and nurses are both concerned about and share a deep sense of responsibility for the infant. As a result, they experienced overlapping roles, and had to continually negotiate their roles, in caring for the infant.

Weingarten, Baker, Manning, and Kutzner (1990) compared White mothers of 28 premature and 37 full-term infants on perceptions of their infants in the immediate postpartum period and 6–8 weeks later. There were no differences in the scores of the two groups on the Broussard Neonatal Perception inventory at both time points. However, when the mothers of preterm infants compared their infant to a typical preterm infant, rather than an average baby, their scores were much higher, suggesting that mothers of preterm infants have a negative perception of the typical behaviors of preterm infants.

Finally, Zahr and Cole (1991) developed an instrument for neonatal nurses to rate the quality of mother–infant interactions during each hospital visit. Seven items measured parental sensitivity to the infant, and five measured the parent's competence in caretaking. Each item was rated on a 6-point scale, from "not observed" to "superior." This instrument was tested on a sample of 49 low-socioeconomic status, minority preterm infants. Although the tool was flawed, with very low inter-rater reliability, it did exhibit significant though low correlations with maternal parity and with ratings of maternal caretaking skills and affective behaviors during a play situation at 8 months. It was not related to infant behaviors in the play situation, infant medical variables, or socioeconomic status variables.

Thus, there has been extensive nursing interest in parenting during the initial hospitalization. These studies indicate that significant amounts of parent–infant interaction occur during hospitalization (L. L. Harrison et al., 1990, 1991; Miller & Holditch-Davis, 1992; Oehler, 1995; Oehler et al., 1993; Yu et al., 1981) and that interaction patterns developed during hospitalization affect later interactions and caregiving (Kaufman & Hall, 1989; Mead et al., 1992; Oehler, 1995). Parents generally value the times they interact with hospitalized infants (Eckerman & Oehler, 1992; Hayes et al., 1993; Lasby et al., 1994). These interaction patterns are affected by a number of factors, including nurses, socioeconomic status, marital status, distance from the hospital, parental gender, and social support (Brown et al., 1989; Giacoia et al., 1985; L. L. Harrison & Woods, 1991; Kaufman & Hall, 1989; Lasby et al.,

1994; Mead et al., 1992; Miles & Frauman, 1993; Miller & Holditch-Davis, 1992; Scharer & Brooks, 1994; Yu et al., 1981). However, more research is still needed to clarify these findings.

The most important area for future research concerns the changes in the relationship between parents and their preterm infants that occur throughout hospitalization and during the transition to the home. More research is also needed on the role of nurses in promoting—and at times hindering—interactions between parents and their preterm infants. Although fathers have been included in many of the studies conducted during hospitalization, this data has tended either to be compared or combined with that of mothers (e.g., L. L. Harrison & Woods, 1991; Miller & Holditch-Davis, 1992; Yu et al., 1981). Very few of the studies that examined interactive patterns in detail included fathers, and none were focused on identifying the interaction patterns of fathers. Research is needed that examines the unique role that fathers fulfill while their preterm infant is hospitalized. Moreover, only one study investigated the relationship of other family members to the hospitalized preterm infant (L. L. Harrison & Woods, 1991). Finally, more attention needs to be paid to the psychometric properties of the instruments used. Although most studies used strong measures, including observation and physiological measures, two studies were fatally flawed with unreliable measures (Weingarten et al., 1990; Zahr & Cole, 1991).

CONCERNS OF MOTHERS ABOUT INFANT DISCHARGE

Parents are often relieved and happy when the time comes for discharge from the hospital, but they also experience many distressing responses when they assume total responsibility for their preterm infant. Thus a number of nurse researchers have focused on parents at or following discharge. Most of these studies have evaluated the adequacy of discharge teaching and the concerns of mothers.

In a descriptive study, Kenner and Lott (1990) found that 10 parents were unprepared for their infant's discharge. Feeling little support for their parental role in the NICU, they were not prepared to take on their parental responsibilities at discharge. They felt they did not have enough information about infant care and that they did not know their baby very well. Furthermore, they experienced shock at discharge due to their continued fear that their infant would die and their perceived lack of preparation to care for a baby whom they still viewed as sick.

McKim (1993) conducted a descriptive survey focused on information and support available to 61 mostly White, Canadian mothers of premature infants. Mothers received much of the information they wanted. However, many did not receive needed information on infant colic, noisy breathing, "spitting up," "fussy periods," recognition of illness, when to take the baby outside, behavioral responses, and other relatively normal child care information. Maternal confidence in caregiving and anxiety level were significantly related.

Butts et al. (1988) studied parent-initiated telephone calls after the discharge, using a primarily African American sample. The 36 mothers in the study called because of concerns about infant health, normal infant care, reporting and soliciting information about the infant's condition, and parenting. These mothers wanted reassurance that what they observed in their infants was normal and that their care was appropriate. The same researchers reported on concerns expressed by 65 primarily African American mothers during interviews conducted from discharge to 6 months postterm (Gennaro, Zukowsky, Brooten, Lowell, & Visco, 1990). Infant health was by far the most frequent concern, followed by infant weight and development. The number of health concerns was highest at birth, with a slow decline until 6 months. Mothers with less education expressed significantly fewer concerns.

The concerns about their infants expressed by mothers of prematures and full-terms also differed. At 2 weeks after hospital discharge, Goodman and Sauve (1985) found that although 30 mostly White mothers of full-term infants had concerns similar to those of 30 mostly White mothers of prematures, the latter had more concerns and a higher level of concerns. All mothers were concerned about feeding, gastrointestinal problems, sleeping, crying, attachment, and rashes. However, only mothers of preterms were concerned about the infant's appearance, and mothers of normal newborns tended to have more positive perceptions of their child.

Drake (1995) studied the discharge teaching needs of 10 mothers of premature infants (75% of whom were White). The mothers' priorities for discharge teaching included a response to infant apnea, temperature-taking, identification of illness, long-term health problems, and feeding. Nurses also identified all of these except temperature-taking as priorities, and also felt that teaching mothers where to call with questions was a priority.

Except for the work of Butts et al. (1988) and Gennaro, Zukowsky et al. (1990), most of the studies on concerns and needs of parents following discharge were small descriptive studies. However, the findings suggest that parents experience many concerns and related needs when the infant is discharged to their care. Mothers' concerns focus both on normal infant care and on the special health needs of premature infants. On the other hand, much additional research is needed to determine how mothers handle their concerns and how these concerns change over the first weeks and months after discharge.

In addition, these studies rarely included fathers or other family members, suggesting that researchers do not view fathers as involved with the infant's care at discharge or view father's concerns as affecting the family. Moreover, no study examined parental concerns and needs to determine difference by ethnic group or by socioeconomic status. Clearly, larger, multisite, and longitudinal studies are needed to further identify parental discharge needs and to develop and evaluate effective interventions for parents at discharge.

Fathering in the First 2 Years After Term

Although the mothers of prematures have generally been found to provide less stimulation than mothers of full-terms (Barnard et al., 1984; Holditch-Davis & Thoman, 1988), less is known about the stimulation provided by fathers. Parke and Anderson (1987), nonnurses, suggested that father involvement increases in circumstances, such as premature birth, in which an infant's illness leads to moderately difficult circumstances that impair the mother's ability to care for the infant. The findings of nursing researchers support this suggestion.

M. J. Harrison (1990) compared married, English-speaking Canadian parents of 28 premature and 31 full-term infants on the Nursing Child Assessment Teaching Scale (NCATS) 3 months after the infant's discharge from the hospital. Fathers of prematures had significantly more positive interactions than fathers of full-term infants, but the interactive scores of the mothers did not differ. In addition, mothers reported that fathers of prematures provided more caregiving, although this difference was not significant.

Using a self-report questionnaire, Brown, Rustia, and Schappert (1991) found that 18 fathers of prematures performed more infant care activities and were better adjusted to fatherhood than 18 fathers of full-term infants in the first month after hospital discharge. By 3 months after discharge, the amount of care provided by the two groups of fathers and their adjustment to parenting did not differ. All fathers were cohabiting with the mothers of their infants; their ethnic backgrounds were not specified.

Thus, the findings of the two nursing research studies on fathers' relationships with premature infants support Parke and Anderson's (1987) hypothesis that fathers are more involved with premature infants than with full-terms. However, in view of the small sample sizes of these studies, their reliance on self-report measures, and the limited time periods covered by the studies, additional studies are clearly needed. Studies need to utilize the same complex interactive measures used in studies of mother–premature infant interactions, rather than just screening tools, such as the NCATS, or paternal perception scales. These studies need be longitudinal throughout the first year and to examine how mothers and fathers interact together to care for their infants, rather than merely comparing mothers and fathers. In addition, studies are needed on the roles of both married and unmarried fathers. If Parke and Anderson's (1987) hypothesis about the importance of fathers to the care of premature infants proves correct, the ways nurses relate to fathers during the infant's hospitalization will need to be altered.

INTERACTIONS IN SPECIAL SUBPOPULATIONS OF PREMATURE INFANTS AND PARENTS

There is widespread agreement that premature infants and their parents make up a very heterogeneous population. The infants differ widely on gestational age at birth, birth weight, severity of neonatal illnesses, medical complications, and presence of chronic complications after discharge. Premature infants are more likely to be the result of multiple births than are full-term infants. Their parents differ on age, socioeconomic backgrounds, ethnic and cultural backgrounds, race, parenting experiences, and reproductive experiences. Each of these factors may have an important influence on parenting, but very few nursing studies have examined specific subpopulations of premature infants or their parents.

One exception is the work of Pridham on infants with bronchopulmonary dysplasia. Pridham, Martin, Sondel, and Tluczek (1989) videotaped the parents of 11 children under 36 months receiving followup care for bronchopulmonary dysplasia while they were feeding their child, and used the videotape as a stimulus for interviewing the parents. The ethnic backgrounds of these families were not specified. All parents had at least one feeding concern, including concerns about the child's tolerance of food, child's dietary adequacy, parent's adequacy as feeder, responsibility of feeding, normality of feeding, and enjoyment of feeding by parent and child. The parents mentioned that, in general, they became involved with their infant's feeding at the suggestion of nurses (Martin & Pridham, 1992). Although these parents used several strategies to prepare themselves for feeding at home, and believed they were ready for discharge, more than half reported that they were totally unprepared for their child's feeding difficulties at home. Neonatal nurses and physicians were the primary sources of help for these problems.

Leonard, Scott, and Erpestad (1992) examined the effect of home apnea monitoring on mothers' perceptions of their premature infants of unspecified ethnic backgrounds. At 2 weeks after hospital discharge, 19 mothers of premature infants on monitors had significantly more positive views of their infant on the Broussard Neonatal Perception Inventory than 13 mothers of nonmonitored premature infants. Their NPI scores were also slightly higher than those of 14 mothers of full-terms. The psychological distress scores of the mothers of nonmonitored infants were higher than those of the other two groups of mothers, though not significantly so. At 6 months after discharge, maternal ratings of their infant's social and intellectual development were significantly higher for the monitored infants than for the nonmonitored premature infants. The reasons for these differences between monitored and nonmonitored infants were not determined, although the monitored infants were 10 days older than nonmonitored infants at the time of discharge, and the apnea monitors might have reduced maternal anxiety about caring for their infant after discharge. The ethnic backgrounds of these infants were not specified.

Clearly, the area of special subpopulations needs much additional research. These three studies provide only a beginning. Much additional research is needed to determine the extent to which special subpopulations of premature infants are similar to or differ from other prematures. Although clinicians assume that certain types of premature infants elicit more negative responses in parents and are more difficult for parents to care for—for example, infants who have chronic lung disease, who are technologically dependent, who were very immature at birth, or who experienced neurological insults—there is virtually no nursing research to support these assumptions. It is possible that premature birth itself is so far from most parents' expectations that until they have an opportunity to see other infants, they can not conceive of infants who are sicker than theirs. Catlett, Miles, and Holditch-Davis (1994) found that, on admission to the NICU, virtually all mothers of preterm infants rated their infants as being as severely ill as it was possible to be. Likewise, certain groups of parents—for example, those who are young, poor, unmarried and/ or minority—are assumed to be less able to adequately parent premature infants. Research is needed not only to confirm or deny these assumptions, but also to identify positive parenting patterns within these populations, so that nurses can intervene more effectively. In addition, families experiencing multiple births need to be studied, because their needs and parenting practices may differ markedly from those of families of singletons.

PARENTING AFTER THE FIRST 2 YEARS

Relatively little is known about how preterm birth affects parenting after infancy. O'Mara and Johnston (1989) found that 47 English-speaking Canadian mothers of 3-year-olds who were born prematurely were more likely to be overindulgent, but not overprotective, than 47 mothers of children born at term. Twenty-four primarily White parents of preschool children who were born prematurely also expressed a number of concerns about the child's health and developmental outcomes and their difficult personalities (McCain, 1990).

In a recent study, Miles and Holditch-Davis (1995) explored how prematurity influenced mothers' perceptions of their parenting when their children were 3 years postterm. Twenty-seven primary caregivers of 30 children who were born prematurely (40% of whom were White) were interviewed about parenting experiences. These mothers were found to use a "Compensatory Parenting Style" in which they attempted to compensate the child for the neonatal experiences. Mothers viewed the child born prematurely as both "special" and "normal," and this parenting style was a way of resolving these apparently paradoxical attitudes.

Huber, Holditch-Davis, and Brandon (1993) examined the use of early intervention services by parents of 24 3-year-old prematurely born children (55% of whom were White). Although all but one child showed some developmental or health concerns, only four children were receiving adequate early intervention services at the time of the 3-year followup. Many had dropped out of developmental surveillance programs because of long travel times and long waits in the clinic. The rest had been discharged when their child reached a year of age without showing any major handicaps. Several mothers reported that they interpreted this discharge as evidence that their child was completely normal and would have no future developmental problems. Fifteen of these children were referred for further intervention, but only three families followed the recommendations. Most of the other 12 families said that they did not think the referral was appropriate for their child. Family problems—such as maternal depression and marital discord—were also a factor in the failure to follow recommendations.

Holditch-Davis and Belyea (1994) showed that the developmental status of 3-year-old prematurely born children (43% of whom were White) is related to the quality of parenting. Children showing normal IQ, language, or attentional status on average had more optimal behaviors during free play, received more social stimulation from their mothers during free play, and had higher Nursing Child Assessment Teaching Scale (NCATS) and HOME scores than children with developmental concerns. Both NCATS and HOME scores were higher for children with normal language abilities; only NCATS was significantly higher for children with normal IQs. Neither was higher in children with normal attention spans. Maternal behaviors during free play differed for children with and without developmental concerns only in the language domain, although child behaviors during free play discriminated between normal and low-IQ children and between children with and without attention problems.

Thus, the few studies conducted in the preschool period indicate that prematurity continues to affect parenting. In particular, mothers of prematurely born children perceive their parenting style differently than do mothers of full-terms (McCain, 1990; Miles & Holditch-Davis, 1995; O'Mara & Johnston, 1989), but there is no research to indicate whether parenting behaviors are also altered or whether any changes in parenting behaviors affect child outcomes. However, there continues to be a relationship between child developmental status and parenting. Not only are child developmental problems associated with poorer parenting (Holditch-Davis & Belyea, 1994) but parents may actually worsen developmental problems through denial and unwillingness to deal with them (Huber et al., 1993). Additional research is needed to clarify these issues. Research is also needed to examine the extent to which premature birth may continue to influence parenting through school-age years and adolescence.

INTERVENTIONS TO IMPROVE PARENTING

Nurse researchers have tested a number of interventions to improve the interactions between premature infants and their parents. "Kangaroo care," in which mothers hold their hospitalized preterm infants in skin-to-skin contact for prolonged periods, has been found to be safe (Gale, Franck, & Lund, 1993; Ludington, Thompson, & Swinth, 1992) and to have a number of beneficial effects for infants, including increasing the amount of quiet sleep over periods when the infant is alone in the incubator, early breast-feeding, and improvement in respiratory patterns (Ludington, 1990; Ludington et al., 1992; Ludington-Hoe et al., 1993). However, intubated infants weighing less than 1220 gm or with a postconceptional age of less than 30 weeks are only able to tolerate brief (20–30 minute) periods of kangaroo care (Gale et al., 1993).

Kangaroo care has also been shown to benefit parents. Affonso, Wahlberg, and Persson (1989) interviewed 66 mothers of premature infants in Sweden, 33 who experienced kangaroo care and 33 who had not. The control group's infants had been in the unit prior to the initiation of kangaroo care, and they were interviewed about a year and a half after the infants' discharge. The kangaroo care mothers were interviewed while their infants were still hospitalized. The control group mothers focused on trying to understand the things that had happened in the NICU, whereas the kangaroo care mothers were more concerned with getting to know their infant and developing a maternal identity. Kangaroo care mothers were ready to discuss their emotional reactions to the NICU while their infants were still hospitalized, whereas control group mothers reported that they were not ready to discuss their feelings for several months after their infants' discharge. Kangaroo care mothers were more likely to be breast-feeding at discharge than were control mothers (77% versus 43%).

Although these group differences are striking, they must be interpreted with caution because of the much longer time that the control mothers had had to reflect on their infants' hospitalizations and their greater experience in caring for their infants.

Gale and colleagues (1993) interviewed the primarily White parents of 25 infants who had received kangaroo care while still intubated. Both mothers and fathers felt that their experiences with kangaroo care were positive. About a quarter of the parents engaged in kangaroo care only once. Although they did not express negative reactions, they declined further offers of kangaroo care, citing inconvenience, feelings of embarrassment, or inability to see the infant's face. Fathers were more reluctant initially than mothers to engage in kangaroo care and spent less time in kangaroo care overall.

Although these findings indicate that kangaroo care has the potential to improve parent–preterm infant interactions, additional research is needed to confirm its benefits. In particular, it is not known whether kangaroo care has special advantages for parents and infants, or whether prolonged periods of parental holding would have similar effects. Also, research is needed to determine the degree to which kangaroo care is acceptable to parents and to identify strategies to increase its acceptability.

Another intervention tested by nurse researchers was active involvement of the mother in providing stimulation for the infant during hospitalization. White-Traut and Nelson (1988) studied 33 primarily African American mother–preterm infant pairs, divided into three groups. In the routine care group, mothers received instruction on premature infants' clothing; mothers in the talking group received the same instruction about infant clothing and were instructed to talk or sing to their infants for 15 minutes at specified time intervals; and a final group of mothers were trained to massage their infants for 10 minutes and to follow the massage with 5 minutes of rocking. There were significant differences between the groups in the amount of maternal behavior exhibited on a Nursing Child Assessment Feeding Scale administered a day prior to hospital discharge. The infant massage mothers exhibited the most maternal behaviors and the routine care group the fewest. Infant behaviors did not differ between groups.

In a series of reports, Zahr examined the effectiveness of providing a group of mostly African American mothers of preterm infants with weekly sessions with an infant development specialist throughout hospitalization (Parker, Zahr, Cole, & Brecht, 1992; Zahr, Parker, & Cole, 1992). During the sessions, the mother and developmental specialist observed the infant's behaviors using the NIDCAP and APIB tools (Als, Lester, Tronick, & Brazelton, 1982) and related them to the infant's needs. Control infants received developmental care plans without maternal involvement. Twenty-six experimental mothers and 15 control mothers were studied concurrently, but were not assigned randomly. The experimental group scored significantly higher on the Bayley mental scale at 4 and 8 months and on the Bayley motor scale at 4 months. The Home Inventory score for the experimental group was higher at 4 months.

Provision of education about the characteristics of preterm infants was another intervention tested by nurse researchers. L. L. Harrison and Twardosz (1986) compared three groups of 10 White mothers of preterm infants. The control group received standard nursery care; the instruction group received an hour's instruction about the behavioral characteristics of preterm infants; and the attention group received an opportunity to discuss nonmedical aspects of their infant's care with a nurse. The three groups did not differ on their perception of the infant as measured by the Broussard Neonatal Perception Inventory, the number of calls and visits they made to the nursery, their score on the HOME Inventory after discharge, or three measures of the quality of mother–infant interactions after discharge.

L. L. Harrison, Sherrod, Dunn, Olivet, and Jeong (1991) compared the effectiveness of instruction on the behavioral characteristics of preterm infants (about an hour in length), having the parent observe a researcher assess the infant on the Neonatal Behavioral Assessment Scale, and having the parent complete a rating of the infant's behavioral scale. Ten mothers received the entire intervention; 10 simply completed their own ratings of the infant's behavior; and 12 were in a control group. Two thirds of these mothers were African American. There were no differences among the groups on the quality of maternal behaviors during the Nursing Child Assessment Feeding Scale, though the total score for mothers who received the combined intervention group was somewhat higher than that of the other two groups. The two intervention groups did not differ in how they rated their infants' behavioral styles.

Another strategy was to provide nursing support for parenting along with education in the first few weeks after hospital discharge. Barnard et al. (1987) conducted a field test of the Nursing Systems Toward Effective Parenting-Premature (N-Step) program using 23 nurses in 6 states. They used the program with 76 mothers of premature infants, 72% of whom were White. Public health nurses made 8 visits to the mother's home between 37 weeks postconceptional age and 20 weeks after term. A specific curriculum was taught at each visit that included age-appropriate discussion of state regulation, infant behavioral responses, infant health, and family and community resources. Specific assessments were also made at each visit. At each visit, the nurses completed 90–98% of the protocol items. The mother's perceived social support did not change over the program period. There was a small but significant decrease in the mother's perception of family functioning over time. Significant increases in the mothers' sensitivity to cues and response to distress during a feeding observation, the mothers' cognitive growth fostering during a teaching observation, and the overall HOME Inventory scale occurred over time. Although these results suggest that the N-Step program is a promising intervention for mothers of premature infants, the lack of information from a control group makes any conclusions about the effectiveness of this program premature.

Kang et al. (1995) conducted a further field test of the N-STEP program with 327 mothers of preterm infants, 56% of whom were White, 21% Hispanic, 16% African American, and 5% of other backgrounds. Two thirds were married. These mothers were divided into high and low education groups based on whether they had more than 12 years of education. In the hospital, half of each group was assigned to an experimental group (instruction in providing appropriate stimulation for their infant) or a control group (instruction about car seats). After discharge, high-education mothers received no further intervention, but low-education mothers in the experimental group were randomly assigned to either routine public health nurse followup or the N-Step program; control group mothers received public health nurse followup. For the high-education group, scores on the feeding scale at 1.5 months postterm were better for the experimental infants, although maternal scores did not differ. At 5 months, both experimental mothers and infants scored better on the teaching scale. For the low-education group, the infants of both experimental groups scored better on the feeding scale at 1.5 months. At 5 months, mothers in the experimental group that received the N-Step followup scored significantly higher on a teaching observation than either control group mothers or the experimental mothers receiving public health nurse followup. Infant scores did not differ. These results suggest that the N-Step program may lead to a more sustained improvement in the quality of parenting for premature infants, at least for a mother with no more than a high school education, than does in-hospital teaching.

Kirgis, Godfrey, and McNeal (1991) provided a 4-week intervention to 43 predominantly White mothers of low-risk preterm infants. Nurses provided an opportunity for mothers to discuss their experience with the infant, provided education about preterm infant behaviors and activities to promote infant communicative abilities, and reassured the mothers about their ability to successfully parent the infant. The nurses used 10 different supportive acts, with active listening and sounding boards being the most frequent. The highest number of supportive acts occurred at the visit immediately after the infant's hospital discharge.

The research on interventions to improve the parenting of premature infants is quite fragmented, with most interventions being tested only in a single, small sample study. Thus, it is difficult to summarize these findings. These studies were also marred by methodological problems. Many of these studies either lacked control groups (Barnard et al., 1987; Gale et al., 1993; Kirgis et al., 1991) or did not use an appropriate random procedure for assigning experimental and control membership (Affonso et al., 1989; Parker et al., 1992; Zahr et al., 1992). All of the studies using experimental or quasiexperimental designs, except Kang et al. (1995), had small sample sizes (less than 20 per group) with inadequate power.

Also, most of the studies used outcome measures lacking in sensitivity (Barnard et al., 1987; L. L. Harrison & Twardosz, 1986; L. L. Harrison et al., 1991; Kang et al., 1995; Parker et al., 1992; White-Traut & Nelson, 1988; Zahr et al., 1992). The HOME Inventory and NCATS tools are designed to differentiate between inadequate and adequate parenting, but in many cases the goal of the nurse researcher is to improve already adequate parenting. Use of these tools by Barnard et al. (1987), Kang et al. (1995), Parker et al. (1992), White-Traut and Nelson (1988), and Zahr et al. (1992) may not have been appropriate. Both the validity and reliability of Broussard's NPI have been seriously questioned, and there is no reason to believe this tool is sensitive to change. Yet L. L. Harrison and Twardosz (1986) used this tool as a major outcome variable.

Few of the studies were clear about the theoretical bases of the interventions, including the specific parenting problems they were addressing and how the intervention would improve these problems. With the exception of the postterm education/support interventions, few investigators made any attempt to determine the extent to which the mothers actually took part in the intervention. All of the studies were focused exclusively on mothers. Intervention studies for fathers are needed. Thus, it would be premature to make any definitive statements about the value of these interventions.

There is one especially promising lead for future research. A variety of studies, including those on kangaroo care, massage therapy, and developmental care, suggested that when the mother is given a specific and ongoing role in the care of her premature infant in the hospital, parenting is improved. This needs further research. Also, the effects of other activities, such as breast-feeding, that might promote ongoing maternal involvement during the preterm hospitalization need to be explored.

DIRECTIONS FOR FUTURE RESEARCH

The amount and scope of nursing research on parenting prematurely born children parallels the intense clinical interest and concern of nurses in working with and helping these parents. The strongest and largest body of research focused on the mother–infant relationship and on parenting in the NICU. Research focusing on fathers, on parents from low-income and ethnic and cultural minority groups, and on parents whose infants have special health problems and complications was limited. Although on the surface it seems that nurses either intuitively or through experience know what parents of prematurely born children need and experience, there are, in fact, many avenues of research that need much exploration. It may be that this reflects a "failure to study what everybody already knows."

The quality of this body of research varies. Many studies reflected a strong theoretical base, strong designs, adequate sampling, and valid and reliable data-collection methodologies. Others were inadequately conceptualized, had small numbers of subjects, used weak data-collection methods, and had other methodological flaws.

Although there is extensive research, it is generally fragmented, and there is no cohesive body of knowledge. The research articles we reviewed were published in a wide variety of clinical and research journals within nursing and in other fields, particularly developmental psychology and neonatology, as well as interdisciplinary journals. Researchers generally developed their own individual directions, often influenced by other disciplines more than by nursing, and there was limited evidence of nurse scholars building on the work of others. In evaluating the overall body of research, we identified a number of major areas and approaches for future research, which are described below.

Because the assumption and attainment of the parental role with newborn infants is known to be a process that occurs over time, it is essential to study parental behaviors and responses of these parents over time to really understand the process and outcomes of this experience. Likewise, we need to link parents and infants conceptually or methodologically in the design of these studies. Studies are needed to investigate how parental responses affect parenting behaviors with the child both in the hospital and following discharge.

A major weakness of much of this research was the lack of repeated measures or longitudinal designs. Many of the researchers collected data at only one or two points. It is essential to use longitudinal designs that facilitate the study of the process of parenting, rather than looking only at brief windows of time. Links need to be made between parenting behaviors in the critical care period and parenting and the parent–child relationship during early and middle childhood. Studies are needed that follow parents from the NICU to community hospital care, if used, and to the home. Given that parents themselves are requesting that research on prematures continue through the young adult years (H. Harrison, 1993), it is essential that these parents and children be followed for longer periods of time.

Longitudinal studies would be strengthened by using more sensitive outcome measures for both parent and child outcomes. Given the importance and complexity of studying parenting over time, it is highly recommended that mixed methods of data collection be used; this might include, for example, several observational methods, self-report questionnaires, interviews, and assessment approaches.

Influenced by the theory of maternal role attainment (Koniak-Griffin, 1993; Mercer, 1985; Rubin, 1967; Walker, Crain, & Thompson, 1986), most studies have been focused on mothers. The study of fathers both in the hospital and after discharge has largely been neglected. Fathers are left out of the sample, are combined with the mothers for analysis, or are compared to mothers as if mothers were the standard for all parents. Conceptualization, data collection, and analysis need to be based on a fuller understanding of fathering in general and of fathering high-risk infants in particular. Again, well-designed descriptive studies would be helpful in delineating the father's unique responses and roles with the preterm infant. In studying fathers, tools that are appropriate and meaningful need to be used. Sampling should include both single and married fathers, and fathers from various socioeconomic and ethnic minority groups. However, careful analysis is important to appropriately evaluate possible differences in response and needs based on these variables and to use mother–father dyads when comparing responses.

There has been limited attention to the interplay between nurses and parents. Of particular interest is the nurse's role and relationships with the infant and parents, and how nurses influence parental responses and parenting. Finally, it is essential that we learn more about communication issues between parents and the entire health care team that may influence their responses, their needs, and their parenting.

Although research on the parent–infant relationship has generally been based on conceptual models related to parenting, there was a wide diversity in the frameworks used. Most investigators used frameworks developed for full-term infants. It would strengthen this body of research if conceptualizations appropriate for the parenting of premature infants were developed and tested. Well-designed descriptive studies would help us identify such frameworks.

Although many preterm births involve multiple births, no studies focused on any aspect of parental responses or parenting in the case of multiple births. Research is needed that explores both the impact of this experience on parents and the issues surrounding the parent–infant relationships and parenting of these children. Also needed is research that explores how the death of one or more infants in a multiple birth affects parents and parenting.

More and better intervention research is essential. Interventions during the critical care period in the NICU, at discharge, and following discharge are needed, with clear theoretical rationales for both the intervention and the outcome measures. The intervention must be carefully designed and measured, including the amount of intervention received. Outcome measures need to assess the effects on parental responses, on parenting behaviors, on the parent–child relationship, and on the child's health, behavior, and development. It is essential that outcomes be tracked to evaluate both short- and long-term effects.

A number of variables that may influence parental responses and parenting have not been adequately examined, particularly the child's health status both in the hospital and after discharge. It is assumed that infants who are sicker, smaller, and more handicapped are harder to parent (Koniak-Griffin, 1993). However, there is virtually no data to support this assumption. Thus, during the initial hospitalization, the infant's acuity, length of stay, and specific complications and critical events along with birth weight need to be considered carefully in design. Of particular importance is how parents respond to and are influenced by their infant's appearance, criticality, behaviors, and caregiving needs, including technological care. In longitudinal or followup designs, chronic illness or chronic health problems and developmental disabilities need to be evaluated in studying parenting and the parent–child interaction.

A major future direction for research is the cultural, ethnic, and social class differences in parental responses and parenting, and possible differences related to urban versus rural residence. Samples need to include adequate representation of parents from various ethnic minority groups, cultures, social classes, and places of residence. A surprisingly large percentage of studies of parenting the premature infants failed to even specify the racial and/or ethnic backgrounds of the participants. To date, no study has examined how cultural background influences parenting of premature infants. In addition, the analysis needs to be more sensitive to possible differences based on these variables. Using the White, middle-class mother as the comparative group or norm for these populations is no longer relevant. Cultural and ethnic differences and differences based on socioeconomic status and place of residence need to be explored carefully using ethnographic and other nonbiased approaches in design, data collection, and analysis. Advisory or focus groups of parents from these populations could be used also.

In conclusion, nurse researchers have made major contributions to the study of parental responses and parenting the prematurely born child. Within this field of research, their contributions have been important and substantial across disciplines. Still, there is a need to strengthen the design and conceptualization of these studies, to move toward more intervention research, and to do research that is more culturally sensitive, especially towards fathers, ethnic and cultural minority groups, the poor, and the rural poor. There is a particular need to develop sound conceptualizations, build on previous research, and develop a cohesive body of nursing knowledge that can guide practice. Neonatal, public health, pediatric, and other nurses working in a variety of settings and nurse educators who are teaching future nurses need to work together to develop approaches for using this research to improve practice.

ACKNOWLEDGMENTS

The preparation of this paper was supported in part by grants from the National Institute of Nursing Research, National Institutes of Health: Grant No. R01 NR02868—Parental Role Attainment with the Medically Fragile Infant, and Grant P30 NR03962—Nursing Support Intervention for Mothers of Preterm Infants, a pilot/feasibility study.

REFERENCES

Affonso, D. D., Wahlberg, V., & Persson, B. (1989). Exploration of mothers' reactions to the kangaroo method of prematurity care. *Neonatal Network, 7*, 43–51.

Als, H., Lester, B. M., Tronick, E. C., & Brazelton, T. B. (1982). Manual for the assessment of preterm infants' behavior (APIB). In H. E. Fitzgerald, B. M. Lester, & M. W. Yogman (Eds.), *Theory and research in behavioral pediatrics* (Vol. 1, pp. 65–132). New York: Plenum.

Aylward, G. P. (1992). The relationship between environmental risk and developmental outcome. *Journal of Developmental and Behavioral Pediatrics, 13*, 22–29.

Aylward, G. P., Pfeiffer, S. I., Wright, A., & Verhurst, S. T. (1989). Outcome studies of low birth weight infants published in the last decade: A metaanalysis. *The Journal of Pediatrics, 115*, 515–520.

Barnard, K. E. (1984). Nursing research related to infants and young children. In H. H. Werley & J. J. Fitzpatrick (Eds.), *Annual Review of Nursing Research* (Vol. 1, pp. 3–26). New York: Springer Publishing Co.

Barnard, K. E., Bee, H. L., & Hammond, M. A. (1984). Developmental changes in maternal interactions with term and preterm infants. *Infant Behavior and Development, 1*, 101–113.

Barnard, K. E., Hammond, M. A., Sumner, G. A., Kang, R., Johnson-Crowley, N., Snyder, C., Spietz, A., Blackburn, S., Brandt, P., & Magyary, D. (1987). Helping parents with preterm infants: Field test of a protocol. *Early Child Development and Care, 27*, 255–290.

Beck, C. T. (1988). Pediatric nursing research from 1977 to 1986. *Issues in Comprehensive Pediatric Nursing, 11*, 261–270.

Beck, C. T. (1989). Maternal-newborn nursing research published from 1977 to 1986. *Western Journal of Nursing Research, 11*, 621–626.

Brandt, P., Magyary, D., Hammond, M., & Barnard, K. (1992). Learning and behav-
ioral-emotional problems of children born preterm at second grade. *Journal of
Pediatric Psychology, 17,* 291–311.

Brown, L. P., York, R., Jacobsen, B., Gennaro, S., & Brooten, D. (1989). Very
low birth-weight infants: Parental visiting and telephoning during initial infant
hospitalization. *Nursing Research, 38,* 233–236.

Brown, P., Rustia, J., & Schappert, P. (1991). A comparison of fathers of high-
risk newborns and fathers of healthy newborns. *Journal of Pediatric Nursing,
6,* 269–273.

Butts, P. A., Brooten, D., Brown, L., Bakewell-Sachs, S., Gibbons, A., Finkler, S.,
Kumar, S., & Delivoria-Papadapoulos, M. (1988). Concerns of parents of low
birth-weight infants following hospital discharge: A report of parent-initiated
telephone calls. *Neonatal Network, 7,* 37–42.

Catlett, A. T., Miles, M. S., & Holditch-Davis, D. (1994). Maternal perception of
illness severity in premature infants. *Neonatal Network, 13,* 45–49.

Censullo, M. (1994). Developmental delay in healthy premature infants at age two years:
Implications for early development. *Journal of Developmental and Behavioral
Pediatrics, 15,* 99–104.

Censullo, M., Lester, B., & Hoffman, J. (1985). Rhythmic patterning in mother-newborn
interaction. *Nursing Research, 34,* 324–346.

Drake, E. (1995). Discharge teaching needs of parents in the NICU. *Neonatal Network,
14,* 49–53.

Eckerman, C. O., & Oehler, J. M. (1992). Very-low-birth-weight newborns and parents
as early social partners. In S. L. Friedman & M. D. Sigman (Eds.), *The psychological development of low birth-weight infants* (pp. 91–124). Norwood, NJ: Ablex.

Engelke, M. K., & Engelke, S. C. (1992). Predictors of the home environment of high-
risk infants. *Journal of Community Health Nursing, 9,* 171–181.

Feingold, C. (1994). Correlates of cognitive development in low-birth-weight infants
from low-income families. *Journal of Pediatric Nursing, 9,* 91–97.

Gale, G., Franck, L., & Lund, C. (1993). Skin-to-skin (kangaroo) holding of the
intubated premature infant. *Neonatal Network, 12,* 49–57.

Gennaro, S. (1986). Anxiety and problem-solving ability in mothers of premature
infants. *Journal of Obstetric, Gynecologic, and Neonatal Nursing, 15,* 160–164.

Gennaro, S., York, R., & Brooten, D. (1990). Anxiety and depression in mothers of
low birth-weight and very low birth-weight infants: Birth through 5 months.
Issues in Comprehensive Pediatric Nursing, 13, 97–109.

Gennaro, S., Zukowsky, K., Brooten, D., Lowell, L., & Visco, A. (1990). Concerns
of mothers of low birth-weight infants. *Pediatric Nursing, 16,* 459–462.

Giacoia, G. P., Rutledge, D., & West, K. (1985). Factors affecting visitation of sick
newborns. *Clinical Pediatrics, 24,* 259–262.

Goodman, J. R., & Sauve, R. S. (1985). High risk infant: Concerns of the mother after
discharge. *Birth, 12,* 235–242.

Gross, D., Rocissano, L., & Roncoli, M. (1989). Maternal confidence during tod-
dlerhood: Comparing preterm and full-term groups. *Research in Nursing &
Health, 12,* 1–9.

Hack, M. M., Breslau, N., Aram, D., Weissman, B., Klein, N., & Borawski-Clark, E. (1992). The effect of very low birth weight and social risk on neurocognitive abilities at school age. *Journal of Developmental and Behavioral Pediatrics*, *13*, 412–420.

Harrison, H. (1993). The principles for family-centered neonatal care. *Journal of Pediatrics*, *82*, 643–650.

Harrison, L. L., Leeper, J. D., & Yoon, M. (1990). Effects of early parental touch on preterm infants' heart rates and arterial oxygen saturation levels. *Journal of Advanced Nursing*, *15*, 877–885.

Harrison, L. L., Leeper, J., & Yoon, M. (1991). Preterm infants' physiologic responses to early parent touch. *Western Journal of Nursing Research*, *13*, 698–713.

Harrison, L., Sherrod, R. A., Dunn, L., Olivet, L., & Jeong, J. (1991). Effects of hospital-based instruction on interactions between parents and preterm infants. *Neonatal Network*, *9*, 27–33.

Harrison, L. L., & Twardosz, S. (1986). Teaching mothers about their preterm infants. *Journal of Obstetric, Gynecologic, and Neonatal Nursing*, *15*, 165–172.

Harrison, L. L., & Woods, S. (1991). Early parental touch and preterm infants. *Journal of Obstetric, Gynecologic, and Neonatal Nursing*, *20*, 299–306.

Harrison, M. J. (1990). A comparison of parental interactions with term and preterm infants. *Research in Nursing & Health*, *13*, 173–179.

Hayes, N., Stainton, M. C., & McNeil, D. (1993). Caring for a chronically ill infant: A paradigm case of maternal rehearsal in the neonatal intensive care unit. *Journal of Pediatric Nursing*, *8*, 355–360.

Holditch-Davis, D. (1990). Development of sleeping and waking states in high-risk preterm infants. *Infant Behavior and Development*, *13*, 513–531.

Holditch-Davis, D., & Belyea, M. (1994, June). *Prematurely born children at 3: Developmental status and interactions with mothers*. Poster session presented at the biennial International Conference on Infant Studies, Paris.

Holditch-Davis, D., & Thoman, E. B. (1987). Behavioral states of premature infants: Implications for neural and behavioral development. *Developmental Psychobiology*, *20*, 25–38.

Holditch-Davis, D., & Thoman, E. B. (1988). The early social environment of premature and full-term infants. *Early Human Development*, *17*, 221–232.

Huber, C., Holditch-Davis, D., & Brandon, D. (1993). High-risk preterms at three years of age: Parental response to the presence of developmental problems. *Children's Health Care*, *22*, 107–122.

Kang, R., Barnard, K., Hammond, M., Oshio, S., Spencer, C., Thibodeaux, B., & Williams, J. (1995). Preterm infant follow-up project: A multi-site field experiment of hospital and home intervention programs for mothers and preterm infants. *Public Health Nursing*, *12*, 171–180.

Kaufman, K. J., & Hall, L. A. (1989). Influences of the social network on choice and duration of breast-feeding in mothers of preterm infants. *Research in Nursing & Health*, *12*, 149–159.

Kenner, C., & Lott, J. W. (1990). Parent transition after discharge from the NICU. *Neonatal Network*, *9*, 31–38.

Kirgis, C. A., Godfrey, A. B., & McNeal, C. (1991). Nurse supportive acts for mother-preterm infant pairs. *Children's Health Care, 20,* 144–149.

Koniak-Griffin, A. (1993). Maternal role attainment. *Image: The Journal of Nursing Scholarship, 25,* 257–262.

Lasby, K., Newton, S., Sherrow, T., Stainton, M. C., & McNeil, D. (1994). Maternal work in the NICU: A case study of an "NICU-Experienced" mother. *Issues in Comprehensive Pediatric Nursing, 17,* 147–160.

Leonard, B. J., Scott, S. A., & Erpestad, N. (1992). Maternal perception of first-born infants: A controlled comparative study of mothers of premature and full-term infants. *Journal of Pediatric Nursing, 7,* 90–96.

Ludington, S. M. (1990). Energy conservation during skin-to-skin contact between premature infants and their mothers. *Heart and Lung, 19,* 445–451.

Ludington, S. M., Thompson, C., & Swinth, J. (1992). Efficacy of Kangaroo Care with preterm infants in open-air cribs. *Neonatal Network, 11,* 101.

Ludington-Hoe, S. M., Anderson, G. C., Simpson, S., Hollingshead, A., Argote, L. A., Medellin, G., & Ray, H. (1993). Skin-to-skin contact beginning in the delivery room for Colombian mothers and their preterm infants. *Journal of Human Lactation, 9,* 241–242.

Magyary, D. (1983). Cross-time and cross-situational comparisons of mother-preterm infant interactions. *Communicating Nursing Research, 16,* 15–25.

Martin, R. J., & Pridham, K. F. (1992). Early experiences of parents with their infants with bronchopulmonary dysplasia. *Neonatal Network, 11,* 23–29.

McCain, G. C. (1990). Family functioning 2 to 4 years after preterm birth. *Journal of Pediatric Nursing, 5,* 97–103.

McBride, A. B. (1984). The experience of being a parent. In H. H. Werley & J. J. Fitzpatrick (Eds.), *Annual Review of Nursing Research* (Vol. 2, pp. 63–81). New York: Springer Publishing Co.

McKim, E. M. (1993). The information and support needs of mothers of premature infants. *Journal of Pediatric Nursing, 8,* 233–244.

Mead, L. J., Chuffo, R., Lawlor-Klean, P., & Meier, P. (1992). Breast-feeding success with preterm quadruplets. *Journal of Obstetric, Gynecologic, and Neonatal Nursing, 21,* 221–227.

Medoff-Cooper, B., & Schraeder, B. D. (1982). Developmental trends and behavioral styles in very low birth weight infants. *Nursing Research, 31,* 68–72.

Meier, P. (1988). The effects of breast-feeding and bottlefeeding on transcutaneous oxygen pressure in small premature infants. *Nursing Research, 37,* 35–41.

Meier, P., & Anderson, G. C. (1987). Responses of small preterm infants to bottle- and breast-feeding. *MCN: The American Journal of Maternal-Child Nursing, 12,* 97–105.

Meier, P., & Pugh, E. J. (1985). Breast-feeding behavior of small preterm infants. *MCN: The American Journal of Maternal-Child Nursing, 10,* 396–401.

Meier, P., & Wilks, S. (1987). The bacteria in expressed mothers' milk. *MCN: The American Journal of Maternal-Child Nursing, 12,* 420–423.

Mercer, R. T. (1985). The process of maternal role attainment over the first year. *Nursing Research, 34,* 198–204.

Miles, M. S., & Frauman, A. C. (1993). Nurses' and parents' negotiation of caregiving roles for medically fragile infants: Barriers and bridges. In S. G. Funk, E. M. Tornquist, M. T. Champagne, & R. A. Weiss (Eds.), *Key aspects of caring for the chronically ill: Hospital and home* (pp. 239–250). New York: Springer Publishing Co.

Miles, M. S., Funk, S., & Kasper, M. A. (1992). The stress response of mothers and fathers of preterm infants. *Research in Nursing & Health, 15*, 261–269.

Miles, M. S., & Holditch-Davis, D. (1995). Compensatory parenting: How mothers describe parenting their 3-year-old prematurely born children. *Journal of Pediatric Nursing, 10*, 243–253.

Miller, D. B., & Holditch-Davis, D. (1992). Interactions of parents and nurses with high-risk preterm infants. *Research in Nursing & Health, 15*, 187–197.

O'Mara, L., & Johnston, C. (1989). Mothers' attitudes and their children's behavior in three-year-olds born prematurely and at term. *Journal of Developmental and Behavioral Pediatrics, 10*, 192–197.

Oehler, J. M. (1995). Development of mother-child interaction in very low birth weight infants. In S. G. Funk, E. M. Tornquist, M. T. Champagne, & R. A. Wiese (Eds.), *Key aspects of caring for the acutely ill: Technological aspects, patient education, and quality of life* (pp. 120–133). New York: Springer Publishing Co.

Oehler, J. M., Hannan, T., & Catlett, A. (1993). Maternal views of preterm infants' responsiveness to social interaction. *Neonatal Network, 12*, 67–74.

Parke, R. D., & Anderson, E. R. (1987). Fathers and their at-risk infants: Conceptual and empirical analysis. In P. W. Berman & F. A. Pederson (Eds.), *Men's transitions to parenthood: Longitudinal studies of early family experience* (pp. 197–215). Hillsdale, NJ: Erlbaum.

Parker, S. J., Zahr, L. K., Cole, J. G., & Brecht, M.-L. (1992). Outcome after developmental intervention in the neonatal intensive care unit for mothers of preterm infants with low socioeconomic status. *Journal of Pediatrics, 120*, 780–785.

Pridham, K. F., Martin, R., Sondel, S., & Tluczek, A. (1989). Parental issues in feeding young children with bronchopulmonary dysplasia. *Journal of Pediatric Nursing, 4*, 177–185.

Rubin, R. (1967). Attainment of the maternal role: Part I. Processes. *Nursing Research, 16*, 237–245.

Scharer, K., & Brooks, G. (1994). Mothers of chronically ill neonates and primary nurses in the NICU: Transfer of care. *Neonatal Network, 13*, 37–47.

Schraeder, B. D. (1986). Developmental progress in very low birth weight infants during the first year of life. *Nursing Research, 35*, 237–242.

Schraeder, B. D., Heverly, M. A., O'Brien, C., & McEvoy-Shields, K. (1992). Finishing first grade: A study of school achievement in very-low-birth-weight children. *Nursing Research, 41*, 354–361.

Schraeder, B. D., Heverly, M. A., & Rappaport, J. (1990). The value of early home assessment in identifying risk in children who were very low birth-weight. *Pediatric Nursing, 16*, 268–272.

Schraeder, B. D., & Medoff-Cooper, B. (1983). Development and temperament in very low birth weight infants: The second year. *Nursing Research, 32*, 331–335.

Schraeder, B. D., Rappaport, J., & Courtwright, L. (1987). Preschool development of very low birth-weight infants. *Image: Journal of Nursing Scholarship, 19,* 174–178.

Thompson, R. J., Jr., Goldstein, R. F., Oehler, J. M., Gustafson, K. E., Catlett, A. T., & Brazy, J. E. (1994). Developmental outcome of very low birth-weight infants as a function of biological risk and psychosocial risk. *Journal of Developmental and Behavioral Pediatrics, 15,* 232–238.

Tobey, G. Y., & Schraeder, B. D. (1990). Impact of caretaker stress on behavioral adjustment of very low birth-weight infants. *Nursing Research, 39,* 84–89.

Vasquez, E. (1995). Creating paths: Living with a very-low-birth-weight infant. *Journal of Obstetric, Gynecologic, and Neonatal Nursing, 24,* 619–624.

Walker, L. O. (1992). *Parent-infant nursing science: Paradigms, phenomena, methods.* Philadelphia: Davis.

Walker, L. O., Crain, H., & Thompson, E. (1986). Mothering behavior and maternal role attainment during the postpartum period. *Nursing Research, 35,* 352–355.

Weingarten, C. T., Baker, K., Manning, W., & Kutzner, S. K. (1990). Married mothers' perceptions of their premature or term infants and the quality of their relationships with their husbands. *Journal of Obstetric, Gynecologic, and Neonatal Nursing, 19,* 64–73.

White-Traut, R. C., & Nelson, M. N. (1988). Maternally administered tactile, auditory, visual, and vestibular stimulation: Relationship to later interactions between mothers and premature infants. *Research in Nursing & Health, 11,* 31–39.

Yu, V. H., Jamieson, J., & Astbury, J. (1981). Parents' reactions to unrestricted parental contact with infants in the intensive care nursery. *The Medical Journal of Australia, 1,* 294–296.

Zahr, L. (1991). Correlates of mother-infant interaction in premature infants from low socioeconomic backgrounds. *Pediatric Nursing, 17,* 259–264.

Zahr, L., & Cole, J. (1991). Assessing maternal competence and sensitivity to premature infants' cues. *Issues in Comprehensive Pediatric Nursing, 14,* 231–240.

Zahr, L. K., Parker, S., & Cole, J. (1992). Comparing the effects of neonatal intensive care unit intervention on premature infants at different weights. *Journal of Developmental and Behavioral Pediatrics, 13,* 165–172.

Chapter 2

Interventions for Cognitive Impairment and Neurobehavioral Disturbances of Older Adults

Diane Cronin-Stubbs
College of Nursing
Rush University

ABSTRACT

This synthesis of the research literature includes a discussion of selected neurobehavioral disturbances that accompany impairments in cognitive functioning in older adults. A combination of computerized and manual searches was used to access interdisciplinary and nursing research reports on the care and treatment of older adults who are cognitively impaired. The results demonstrated that protocols are needed that systematically integrate and evaluate extant working knowledge and evolving research bases for proactive preventive approaches to the care of cognitively impaired older adults with neurobehavioral disturbances.

Keywords: Integrative Research Review, Cognitive Impairment, Neurobehavioral Disturbances, Interdisciplinary, Nursing, Interventions

Interest in cognitive impairment among researchers coincides with the growth in the population of older adults, the decline in cognitive functioning attending cerebral degenerative diseases, and challenges to caregivers. This review is a synthesis of the research literature on the care and treatment of older adults who are cognitively impaired. After a general orientation to the field, with a discussion of selected neurobehavioral disturbances that accompany impairments in cognition, the past generation of intervention research is summarized and the current generation of studies on dementia and delirium is highlighted.

For this review, a combination of computerized and manual searches and a broad definition of cognitive impairment were used. Because both interdisciplinary and nursing studies were of interest, diverse databases were searched using the following keywords: cognitive impairment, confusion, dementia, delirium, pseudodementia, aged, older adult, elderly, geriatric, care, treatment, and intervention. Manual searches were done of the journals that were not indexed in computer databases; reference lists of reports that had been uncovered were scanned; and unpublished manuscripts were solicited from researchers in the field. From all sources, 332 reports were the basis for this review. For a detailed description of methods for searching and integrating the research literature, readers are referred to Cook and colleagues (1992) and Cooper (1989).

BACKGROUND

Dementia and delirium are the most common of the nine types of organic brain syndrome found in the older adult (Gomez & Gomez, 1989). Dementia and delirium are the descriptors of cognitive impairment in this review. Agitation and aggression occur in both dementia and delirium—agitation with greater frequency and aggression with potential harm to patients and caregivers. Agitation and aggression are the neurobehavioral disturbances reviewed.

Cognitive Impairment

Cognitive impairment, or disordered information processing due to alterations in brain physiology, affects the higher cortical functions of perception ("the ability to attend and meaningfully interpret sensory information"), memory ("the retention and recall of previous experience and knowledge . . . and the ability to store new information"), and thinking ("a conscious process that . . . includes abilities to understand, reason, make decisions, and apply judgment") (Neelon & Champagne, 1992, pp. 239–240).

Cognitive impairment affects from 24% to 80% of hospitalized elderly patients (Foreman, 1991, 1993), is a risk factor for hospitalization and nursing home placement (Weiler, Lubben, & Chi, 1991), and often is underrecognized by health professionals (Gutmann, 1988; Lipowski, 1989) and understudied by health care researchers (Foreman, 1989). Often signifying physical illness and functional disability (Lueckenotte, 1990), cognitive impairment predisposes patients to iatrogenic complications (Johnson, 1990; Williams, Campbell, Raynor, Mlynarczyk, & Ward, 1985). Costs, intensity of care, lengths of stay, and rates of institutionalization and mortality are greater for elders with cognitive impairment than for those who are not cognitively impaired (Francis, Martin, & Kapoor, 1990; Lipowski, 1989; Rockwood, 1989).

Neurobehavioral Disturbances

Neurobehavioral disturbances are frequent concomitants or sequelae of cognitive impairment (Folstein, Anthony, Parhad, Duffy, & Gruenberg, 1985; Kaplan & Sadock, 1991; Neelon & Champagne, 1992; Rasin, 1990). Patients' behavioral responses to changes in cognition, such as becoming agitated or aggressive, often retard health professionals' efforts to restore functional status or promote physical recovery (Kafonek et al., 1989; Larson et al., 1989; Lindesay, Briggs, & Murphy, 1989).

PROTOTYPES OF COGNITIVE IMPAIRMENT: DEMENTIA AND DELIRIUM

Dementia

An insidious, progressive, global degeneration of intellectual functioning with multiple cognitive deficits, dementia is due to degenerative cerebral pathology. Neurons of the brain are lost and the brain atrophies, particularly in the frontal and temporal lobes, sites of memory retrieval and integration of new information (Ugarriza & Gray, 1993; Wise & Brandt, 1992). The loss of intellectual functioning is so great that patients become socially isolated and physically dependent (Gomez & Gomez, 1989).

Some forms of dementia are reversible (e.g., hypothyroid dementia) or treatable, stalling further intellectual loss (e.g., vascular dementia). Senile dementia of the Alzheimer's type (AD), an irreversible dementia, is the most common dementing illness of the elderly. From their East Boston study of a stratified random sample of 467 community elderly, Evans and colleagues (1989) demonstrated increasing prevalence rates of AD with age. Three percent in the 65 to 74 age range, 18.7% between 75 and 84, and 47.2% over 85 were diagnosed with probable AD. The authors concluded that the public health impact of AD will increase as the longevity of the population increases.

Delirium

Delirium, a reversible encephalopathy related to malfunction in brain physiology, is characterized by transient, often abrupt and fluctuating, global disturbances of consciousness, with an acute or subacute onset (Wise & Brandt, 1992) and mild to severe confusion (Watt, 1993); dysfunctions of the reticular activating system with disturbances in attention and the sleep–wake cycle; disturbances in short-term memory, language, perception, and orientation; and dysfunction of the autonomic nervous system with neurobehavioral disturbances. The final common pathway appears to be at the neuronal level, involving an impairment in cellular oxidative metabolism and/or neurotransmitter deficiencies (Champagne & Wiese, 1992; Wise & Brandt, 1992). Patients with delirium appear bewildered and disoriented and sometimes experience fearful hallucinations (Champagne & Wiese, 1992; Folstein et al., 1985; Kaplan & Sadock, 1991; Levkoff, Besdine, & Wetle, 1986; Neelon & Champagne, 1992; Rasin, 1990; Task Force on DSM–IV, 1993; Watt, 1993).

Incidence and prevalence rates of delirium range from 4% to 80% among hospitalized medical and surgical patients (Conn, 1991; Johnson, 1990; Levkoff et al., 1986; Levkoff, Cleary, Liptzin, & Evans, 1991), with mortality rates reported at 26.4% and 30% (Johnson, 1990; Levkoff et al., 1992). Delirium also occurs posthospitalization in patients with iatrogenic complications (Rockwood, 1989).

Delirium may be the first indication of serious illness, (Rockwood, 1989), but any illness can precipitate delirium in older adults. Common precipitants include exogenous toxins; metabolic imbalances; primary cerebral diseases; systemic diseases, especially acute infections, secondarily affecting the brain; and drug reactions, either from substance abuse, polypharmacy, or withdrawal (Lipowski, 1992). Using computerized tomography, Koponen and colleagues (1989) identified structural brain changes (e.g., ventricular dilatation, cortical atrophy) in their 69 patients with delirium, "suggesting a marked predisposing role for the structural brain diseases (primary degenerative and multi-infarct type dementias, Parkinsonism) in the development of delirium in elderly patients" (p. 226). According to Lipowski (1989, 1990), delirium is a more common sign of illness in older adults than fever and pain and an important form of psychopathology in later life. For reviews of precipitants of delirium, interested readers are referred to Foreman (1993), Johnson (1990), Koponen and Riekkinen (1989), and Rockwood (1989).

Delirium, Dementia, and Pseudodementia

The presence of preexisting brain damage, such as dementia, can predispose patients to delirium by lowering neurophysiological thresholds in response to diverse central nervous system insults, such as toxic-metabolic problems (liver or renal impairment or failure) (Watt, 1993; Wise & Brandt, 1992). Because delirium can mask dementia and those with dementia are at increased risk for developing delirium, evaluation of dementia should occur once delirium has been successfully treated. Without treatment of reversible causes and underlying diseases, delirium can cause death or do permanent damage, "turning treatable delirium into chronic dementia" (Gomez & Gomez, 1989, p. 141).

Although organic bases for depression have been documented (see Krishnan, 1991, for a review), and cognitive impairment has been associated with major depression in late life (Blazer, 1989), controversy exists about the diagnosis *pseudodementia*. This depression-related cognitive dysfunction mimics dementia with psychomotor retardation and impairment of intellectual functioning. However, dysphoric mood and response to treatment with antidepressants differentiate depression from dementia and delirium (Campbell, 1988; Tavani, 1990). For reviews of depression research in older adults, readers are referred to *Diagnosis and Treatment of Depression in Late Life* (N. I. H. Consensus Development Panel on Depression in Late Life, 1992), Rapp, Flint, Hermann, and Proulx (1992), Salzman (1987), Schneider, Martinez, and Lebowitz (1993), Schneider and Sobin (1992), Teri and colleagues (1992), and Weiss and Lazarus (1993). Additional comparisons of delirium, dementia, and depression can be found in Foreman and Grabowski (1992).

PROTOTYPES OF NEUROBEHAVIORAL DISTURBANCES: AGGRESSION AND AGITATION

Care providers are challenged by the neurobehavioral disturbances associated with cognitive impairment, such as aggression, agitation, resistance to care, and the psychiatric symptoms, hallucinations and delusions. Agitation and aggression are considered particularly threatening to the older adult or others in their immediate environments (Sternberg, Whelihan, Fretwell, Bielicki, & Murray, 1989; Watt, 1993). In their review of behaviors associated with dementia, Taft and Cronin-Stubbs (1995) found that agitated and aggressive behaviors were more stressful to caregivers than other behaviors and that these behaviors interfered with quality of life.

Aggression

Cognitive impairment "minimizes the use of rational problem-solving," reduces inhibitions, increases frustrations, and can result in "destructive aggression" (Beck, Baldwin, Modlin, & Lewis, 1990, p. 169). Giancola and Zeichner (1993) noted "a paucity of published studies" (p. 8) in their review of theories and etiological explanations for aggressive behavior in the elderly. They offer diverse explanations from neuropsychological, neurochemical, social, psychological, and medical perspectives. In addition to their review, readers are referred to the Patel and Hope (1993) review of biological, psychological, and environmental perspectives.

Agitation

Although the intensity of aggressive episodes is frightening to caregivers, agitation, or "severe anxiety associated with motor restlessness" (Kaplan & Sadock, 1991, p. 217) occurs more frequently. Cohen-Mansfield (1986) found 73% of her nursing home sample of patients with dementia demonstrating agitation on a daily basis. Readers are referred to reviews by Cohen-Mansfield and Billig (1986), Cohen-Mansfield, Marx, and Rosenthal (1989), Cohen-Mansfield, Marx, and Werner (1992), and Taft and Cronin-Stubbs (1995) for additional perspectives on agitation.

Agitation and aggression have been studied typically in long-term care patients with dementia (see Szwabo & Grossberg, 1993, for a review). For example, in a survey of nurses working in nursing homes, Taft (1989) found that (chronic) confusion was the number one patient-care problem and agitation and aggression were of priority concern to nursing home staff. But agitation and aggression are also of concern to clinicians caring for patients with delirium in acute care settings. From his work in a large community general hospital, Watt (1993) was struck with "how much clinicians weight agitation and hallucinations above attentional collapse in arriving at the diagnosis of delirium" (p. 459). Older adults also can experience agitated depression, characterized by pacing and irritability (Smith, Buckwalter, & Mitchell, 1993).

INTERVENTIONS FOR COGNITIVE IMPAIRMENT

Developing and testing biological, behavioral, and environmental approaches to remediating cognitive impairment was recently recommended as a research priority for 1997 at the Second Conference on Research Priorities and approved by the National Advisory Council for Nursing Research of the National Institute of Nursing Research (Zusy, 1993). However, the coexistence of delirium, dementia, and depression in the elderly (Reynolds et al., 1988), and the exacerbations that occur when patients are hospitalized (Folstein et al., 1985), make treatment of cognitive impairment (Koenig, Meador, Cohen, & Blazer, 1988; Zubenko, 1990) and the nursing care of cognitively impaired older adults difficult (Foreman, 1986, 1990; Nagley & Dever, 1988; Rasin, 1990; Wolanin & Phillips, 1981).

In the following section, the intervention research for treating patients with dementia and delirium is summarized. Interventions that are delivered by professional rather than personal caregivers that were tested and evaluated in the review studies are emphasized. Outcomes of these studies pertained to patient-related outcomes (e.g., cognitive and social functioning, behavioral and psychiatric signs and symptoms, quality of life), patient care outcomes (e.g., complications, use of chemical or physical restraints), or health care delivery outcomes (e.g., cost, labor intensivity, length of stay, posthospital institutionalization).

Dementia Intervention Research

Generally, the aims of these studies were to stall declines in cognition (e.g., orientation, memory), maintain performance of physical and instrumental activities of daily living, or to reduce, manage, and, in some cases, prevent patients' behavioral and psychiatric symptoms that were considered by caregivers or the investigators to be dysfunctional (interfering with the patients' functioning), disruptive to the patient's care, disruptive or destructive to the patient care environment, or harmful to the patient or others in the patient's environment.

Interdisciplinary and nursing reviews of interventions reveal that the most commonly used methods for reducing or managing behavioral symptoms of dementia patients are physical and chemical restraints (Rovner et al., 1990; Taft & Cronin-Stubbs, 1995). There have been recent attempts at targeting interventions for cognitive and noncognitive symptoms and using nonrestrictive, behavioral methods for caring for cognitively impaired patients with dementia.

Interdisciplinary treatment research.   Interventions for caring for cognitively impaired older adults typically have been focused on the pharmacologic and nonpharmacologic approaches to maintain or prevent the loss of cognitive functioning and to reduce or manage behavioral and psychiatric symptoms in dementia (Maletta, 1992; Reisberg, Ferris, Torossian, Kluger, & Monteiro, 1992; Risse & Barnes, 1986; Smith & Perry, 1992; Teri et al., 1992). Reisberg and colleagues (1992) distinguished cognitive and noncognitive (behavioral) symptoms of AD and recommended that these be separated in pharmacologic prevention and treatment trials because interventions for remediating behavioral symptoms would be expected to be different than those for improving cognitive symptomatology. Reviewing the interventions for improving cognitive symptoms and related performance of activities of daily living, they found that none were effective. Results of studies of pharmacologic interventions for ameliorating behavioral symptoms showed either that the symptoms remitted spontaneously or improved over the course of the disease or that the studies had methodological problems.

Schneider et al. (1993) summarized the AD research and identified the following prominent areas: pharmacologic and nonpharmacologic treatment of cognitive impairment and behavioral symptoms, the development and testing of cognition-enhancing cholinesterase inhibitors, and a recent increase in clinical trials using combinations of neurotransmitter-targeting agents. Although results of studies of cognition-enhancing pharmacologic agents, such as the cholinesterase inhibitor tacrine, have not demonstrated consistent efficacy, interventions studies of behaviors associated with AD have yielded more consistent results. Of the pharmacologic treatments, neuroleptics, especially low doses of haloperidol, showed ''modest efficacy in the treatment of [psychiatric manifestations] and agitation in dementia'' (Schneider et al., 1993, p. 91). The results of these treatments can affect both cognition and behaviors. Controlling psychotic symptoms, for example, helps manage not only the behaviors associated with AD, but also stalls some of the acceleration of cognitive decline associated with psychotic symptoms.

In a review of pharmacologic nonneuroleptic treatment of behavior disturbances in organic mental syndromes, Smith and Perry (1992) concluded that beta blockers lessen aggressive behaviors of patients with dementia. Benzodiazepines also were helpful in modulating behaviors associated with dementia. However, this author has identified several methodological problems that temper the reviewers' conclusions. First, random variance in heterogeneous samples, which threatens the statistical conclusion validity of the findings, occurs when data are combined from patients younger and older than the population of interest. Across the Smith and Perry review, age ranged from 22 to 81 years (mean = 48). Because the pharmacokinetics and pharmacodynamics of medications differ in the young and old, age-controlled trials are needed on the effectiveness of beta blockers and benzodiazepines on lessening aggressive behaviors in the different age groups. Despite noting that the studies were poorly designed and that interpretations were difficult to make, Smith and Perry recommended treating behavior disturbances with benzodiazepines. In their eagerness to find solutions to pressing problems, it is not uncommon for reviewers to recommend treatments from available research. Statements about treatment efficacy, deduced from studies lacking in interpretable causal relationships, however, are not supported by the evidence.

Dietary manipulation of neurotransmitter precursors, such as administering the amino acid, L-tryptophan, to increase brain levels of serotonin, is receiving attention recently as a way of curbing aggressive behaviors. In a recent review of animal and human studies (Joyal, Lalonde, Vikis-Freibergs, &

Botez, 1993), dietary supplements of vitamins, especially folates, were found to decrease age-related behavioral dysfunctions related to cognitive and mood disturbances. Deficiencies of this vitamin in the general population, and especially in the institutionalized elderly, have been found to be associated with low levels of serotonin. However, research on the utility of folate therapy in managing behaviors associated with dementia is just beginning.

Maletta (1992) delineated behavioral or psychiatric disorders that are amenable to pharmacologic treatment of the elderly from nonpsychiatric disorders that are not amenable to pharmacotherapy. He concluded that effective treatment for psychiatric behavior disorders, such as aggression and assaultive behavior, combines both pharmacologic and nonpharmacologic (behavioral and environmental) methods. Although others have drawn the same conclusion (e.g., Teri et al., 1992), Maletta's underlying assumption that "all currently accepted modalities of psychiatric treatment are efficacious in the treatment of nursing home residents with behavioral/emotional disorders, including psychopharmacological, behavioral, and psychotherapeutic approaches" (p. 118) was not supported by the studies he reviewed.

In their extensive review of nonpharmacologic approaches for the treatment of agitation in AD patients, Teri and colleagues (1992) concluded that "behavioral manipulations (e.g., physical contact, pet therapy, stimulus control, behavior modification techniques, and simple communication practices) are often neglected despite the growing opinion that there is a definite place for the nonpharmacologic management of behavioral disturbances in AD" (p. 79). Perhaps, as noted by Carstensen (1988), behavioral techniques are used less often to modify behavioral symptoms of older adults who have irreversible cognitive impairment, because "if a person cannot *learn*, behavioral intervention would be expected to yield few gains" (p. 268). In her review, Carstensen reported the results of several projects where behavioral techniques successfully influenced verbal, social, self-care, self-stimulation, and wandering behaviors.

Some success has been reported for the use of operant conditioning techniques (reward and punishment) for decreasing aggressive behaviors in nursing home patients (Vaccaro, 1988a, 1988b, 1990). In addition to the controversial use of punishment for influencing behavior, Vaccaro's samples were exceptionally small. Also, his behavioral interventions were labor-intensive, requiring ongoing monitoring by objective and well-trained observers. Interpretations of single subject research (Vaccaro, 1988b), especially the less systematic case study approaches, are limited. Both sample sizes and labor intensity limit the external validity of the findings.

Interpretations of single-subject research, especially the less systematic case study approaches, are limited. Both sample size and labor-intensivity limit the external validity of the findings. However, information about the internal validity of the relationship between the treatment and targeted outcomes are probed in such well-controlled studies. With internal validity estimated, replications in controlled clinical trials with larger samples promotes the generalizability of the findings.

Labor-intensivity also characterized a recent approach for managing acute agitated behavior in elderly demented patients advanced by Mintzer and colleagues (1993). Using both behavioral and environmental approaches to individualized treatment of agitated behaviors, the authors evaluated their 3-week inpatient Geriatric Behavioral Intensive Care program and found lower rates of both posthospital institutionalization and use of pharmacologic controls of behaviors in 55 patients. The authors identified the need for systematic evaluation of the treatment efficacy and cost-effectiveness of their program. Key to demonstrating the effectiveness of their program in less controlled environments would be to minimize self-selection bias, a threat to validity in their study. For detailed reviews of the application of behavioral methods in the care of older adults with dementia, interested readers are referred to Burgio and Burgio (1986) and Carstensen (1988). For a review of cognitive intervention research in dementia, readers are referred to Camp (1993). The results of an experiment on memory training were reported by Camp and colleagues (1993).

Maas and Buckwalter (1991) reviewed the efficacy of special care units (SCU) for minimizing behavioral dysfunctions by tailoring health care environments to patients' physical and psychosocial needs. In units designed to eliminate the need for chemical and physical restraints, they found that injuries and falls and the use of chemical restraints increased, whereas the use of physical restraints decreased. Patient's dysfunctional behaviors decreased. Conclusions about these results are tempered by the design and measurement problems noted by the reviewers. Readers are referred to a recent volume of SCU studies by Holmes, Ory, and Teresi (1994).

Nursing care research.   Some progress has been made since Beck and Heacock (1988) concluded that much of the nursing literature is theoretical and general and has not been validated through research. For example, in their 1992 review, Beck, Modlin, Heithoff, and Shue reported improved cognitive and social functioning and decreased disruptive behaviors from the results of two studies on the effects of exercise on behavior problems. However, these results should be interpreted cautiously, pending replication in controlled clinical trials. Taft's (1992) review of validation therapy as a communication technique for disoriented elderly individuals yielded clinical rather than scientific evidence for its efficacy. Beck, Heacock, Rapp, and Shue (1993) reviewed assessment and intervention strategies for cognitive impairment and noted that the majority of studies were descriptive, the tools for measuring the studies' variables required additional psychometric testing, and trials were needed that examined the interface between the biologic sciences and nursing care, such as the role of exercise, lighting, and nutritional status on disruptive behavior. A more recent review by Beck and Shue (1994) summarized diverse biopsychosocial nursing interventions for treating disruptive behaviors, such as behavioral techniques, environmental modifications, group and social interaction programs, and educational programs. Although the reviewers expressed concern about the lack of conceptual frameworks to guide interventions, they did not include an evaluation of other scientific aspects of the review studies. For example, the majority of the studies had outcome measures that relied on anecdotal evidence or self-reports by caregivers. Direct and objective observations to validate that desired changes occurred in patients' and caregivers' behaviors are needed to modulate biases, such as acquiescence response set, social desirability response set, selective recall by the respondents, and selective reporting by the researchers.

In her recent qualitative study, Taft (1994) described social and psychological approaches that professional and family caregivers ($N = 40$) described in open-ended questions about dementia care. Maintaining involvement, providing emotional support, and seeing the world from the perspective of the person with dementia were the most frequently reported caregiving approaches. Controlled trials to determine the relative efficacy of those approaches on outcomes pertaining to patient care, patient-related symptoms and functioning, and health care delivery would guide future caregivers in their care of dementia patients.

In summary, it is difficult to identify effective interventions for behavioral symptoms because the underlying causes of behavioral dysfunctions in AD are not yet known. Although behavioral symptoms may be secondary to the AD disease process and may be an early sign of dementia, Spector (1991) estimated that only 57% of patients with disruptive behaviors in the 1984 National Long-Term Care Survey also were impaired cognitively: "Behavioral problems are not generally included as a subset of cognitive impairment because they may be caused by mental disorders as well as cognitive deficits" (p. 52). In addition, "behavioral problems may also represent acting out behavior as a consequence of improper treatment by caregivers or inappropriate setting" (p. 54). Interventions, then, need to be targeted to specific etiologies for cognitive and noncognitive symptoms.

Summarizing the dementia intervention research, Teri and colleagues (1992) concluded, "Significantly more attention needs to be paid to the clinical management of behavioral problems in patients with AD. Both pharmacologic and nonpharmacologic interventions focusing on improving behavior and controlled clinical trials of these treatments are desperately needed'' (p. 77). Although pharmacotherapy is the most frequent treatment for aggressive behaviors in the elderly, Giancola and Zeichner (1993) projected that, with continued increases in the elderly population, nonpharmacological treatments ''may become extremely laborious, increasing burden on staff time and energy'' (p. 17). The agenda for the research-based care of AD patients, synthesized by Duffy, Hepburn, Christensen, and Brugge-Wiger (1989) from a 1988 consensus conference of 183 researchers and clinicians, included such priority areas as describing and managing disruptive behaviors, generating alternatives to physical and chemical restraints, and training staff to work with the confused elderly. Although progress is being made in these areas, scientific data about the outcomes of interventions—their efficacy and cost-effectiveness—remains scant.

Delirium Intervention Research

Research on the care and treatment of the cognitively impaired older adult with delirium lags behind dementia intervention research, perhaps related to complex physiologic etiologies and underrecognition of the disorder. Because the causes of delirium often can be identified and delirium is potentially reversible, interventions are targeted not only to reducing behavioral symptoms, but also to ameliorating underlying causes and reversing cognitive impairment.

Interdisciplinary treatment research.   Rabins (1991) found little research on the appropriate treatment of patients with delirium in his review but recommended treatment that included identifying and ameliorating underlying etiologies; frequently orienting patients in safe, predictable environments; telling patients they are confused or disoriented because of their condition; and providing support for patients' and families' fears. Consistent with the management of behaviors associated with dementia, the cautious use of physical restraints and low-dose neuroleptics, such as haloperidol, has been recommended for managing agitated or aggressive behaviors that can harm patients or others in their environment. However, these interventions require systematic testing for their efficacy in randomized clinical trials.

Nursing care research.   Reviewing the nursing research literature, Nagley and Dever (1988) noted that ''nursing actions suggested in the literature are those that reestablish normal physiological status or assist patients in adequate interpretation of their environment'' (p. 81). However, interventions were typically derived from logical inferences from what is known about confusion, rather than from empirical evidence.

In his extensive review of nursing intervention studies, Foreman (1993) found that psychosocial interventions, such as orientation, continuity of care, and anticipatory guidance for confused patients, contributed to lower incidences of confusion, fewer complications, and shortened hospitalizations. However, even with care, "the incidence and consequences of acute confusion persisted at significant levels" (p. 20). Similarly, physiological interventions, such as administering oxygen to prevent or minimize perioperative hypoxia and hypotension, yielded comparable results. Foreman concluded that interventions for acute confusion need to include both psychosocial and physiologic strategies. However, findings about the efficacy of these interventions should be interpreted cautiously, as critical appraisal of the studies' scientific aspects was not apparent.

Cronin-Stubbs (1996) conducted a critical appraisal of the scientific aspects of selected interdisciplinary and nursing intervention studies for delirium that met a priori criteria and that had been conducted in the last 20 years in acute care settings. From the threats to construct validity and statistical conclusion validity that were uncovered, she concluded that the field is in the early phases of developing research-based interventions and that more work is needed on the following: determining the efficacy of interventions in controlled clinical trials, evaluating the validity and reliability of intervention programs, and promoting the use of research findings to improve the care of our medically and mentally ill older adults.

Rasin (1990) identified scant research in her review of the interdisciplinary and nursing literature on caring for patients with confusion. She concluded that proactive, preventive approaches, such as early identification and prompt treatment of patients at risk for confusion, are more effective than waiting for emergent symptoms to occur. However, all current intervention activities warranted confirmatory investigations.

CONCLUSIONS

From the review of the intervention literature, the treatment of older adults for irreversible cognitive impairment, or dementia, includes the use of pharmacologic and nonpharmacologic methods to stall cognitive decline, maintain activities of daily living skills, curb behavioral and psychiatric symptoms, and improve patients' social functioning. Although health care delivery outcomes were reported in some studies, the emphasis in the majority of the review studies was on patient-related outcomes.

Treatment for reversible cognitive impairment, or delirium, includes the identification and treatment of underlying, typically physiological, etiologies and the prevention of complications, such as falls and irreversible dementia. However, the majority of interventions require validation in systematic and controlled evaluations. Behaviorally based interventions have been evaluated in anecdotal case studies, intensive single-subject studies, or nongeneralizable and intensive staff training demonstration projects. Although these represent the ideals in research design and patient care, the cost-effectiveness and replicability of these approaches is not known. Algorithms of pharmacologic and behavioral treatments for the care of the behaviorally involved cognitively impaired have not been evaluated in controlled clinical trials. As recommended by Teri and her colleagues (1992):

> The potential efficacy of each form of intervention, separately and together, must be considered and well-controlled clinical trials encouraged. The likelihood that different treatments will be differentially effective for different behavioral problems in different patients—and the need to begin to understand how best to match patients, behaviors, caregivers, and treatments for maximal efficacy—must be acknowledged and studied. (p. 83)

THE CURRENT GENERATION OF STUDIES

Complementing the review of the past generation of intervention studies were naturalistic studies of selected projects from the current generation of studies. One of this reviewer's aims was to discover current research that was being conducted on the care of cognitively impaired older adults. Through either onsite participant observations of researchers conducting intervention research in the field or interviews of principal investigators of studies funded by the National Institute of Nursing Research (NINR), diverse projects were investigated.

A current study for the management of ''disruptive behaviors'' of nursing home patients with dementia is the multi-site study conducted by Beck in Arkansas and Baldwin in Maryland. They are testing an intervention package that includes psychosocial and activities of daily living interventions and are finding that individualized approaches to patients by highly trained certified nurses' aides result in a decrease in patients' disruptive behaviors. Langley, at a midwest neurological rehabilitation facility, is using behavior modification strategies in therapeutic group settings with traumatically brain-injured young and older adults to modulate aggressive behaviors. Transfer of the skills to the patient care units is attempted by involving patients' personal and professional caregivers in the group activities. Langley is not yet conducting controlled trials to test the efficacy of his clinical approaches.

Delirium intervention research is being conducted by Neelon's research team at the University of North Carolina and Duke University. They are testing protocols for classifying acutely ill elderly patients' risk for acute confusion. In conjunction with patients' scores on the NEECHAM Confusion Scale (Champagne & Wiese, 1992; Neelon & Champagne, 1992), interventions, organized as "care maps," are targeted according to nurses' assessments of patients with symptom checklists (patterns or screens) related to the etiology of delirium (Neelon & Champagne, 1992). "The care maps are protocols of pattern-specific interventions that statistically clustered precipitants into three primary screens: Environmental, Metabolic, & Physiologic" (V. Neelon, personal communication, October 12, 1993). In the Environmental Screen, patients are characterized by low mobility, low function, and impaired cognitive status. Typically, they have a chronic cognitive impairment or dementia. In the Metabolic Screen, patients typically have impaired regulatory function (organ—liver or renal—impairment or failure), with albumin and creatinine abnormalities and possible malnutrition. In the Physiologic Screen, patients typically have oxygen perfusion problems, such as hypoxia and dehydration according to laboratory indicators. From these three primary patterns, there are five risk groups that can be assigned potentially five intervention protocols.

For example, during admission, patients are assessed with the NEECHAM Scale and the General Risk Screen, and then nurses select specific care maps for each patient. Dr. Neelon stated that the more highly confused the patients were, typically, the more care maps they required—"costed out, they would require 24 hours of nursing care" (V. Neelon, personal communication, October 12, 1993). From their preliminary analysis of the data, a treatment effect was found for the first 24 hours in the moderately confused patients who were hypoxic. Neelon believes additional findings may have been impeded by problems with the "dosing of the interventions" (V. Neelon, personal communication, December 2, 1993) or implementation of the intervention protocols.

In their review of the dementia literature on managing behavioral disturbances, Teri and colleagues (1992) concluded that:

> certain overriding concerns exist across studies, including the need for specific definitions of behaviors under investigation; use of established, psychometrically sound, clinically relevant measures; avoidance of global clinical impressions to evaluate change; and integration of multimodal, comprehensive strategies of assessment. (p. 85)

DIRECTIONS FOR THE FUTURE

Given current health care and economic climates, evaluating the scientific merit, clinical usefulness, and cost-effectiveness of interventions is critical

(Cronin-Stubbs et al., 1988; Orsolits, 1989). Protocols that are developed from research results and subsequently tested for their effectiveness in managing behavioral symptoms are needed. Supporting the need for protocols to help nurses care for behaviorally involved, cognitively impaired elderly are the vulnerability of older adults to intensified relationships between medical and mental illnesses, including the impact of acute care environments on cognitive impairment (Foreman, 1991; Roslaniec & Fitzpatrick, 1979); the increasing numbers of medically ill elderly with psychiatric and behavioral disorders; the shortage of health professionals prepared to manage the mental health needs of the elderly (Frazier, Lebowitz, & Silver, 1986); nursing's ability to provide round-the-clock, coordinated, and comprehensive care; and 1987 Omnibus Budget Reconciliation Act (OBRA) requirements that nursing personnel in certified nursing facilities receive training in the care of cognitively impaired older adults.

Synthesizing the research on interventions for caring for and treating cognitively impaired older adults revealed that systematic, rigorously designed interdisciplinary intervention research is needed. In accordance with the review by Teri and colleagues (1992), future studies ''should integrate biomedical and behavioral expertise to develop methodologically rigorous study designs where theoretically sound, clinically judicious, and scientifically rigorous research protocols'' are tested (p. 86). The scientific efficacy of interventions and the effectiveness of the care of patients with dementia and delirium and associated behavioral disturbances have not yet been demonstrated.

ACKNOWLEDGMENT

This review was funded in part by the National Institute of Mental Health, National Institutes of Health (Grant Number 5 K07 MH00953–03). The author gratefully acknowledges Thomas D. Cook, Ph.D., Northwestern University, for enlightenment and direction; Frederick J. Kviz, Ph.D., University of Illinois at Chicago, for scientific and editorial input; Lois B. Taft, D.N.Sc., Rush University, for critical appraisal of earlier drafts of the manuscript; and Maura Capaul, Rush University, and Rachel A. Woodham, University of Iowa, for participation in interrater reliability assessments and preparation of the final manuscript.

REFERENCES

Beck, C., Baldwin, B., Modlin, T., & Lewis, S. (1990). Caregivers' perceptions of aggressive behavior in cognitively impaired nursing home residents. *Journal of Neuroscience Nursing, 22,* 169–172.

Beck, C., & Heacock, P. (1988). Nursing interventions for patients with Alzheimer's disease. *Nursing Clinics of North America, 23*, 95–124.

Beck, C., Heacock, P., Rapp, C. G., & Shue, V. (1993). Cognitive impairment in the elderly. *Nursing Clinics of North America, 28*, 335–347.

Beck, C., Modlin, T., Heithoff, K., & Shue, V. (1992). Exercise as an intervention for behavior problems. *Geriatric Nursing, 13,* 273–275.

Beck, C., & Shue, V. (1994). Interventions for treating disruptive behavior in demented elderly people. *Nursing Clinics of North America, 29*, 143–155.

Blazer, D. (1989). Depression in the elderly. *New England Journal of Medicine, 320*, 164–166.

Burgio, L., & Burgio, K. (1986). Behavioral gerontology: Application of behavioral methods to the problems of older adults. *Journal of Applied Behavior Analysis, 19*, 321–328.

Camp, C. J. (1993). Cognitive interventions in dementia [Special issue 1]. *The Gerontologist, 33*, 51.

Camp, C. J., Foss, J. W., Stevens, A. B., Reichard, C. C., McKitrick, L. A., & O'Hanlon, A. M. (1993). Memory training in normal and demented elderly populations: The E-I-E-I-O Model. *Experimental Aging Research, 19*, 277–290.

Campbell, D. W. (1988). Bedside differentiation of depressive pseudodementia from dementia. *American Journal of Psychiatry, 145*, 1099–1103.

Carstensen, L. L. (1988). The emerging field of behavioral gerontology. *Behavior Therapy, 19*, 259–281.

Champagne, M. T., & Wiese, R. A. (1992). Research on cognitive impairment: Implications for practice. In S. G. Funk, E. M. Tornquist, M. T. Champagne, & R. A. Wiese (Eds)., *Key aspects of elder care: Managing falls, incontinence, and cognitive impairment* (pp. 340–346). New York: Springer Publishing Co.

Cohen-Mansfield, J. (1986). Agitated behaviors in the elderly: Preliminary results in the cognitively deteriorated. *Journal of the American Geriatric Society, 34*, 722–727.

Cohen-Mansfield, J., & Billig, N. (1986). Agitated behaviors in the elderly: A conceptual review. *Journal of the American Geriatric Society, 34*, 711–721.

Cohen-Mansfield, J., Marx, M., & Rosenthal, A. S. (1989). A description of agitation in a nursing home. *Journal of Gerontology, 44*, 77–84.

Cohen-Mansfield, J., Marx, M., & Werner, P. (1992). Agitation in elderly persons: An integrative report of findings in a nursing home. *International Psychogeriatrics, 4*(Suppl. 2), 221–240.

Conn, D. K. (1991). Delirium and other organic mental disorders. In J. Sadavoy, L. W. Lazarus, & L. F. Jarvik (Eds.), *Comprehensive review of geriatric psychiatry* (pp. 311–336). Washington, DC: American Psychiatric Press.

Cook, T. D., Cooper, H., Cordray, D. S., Hartmann, H., Hedges, L. V., Light, R. J., Louis, T. A., & Mosteller, F. (1992). *Meta-analysis for explanation.* New York: Russell Sage Foundation.

Cooper, H. M. (1989). Integrating research: A guide for literature reviews. In L. Bickman & D. J. Rog (Eds.), *Applied social research methods series* (Vol. 2, 2nd ed.). Newbury Park, CA: Sage.

Cronin-Stubbs, D. (1996). Delirium intervention research in acute care settings. In J. J. Fitzpatrick & J. Norbeck (Eds.), *Annual review of nursing research* (Vol. 14, pp. 57–73). New York: Springer Publishing Co.

Cronin-Stubbs, D., Donner, L. L., McFolling, S. D., Kopytko, E. E., Pasch, S. K., & Szczesny, S. G. (1988). Discharge planning for psychiatric inpatients: Evaluation of one technique. *Applied Nursing Research, 1,* 72–79.

Duffy, L. M., Hepburn, K., Christensen, R., & Brugge-Wiger, P. (1989). A research agenda in care for patients with Alzheimer's disease. *IMAGE: Journal of Nursing Scholarship, 21,* 255–257.

Evans, D. A., Funkenstein, H. H., Albert, M. S., Scherr, P. A., Cook, N. R., Chown, M. J., Herbert, L. E., Hunnekens, C. H., & Taylor, J. O. (1989). Prevalence of Alzheimer's disease in a community population of older persons: Higher than previously reported. *Journal of the American Medical Association, 262,* 2551–2556.

Folstein, M., Anthony, J. C., Parhad, I., Duffy, B., & Gruenberg, E. M. (1985). The meaning of cognitive impairment in the elderly. *Journal of the American Geriatric Society, 33,* 228–235.

Foreman, M. D. (1986). Acute confusional states in hospitalized elderly: A research dilemma. *Nursing Research, 35,* 34–38.

Foreman, M. D. (1989). Confusion in the hospitalized elderly: Incidence, onset, and associated factors. *Research in Nursing & Health, 12,* 21–29.

Foreman, M. D. (1990). Complexities of acute confusion. *Geriatric Nursing, 11,* 136–139.

Foreman, M. D. (1991). The cognitive and behavioral nature of acute confusional states. *Scholarly Inquiry for Nursing Practice, 5,* 3–16.

Foreman, M. D. (1993). Acute confusion in the elderly. In J. J. Fitzpatrick & J. S. Stevenson (Eds.), *Annual review of nursing research* (Vol. 11, pp. 3–30). New York: Springer Publishing Co.

Foreman, M. D., & Grabowski, R. (1992). Diagnostic dilemma: Cognitive impairment in the elderly. *Journal of Gerontological Nursing, 18*(9), 5–12.

Francis, J., Martin, D., & Kapoor, W. N. (1990). A prospective study of delirium in hospitalized elderly. *Journal of the American Medical Association, 263,* 1097–1101.

Frazier, S. H., Lebowitz, B. D., & Silver, L. B. (1986). Aging, mental health, and rehabilitation. In S. J. Brody & G. E. Ruff (Eds.), *Aging and rehabilitation* (pp. 19–26). New York: Springer Publishing Co.

Giancola, P. R., & Zeichner, A. (1993). Aggressive behavior in the elderly: A critical review. *Clinical Gerontologist, 13,* 3–22.

Gomez, G., & Gomez, E. A. (1989). Dementia? or delirium?: Here's help in sorting it out. *Geriatric Nursing: American Journal of Care for the Aging, 10,* 141–142.

Gutmann, D. (1988). Late onset pathogenesis: Dynamic models. *Topics in Geriatric Rehabilitation, 3,* 1–8.

Holmes, D., Ory, M., & Teresi, J. (Eds.). (1994). *Special dementia care: Research, policy, and practice issues.* New York: Raven Press.

Johnson, J. C. (1990). Delirium in the elderly. *Emergency Medicine Clinics of North America, 8,* 255–265.

Joyal, C. C., Lalonde, R., Vikis-Freibergs, V., & Botez, M. I. (1993). Are age-related behavioral disorders improved by folate administration? *Experimental Aging Research, 19*, 367–376.

Kafonek, S., Ettinger, W. H., Roca, R., Kittner, S., Taylor, N., & German, P. S. (1989). Instruments for screening for depression and dementia in a long-term care facility. *Journal of the American Geriatric Society, 37*, 29–34.

Kaplan, H. I., & Sadock, B. J. (1991). *Synopsis of psychiatry: Behavioral sciences clinical psychiatry* (6th ed.). Baltimore, MD: Williams & Wilkins.

Koenig, H. G., Meador, K. G., Cohen, H. J., & Blazer, D. G. (1988). Depression in elderly hospitalized patients with mental illness. *Archives of Internal Medicine, 148*, 1929–1936.

Koponen, H., Hurri, L., Stenback, U., Mattila, E., Soininen, H., & Riekkinen, P. J. (1989). Computed tomography findings in delirium. *Journal of Nervous and Mental Disease, 177*, 226–231.

Koponen, H., & Riekkinen, P. J. (1989). Delirium in the elderly: A review. *Psychiatria Fennica, 20*, 129–136.

Krishnan, K. R. (1991). Organic bases of depression in the elderly. *Annual Review of Medicine, 42*, 261–266.

Larson, E. B., Featherstone, H. J., Burton, V., Reifler, C. G., Canfield, C. G., & Chinn, N. M. (1989). Medical aspects of care of elderly patients with cognitive impairment. *Developmental Neuropsychology, 1*, 145–171.

Levkoff, S. E., Besdine, R. W., & Wetle, T. (1986). Acute confusional states (delirium) in the hospitalized elderly. In C. Eisdorfer (Ed.), *Annual review of gerontology and geriatrics* (Vol. 6, pp. 1–26). New York: Springer Publishing Co.

Levkoff, S., Cleary, P., Liptzin, B., & Evans, D. A. (1991). Epidemiology of delirium: An overview of research issues and findings. *International Psychogeriatrics, 3*, 149–167.

Levkoff, S., Evans, D. E., Liptzin, B., Cleary, P. D., Lipsitz, L. A., Wetle, T. T., Reilly, C. H., Pilgrim, D. M., Schor, J., & Rowe, J. (1992). Delirium: The occurrence and persistence of symptoms among elderly hospitalized patients. *Archives of Internal Medicine, 152*, 334–340.

Lindesay, J., Briggs, K., & Murphy, E. (1989). The Guy's/Age Concern Survey: Prevalence rates of cognitive impairment, depression, and anxiety in an urban elderly community. *British Journal of Psychiatry, 155*, 317–329.

Lipowski, Z. J. (1989). Delirium in the elderly patient. *New England Journal of Medicine, 320*, 578–582.

Lipowski, Z. J. (1990). *Delirium: Acute confusional states.* New York: Oxford University Press.

Lipowski, Z. J. (1992). Update on delirium. *Psychiatric Clinics of North America, 15*, 335–346.

Lueckenotte, A. G. (1990). *Pocket guide to gerontologic assessment.* St. Louis: Mosby.

Maas, M. L., & Buckwalter, K. C. (1991). Alzheimer's disease. In J. J. Fitzpatrick & J. S. Stevenson (Eds.), *Annual review of nursing research* (Vol. 9, pp. 19–55). New York: Springer Publishing Co.

Maletta, G. J. (1992). Treatment of behavioral symptomatology of Alzheimer's disease, with emphasis on aggression: Current clinical approaches. *International Psychogeriatrics, 4*(Suppl. 1), 117–130.

Mintzer, J. E., Lewis, L., Pennypaker, L., Simpson, W., Bachman, D., Wohlreich, G., Meeks, A., Hunt, S., & Sampson, R. (1993). Behavioral intensive care unit (BICU): A new concept in the management of acute agitated behavior in elderly demented patients. *The Gerontologist, 33*, 801–806.

Nagley, S. J., & Dever, A. (1988). What we know about treating confusion. *Applied Nursing Research, 1*, 80–83.

N. I. H. Consensus Development Panel on Depression in Late Life. (1992). Diagnosis and treatment of depression in late life. *Journal of the American Medical Association, 268*, 1018–1024.

Neelon, V. J., & Champagne, M. T. (1992). Managing cognitive impairment: The current bases for practice. In S. G. Funk, E. M. Tornquist, M. T. Champagne, & R. A. Wiese (Eds.), *Key aspects of elder care: Managing falls, incontinence, and cognitive impairment* (pp. 239–250). New York: Springer Publishing Co.

Omnibus Budget Reconciliation Act. (1987). 42 United States Code Sections 1396r (f) (2) (A) (i) (I) and 1395I-3 (f) (2) (A) (i) (I).

Orsolits, M. (1989). Reorganizing nursing for the future: Nursing commission recommendations and research implications. *Applied Nursing Research, 2*, 64–67.

Patel, V., & Hope, T. (1993). Aggressive behavior in elderly people with dementia: A review. *International Journal of Geriatric Psychiatry, 8*, 457–472.

Rabins, P. V. (1991). Psychosocial and management aspects of delirium. *International Psychogeriatrics, 3*, 319–324.

Rapp, M. S., Flint, A. J., Hermann, N., & Proulx, G. B. (1992). Behavioral disturbances in the demented elderly: Phenomenology, pharmacotherapy, and behavioral management. *Canadian Journal of Psychiatry, 37*, 651–657.

Rasin, J. H. (1990). Confusion. *Nursing Clinics of North America, 25*, 909–918.

Reisberg, B., Ferris, S. H., Torossian, C., Kluger, A., & Monteiro, I. (1992). Pharmacologic treatment of Alzheimer's disease: A methodologic critique based upon current knowledge of symptomatology and relevance for drug trials. *International Psychogeriatrics, 4*(Suppl. 1), 9–42.

Reynolds, C. F., Hoch, C. C., Kupfer, D. J., Buysse, D. J., Houck, P. R., Stack, J. A., & Campbell, D. W. (1988). Bedside differentiation of depressive pseudodementia from dementia. *American Journal of Psychiatry, 145*, 1099–1103.

Risse, S. C., & Barnes, R. (1986). Pharamacologic treatment of agitation associated with dementia. *Journal of the American Geriatric Society, 34*, 368–376.

Rockwood, K. (1989). Acute confusion in elderly medical patients. *Journal of the American Geriatric Society, 37*, 150–154.

Roslaniec, A., & Fitzpatrick, J. J. (1979). Changes in mental status in older adults with four days of hospitalization. *Research in Nursing & Health, 2*, 177–187.

Rovner, B. W., German, P. S., Broadhead, J., Morriss, R. K., Brant, L. J., Blaustein, J., & Folstein, M. F. (1990). The prevalence and management of dementia and other psychiatric disorders in nursing homes. *International Psychogeriatrics, 2*, 13–24.

Salzman, C. (1987). Treatment of the elderly agitated patient. *Journal of Clinical Psychiatry, 48*(Suppl. 5), 19–22.

Schneider, L. S., Martinez, R. A., & Lebowitz, B. D. (1993). Clinical psychopharmacology research in geriatrics: An agenda for research. *International Journal of Geriatric Psychiatry, 8*, 89–93.

Schneider, L. S., & Sobin, P. B. (1992). Non-neuroleptic treatment of behavioral symptoms and agitation in Alzheimer's disease and other dementias. *Psychopharmacology Bulletin, 28*, 71–79.

Smith, D. A., & Perry, P. J. (1992). Nonneuroleptic treatment of disruptive behavior in organic mental syndromes. *Annals of Pharmacotherapy, 26*, 1400–1408.

Smith, M., Buckwalter, K. C., & Mitchell, S. (1993). *Geriatric mental health training series*. New York: Springer Publishing Co.

Spector, W. D. (1991). Cognitive impairment and disruptive behaviors among community based elderly persons: Implications for targeting long-term care. *The Gerontologist, 31*, 51–59.

Sternberg, J., Whelihan, W. M., Fretwell, M. D., Bielicki, C. A., & Murray, S. L. (1989). Disruptive behavior in the elderly: Nurses' perceptions. *Clinical Gerontologist, 8*, 43–56.

Szwabo, P. A., & Grossberg, G. T. (Eds.). (1993). *Problem behaviors in long-term care: Recognition, diagnosis, and treatment*. New York: Springer Publishing Co.

Taft, L. B. (1989). Conceptual analysis of agitation in the confused elderly. *Archives of Psychiatric Nursing, 3*, 102–107.

Taft, L. B. (1992). Validation therapy. In M. Snyder (Ed.), *Independent nursing interventions* (pp. 137–144). Albany, NY: Delmar.

Taft, L. B. (1994). *Dementia care: Interventions and factors influencing caregiving approaches*. Unpublished doctoral dissertation, Rush University, Chicago, IL.

Taft, L. B., & Cronin-Stubbs, D. (1995). Behavioral symptoms in dementia: An update. *Research in Nursing & Health, 18*, 145–163.

Task Force on DSM-IV. (1993). *DSM-IV draft criteria*. Unpublished manuscript, American Psychiatric Association, Washington, DC.

Tavani, C. A. (1990). Perioperative psychiatric considerations in the elderly. *Clinics in Geriatric Medicine, 6*, 543–556.

Teri, L., Rabins, P., Whitehouse, P., Berg, L., Risberg, B., Sunderland, T., Eichelman, B., & Creighton, P. (1992). Management of behavior disturbance in Alzheimer disease: Current knowledge and future directions. *Alzheimer Disease and Associated Disorders, 6*, 77–88.

Ugarriza, D. N., & Gray, T. (1993). Alzheimer's disease: Nursing interventions for clients and caretaker. *Journal of Psychosocial Nursing and Mental Health Services, 31*(10), 7–10.

Vaccaro, F. J. (1988a). Application of operant procedures in a group of institutionalized aggressive geriatric patients. *Psychology and Aging, 3*, 22–28.

Vaccaro, F. J. (1988b). Successful operant conditioning procedures with an institutionalized aggressive geriatric patient. *International Journal of Aging and Human Development, 26*, 71–79.

Vaccaro, F. J. (1990). Application of social skills training in a group of institutionalized aggressive elderly patients. *Psychology and Aging, 5*, 369–378.

Watt, D. F. (1993). Delirium and DSM-IV [Letter to the editor]. *Journal of Neuropsychiatry, 5,* 459–460.

Weiler, P. G., Lubben, J. E., & Chi, I. (1991). Cognitive impairment and hospital use. *American Journal of Public Health, 81,* 1153–1157.

Weiss, L. J., & Lazarus, L. W. (1993). Psychosocial treatment of the geropsychiatric patient. *International Journal of Psychotherapy, 8,* 95–100.

Williams, M. A., Campbell, E. B., Raynor, W. J., Mlynarczyk, S. M., & Ward, S. E. (1985). Reducing acute confusional states in elderly patients with hip fractures. *Research in Nursing & Health, 8,* 329–337.

Wise, M. G., & Brandt, G. T. (1992). Delirium. In S. C. Yudofsky & R. E. Hales (Eds.), *Textbook of neuropsychiatry* (2nd ed.) (pp. 291–310). Washington, DC: American Psychiatric Press.

Wolanin, M. E., & Phillips, L. R. F. (1981). *Confusion: Prevention and care.* St. Louis: Mosby.

Zubenko, G. S. (1990). Progression of illness in the differential diagnosis of primary dementia. *American Journal of Psychiatry, 147,* 435–438.

Zusy, M. J. (1993, July 12). National Institute of Nursing Research. *Nursing Spectrum,* p. 17.

Chapter 3

Uncertainty in Acute Illness

MERLE H. MISHEL
SCHOOL OF NURSING
UNIVERSITY OF NORTH CAROLINA AT CHAPEL HILL

ABSTRACT

In this chapter, the research on uncertainty in acute illness is reviewed and critiqued. Both qualitative and quantitative studies are included. The review considers the cause and consequences of uncertainty from research on adults and from research on parents of acutely ill children.

Keywords: Uncertainty, Acute Illness, Coping, Adjustment, Interventions

Uncertainty regarding an illness has been identified as the greatest single psychological stressor for the patient with a life-threatening illness (Koocher, 1984). Uncertainty is not the total experience in acute and chronic illness, yet it is a constant occurrence from diagnosis through living with a long-term illness or condition. Study of uncertainty dates back to some of the early work by F. Davis (1960), who detailed the difference between clinical and functional uncertainty and tied the experience to the delivery of care and the agenda of health care providers. From 1960 through 1974, other classic pieces on uncertainty emerged, which included the work by McIntosh (1974, 1976) on the desire for information among patients with cancer. This work provided some of the first ideas about the ambiguity surrounding diagnosis and prognosis and the influence of this ambiguity on the patient's psychological state. Work by Wiener in 1975 explored the topic of uncertainty in chronic illness. This classic work on living with uncertainty brought home the invasion of uncertainty into multiple aspects of life and the strategies to tolerate the uncertainty.

Since the publication of the Mishel Uncertainty in Illness Scale (MUIS) (Mishel, 1981), the Parents Perception of Uncertainty Scale (PPUS) (Mishel, 1983b), the exploration of uncertainty scales for specific populations (Mishel, 1983a) along with early conceptualization of the variable within illness (Mishel, 1981), the study of uncertainty has greatly proliferated. Qualitative and quantitative work, both in nursing and in other fields, added to the knowledge of the experience of uncertainty in illness. The research has spread to practice through clinical publications (Hilton, 1992; Righter, 1995; Wurzbach, 1992).

This chapter is limited to research with acutely ill populations. Areas of research such as uncertainty in pregnancy, training of physicians to manage uncertainty, and environmental or workplace uncertainty were not included. Articles were selected if the investigator focused on acute illness and if uncertainty was one of the major topics under study, was measured in quantitative studies, or emerged as a major theme from qualitative work. If uncertainty was mentioned but not treated as a distinct topic, the research was not included. Information was retrieved through computerized databases, including MEDLINE (1976–1995), Cumulative Index to Nursing and Allied Health Literature (CINAHL) (1982–1995), and PsycLit (1984–1995), along with use of the invisible college approach (Cooper, 1982). The work of investigators known to the author was tracked, along with a search for publications from users of the MUIS. All users of the MUIS are located in a database; names were taken from this list to check for publications. The ancestry approach of tracking citations from published studies also was employed. The personal library of the chapter author was culled for relevant publications on uncertainty in illness.

In this chapter, work on the major conceptualizations of uncertainty in acute illness are reviewed, along with the work on measuring uncertainty. The causes and consequences of uncertainty in acute illness with adults and in parents of acutely ill children are reviewed. Work on interventions to modify uncertainty in acute illness is presented. Inclusion of these topics necessitates citing some studies more than once. The chapter concludes with recommendations for future research.

CONCEPTUALIZATION AND MEASUREMENT OF UNCERTAINTY IN ILLNESS

In an area of investigation, conceptualization of the phenomenon either drives the study or explains the findings. Few frameworks have been offered in nursing to explain uncertainty in illness. The major conceptualization was offered by Mishel (1988) and grew out of work in related fields. Mishel offered a theory of uncertainty in illness that incorporates a number of conceptual ideas from the work on stress and coping by Lazarus and Folkman (1984). Mishel's conceptualization was the first to focus on uncertainty in illness and tie together research from nursing and related fields to support the links in the theoretical model. In Mishel's publication of the uncertainty in illness theory (1988), she detailed specific antecedents of uncertainty, the appraisal of uncertainty, and the management of uncertainty that influences adaptation as the end state. Mishel (1990) stated that the theory has its strongest support among persons who are experiencing the acute phase of illness or are in illnesses with a downward trajectory.

Following the initial work by Mishel, Selder (1989) presented a life transition theory that described how people restructure their lives and resolve uncertainty after a major experiential transition. The theory is described as applicable to events that qualify as disrupting one's view of reality. Such events may include illness, but are not limited to illness experiences, and may include acute loss as well as other individually defined events. Because this theory is not specifically applicable to the experience of acute illness, it will not be reviewed in this chapter.

The original theory offered by Mishel that was targeted to those in an acute illness experience has been used as either the original conceptualization or the basis for explanation of a number of studies that will be reviewed in this chapter. There is continuing support accumulating for many of the linkages in the model; specifically, for the linkages between antecedents of uncertainty, such as symptom pattern, social support, relationship with health care providers, and uncertainty itself; uncertainty and various personality or cognitive factors, such as mastery and self-efficacy; linkages between uncertainty and danger, uncertainty and emotion-focused coping, and uncertainty and adjustment difficulties. Of the 44 published studies on uncertainty in acute illness included in this review, 18 used a portion of Mishel's 1988 conceptualization of uncertainty as the framework for the investigation or as the explanation for the results. In six of the studies, the conceptualization was based on the stress-and-coping framework of Lazarus and Folkman (1984), whereas social comparison theory, along with the illness trajectory framework, was used in a few studies (Corbin & Strauss, 1991). In qualitative investigations, particularly those by Cohen (1993a, 1995a), conceptualizations were offered to explain the experience of parents while waiting for a diagnosis and following diagnosis. Although these conceptualizations may appear to be alternate theories of uncertainty in illness, they are, to date, limited to the experience of parents of acutely ill children and have not been applied to adults. Other various frameworks were used in four of the investigations while the remaining studies lacked any theory or conceptualization of uncertainty.

Measurement of uncertainty is more consistent than the conceptualization of uncertainty. Of the 34 quantitative investigations, 26 used one of the

Uncertainty in Illness scales developed by Mishel, either the total scale, a subscale, or selected items were used (Mast, 1995). There is some initial work on a Swedish version of the MUIS, albeit the definition of uncertainty may not be consistent across language and culture (Hallberg & Erlandsson, 1991; Mishel, 1991). Although the MUIS and the PPUS are scales derived from Mishel's conceptualization of uncertainty, many investigators who used either scale did not use any theory of uncertainty. Most often the studies were atheoretical.

A second instrument on uncertainty in illness was developed by Hilton (1994). This instrument is based on the stress-and-coping framework by Lazarus and Folkman (1984) and is not derived from a nursing theory of uncertainty in illness. Five studies contained an investigator-derived scale. The reliability of these measures was adequate, although the investigators did not provide any information on the validity of these scales.

CAUSES OF UNCERTAINTY IN ADULTS
WITH ACUTE ILLNESS

As noted by Mast (1995) in her review of research on uncertainty in illness, many investigators have explored variables proposed to be causes of uncertainty. The variables most commonly studied as causes of uncertainty included severity of illness, specificity of diagnosis, personality factors, social support, health care providers, and demographic variables. The selection of antecedents of uncertainty was infrequently based on theory or prior research.

Severity of Illness

Although the majority of investigators reported a relationship between uncertainty and illness severity, diversity in measuring illness severity may account for the absence of consistent findings. Recurrence of disease is one index of severity, as recurrence implies the inability to control the disease. Hilton (1994), using a sample of cancer patients, women having breast biopsy, kidney transplant patients, and those waiting for a transplant, found that recurrence of disease predicted 21% of the variance in the Uncertainty Stress Scale. Cancer patients with more extensive disease significantly differed from those with less extensive disease.

A second approach to measuring severity of illness was repeat surgery or repeat hospitalization for the same condition. In a comparison between those hospitalized for initial versus repeat surgery for cardiovascular disease, Ronayne (1985) reported that uncertainty levels were higher in those with repeat surgery. Returning for repeat treatment also was found to increase uncertainty among cancer patients (Van Den Borne, Pruyn, & Van Den Heuvel, 1987). Mishel (1981), reporting on a sample of hospitalized patients with a variety of diagnoses, found that less time between prior and current hospitalization was significantly associated with higher levels of uncertainty. Similar findings for repeated hospitalizations were reported by Andersson-Segesten (1991). Galloway and Graydon (1996), reporting on a sample of patients treated for colon cancer, found that the longer a patient was hospitalized, the higher was their level of uncertainty. It appears that the stand-in measures for seriousness of illness reported in these studies were useful in studying the association between seriousness of illness and uncertainty.

Some objective indices of seriousness of illness have been found to correlate with uncertainty in patients who are in the treatment phase of acute illness. Mishel (1984) reported that uncertainty was associated with seriousness of illness as measured by the Seriousness of Illness Rating Scale (Wyler, Masuda, & Holmes, 1968). Also, among sicker patients, as indicated by the self-report Heart Failure Functional Status Inventory (Dracup, Walden, Stevenson, & Brecht, 1992), uncertainty remained much higher over time as compared to a group of stronger patients (Hawthorne & Hixon, 1994). Yet, these findings were not supported when illness severity was measured by a subjective evaluation among women recently diagnosed with gynecological cancer or by the Peel Diagnostic Index among men following a myocardial infarction (Christman et al., 1988; Mishel, Hostetter, King, & Graham, 1984).

Out of the 10 studies measuring the association between uncertainty and seriousness of illness, investigators in 8 studies reported a positive association, whereas 2 did not find a significant relationship. Because many of the positive findings are based on stand-in measures of seriousness, the findings cannot be considered conclusive, and further work is needed on a measure of seriousness of illness that can be used across a number of studies.

Specificity of Diagnosis

Closely related to seriousness of illness is specificity of diagnosis. Mishel (1988) proposed that uncertainty would be higher when a diagnosis was absent or when the person was undergoing diagnostic procedures. Mishel (1981) found significant differences in uncertainty levels between medical patients and those undergoing a diagnostic workup. This finding was repeated for a diagnostic workup group versus those having a surgical procedure. Further support for higher levels of uncertainty when a diagnosis is absent was reported for men undergoing a cardiac catheterization as compared to men undergoing hemodialysis (Mishel, 1981). Northouse, Jeffs, Cracchiolo-Caraway, Lampman, and Dorris (1995) reported that uncertainty was a significant predictor of emotional distress in women awaiting breast biopsy for possible breast cancer. Further support was offered by Hilton (1993) who reported from qualitative data that families of women with breast cancer rated uncertainty prior to diagnosis higher then uncertainty at treatment or 1 year posttreatment. The findings are consistent for the relationship between lack of a diagnosis and uncertainty across qualitative and quantitative investigations.

Personality Factors

The role of personality factors as an antecedent of uncertainty has received some attention with study of perceived control over illness and meaning in life. Mishel and Braden (1988) conceptualized perceived control over the illness as a measure of the variable of symptom pattern, which is an antecedent of uncertainty in the uncertainty theory (Mishel, 1988). Measured by a one-item scale ranging from 1 as no control to 10 as total control, less control was found to be a significant predictor of ambiguity, a type of uncertainty, at diagnosis and during treatment for women with gynecological cancer. Eight months after treatment ended, women who estimated that their illness was close to being under control had significantly lower levels of uncertainty (Mishel & Braden, 1987, 1988). Lack of control, as indexed by depression, was found to be a significant predictor of uncertainty within 1 week of diagnosis among patients receiving treatment for hematologic malignancies (Richardson et al., 1987). Related to personal control, Hilton (1989) found that meaning in life, or a sense of commitment, was related to lower levels of uncertainty in women receiving treatment for breast cancer. Although the data suggest support for the variable of perceived control as a predictor of uncertainty, a contrary finding of no relationship between control and uncertainty was reported by Christman (1990) in cancer patients receiving radiation treatment. However, at the end of treatment, patients who desired more behavioral involvement in their care reported higher levels of uncertainty.

The inconsistency across studies is likely due to problems in the definition and measurement of control. Mishel and Braden (1987, 1988) used a 1-item measure which is a dubious reflection of the complexity of the concept of control, while other investigators used a variety of measures and labels for control ranging from lack of having control, personal sense of control, preference for control, and preference for involvement in care. Future investigations are needed where the concept of control is clearly and fully defined and appropriately measured.

Social Support

A number of investigators have studied the role of social support and uncertainty. L. L. Davis (1990) reported that among patients recovering from injury or illness and among their care providers, use of their support system and support network was related to less uncertainty. Similar findings were reported by Bennett (1993), Mishel and Braden (1987, 1988), and Di Iorio, Faherty, and Manteuffel (1991). Mishel and Braden (1987) found that the type of social support needed to reduce uncertainty changed over time among women with gynecological cancer. During diagnosis, affirmation, or the chance to share one's thoughts about the illness with another, was associated with a reduction in ambiguity, a type of uncertainty about the state of the illness. At treatment, affirmation continued, but now reduced a second type of uncertainty, complexity concerning treatment. Eight months later, the support factor of aid reduced the unpredictability of the outcome. Di Iorio et al. (1991) found that it was the intimacy and assistance aspect of social support that reduced unpredictability. Those who were more integrated into a social network experienced less unpredictability about the illness.

The intimacy aspect of social support is likely to come from a patient's spouse, yet Northouse, Laten, and Reddy (1995) reported that uncertainty levels were higher in the spouses of women with recurrent breast cancer then in the women themselves. This finding points out the need to assess uncertainty in the major support persons, as their uncertainty may hamper them in providing support to the patient. As Northouse, Laten, and Reddy noted, there is a need to identify the factors that affect the spouse's uncertainty.

Social support is not limited to family and friends, but it can be extended to include similar others. Molleman, Pruyn, and Knippenberg (1986) reported that cancer patients used fellow patients for social comparison as uncertainty increased. Fellow patients were seen as more informative. There was a preference for interaction with fellow patients who were similar or slightly better in terms of health status. Contact with others was instrumental in reducing uncertainty. Use of others similar in diagnosis, treatment, or health status to reduce uncertainty has been found to be diagnosis-specific. Breast cancer patients who did not receive relevant information from their health care provider used fellow patients to reduce uncertainty about the treatment options. For patients with Hodgkin's disease, such contacts with fellow patients were found to increase uncertainty (Van Den Borne et al., 1987), although the measure of social support was not specified in this study.

Further evidence supporting the specificity of social support in relationship to uncertainty was offered by White and Frasure-Smith (1995) who found that social support mediated the relationship between uncertainty and distress at 1 and 3 months postsurgery for angioplasty patients but not for bypass patients. Differences in the use of social support by diagnostic group seem to be due to the number of questions and the ability of others to provide needed information. Among the diagnostic groups where patients used social support to reduce uncertainty, there were specific questions related to either diagnosis or treatment, and fellow sufferers or significant others could provide concrete information or individually tailored answers (Van Den Borne et al., 1987; White & Frasure-Smith, 1995). At this time, the findings for the use of social support to reduce uncertainty are consistent and the studies provide further information on the type of support that affects specific aspects of uncertainty. Further information on which patients benefitted from the use of social support and the sources of support, such as similar others, to manage uncertainty is beginning to appear in the literature.

Health Care Providers

As experts, health care providers have been proposed to reduce uncertainty by providing information and promoting confidence in their clinical judgement (Mishel, 1988). Desire for information has been associated with higher levels of uncertainty (Galloway & Graydon, 1996). The evidence from four studies supported the proposed relationship. Trust and confidence in the health care provider was found to explain 35% of the variance in uncertainty among women receiving treatment for gynecological cancer (Mishel & Braden, 1988). Van Den Borne et al. (1987), using an investigator-devised measure of uncertainty that demonstrated adequate reliability with 369 breast and lymphoma cancer patients receiving treatment, reported that relevant information from specialists contributed to a decrease in uncertainty about treatment possibilities. When information from specialists was not relevant, contact with fellow patients was initiated. Relevant information for persons with cancer included addressing physical complaints, psychosocial complaints, and treatment (Borgers et al., 1993). Yet, making a distinction between managing uncertainty and managing anxiety, Molleman et al. (1984), in a study of 418 cancer patients, found that contact with experts was the most effective means of reducing uncertainty while the support of the home environment and fellow patients helped to reduce anxiety. Molleman et al. (1986) found support for the patient's choice of experts over nonexperts when patients experience uncertainty. Fellow patients were only a secondary source if the primary source was not available. The most important source of information about the illness and treatment was the medical specialist and, if this information was viewed as useful, uncertainty was reduced (Molleman et al., 1986; Van Den

Borne et al., 1987). All of these studies had an adequate size sample, measures were reliable, and the findings were consistent; the physician has a primary role in reducing the patient's uncertainty.

Demographic Variables

The most common demographic variables investigated for a relationship with uncertainty are education, age, employment, and socioeconomic status. The conceptual rationale for studying education, socioeconomic status, and age as factors influencing uncertainty lies in the experience and knowledge that is likely to be embedded in older age, higher socioeconomic status, and higher education. Experience and knowledge are factors that can reduce uncertainty. There is no conceptual rationale for including employment status.

Lack of support for the relationship between age, marital status, and uncertainty has been reported across varied populations (Andersson-Segersten, 1991; Christman et al., 1988; Mishel, 1984; Mishel et al., 1984; Stetz, 1989; Webster & Christman, 1988; White & Frasure-Smith, 1995; Wong & Bramwell, 1992). The findings for the influence of education are less consistent. Support for the relationship between less education and more uncertainty was found by Mishel et al. (1984) and Hilton (1994) for breast cancer patients and by Christman et al. (1988) at hospital discharge and 1 week later for myocardial infarction patients. Opposite findings were reported by Andersson-Segesten (1991) for patients in intensive coronary care units, by Wong and Bramwell (1992) for breast cancer patients after mastectomy, and by Mishel (1984) among hospitalized medical patients. Fewer investigators have assessed the relationship between socioeconomic status and uncertainty. The findings from two studies are different, with Stetz (1989) reporting that income had no relationship to uncertainty among care-providers and Webster and Christman (1988) finding that patients in lower social classes reported greater uncertainty.

Concerning findings on racial or cultural differences in uncertainty, only one study has been reported in the literature. Among African American cancer patients, including men 3 weeks after treatment for prostate cancer and women 3 months into treatment for breast cancer, uncertainty was reported to be a significant predictor of emotional distress (Mishel, Belyea, et al., 1996). From the results of one study, it appears that uncertainty impacts similarly on White and Black cancer patients.

The results of studies on the relationship between demographic variables and uncertainty show a great deal of inconsistency and are limited to few or no studies on certain demographic variables. Some of this may be due to small sample size, translation of the uncertainty scale into another language, as in the Andersson-Segesten (1991) study, lack of variability in the sample, or excess heterogeneity that masks a possible relationship. All of these methodological problems are found in the studies of demographic variables and uncertainty.

CONSEQUENCES OF UNCERTAINTY

The Impact of Uncertainty on Personality Dispositions

According to the uncertainty theory proposed by Mishel (1988), uncertainty is a neutral cognitive state that is appraised for its value or meaning. In the process of appraisal, a variety of cognitive and personality variables has been proposed by investigators as related to the experience of uncertainty among persons receiving treatment for acute illness. In a report of the proposed relationship between uncertainty and the personality disposition of optimism in women recently diagnosed for cancer, uncertainty had a significant impact on the reduction of optimism (Mishel et al., 1984). Christman (1990) replicated the test of the relationship between uncertainty and optimism using the same instruments with patients receiving radiation therapy at the start of treatment, after the 15th, and after the last treatment. Higher levels of uncertainty were related to a decreased sense of hope at the first and 15th treatment and the direction of the relationship continued by the last treatment, although the relationship was not significant. In further support for the influence of uncertainty on reducing positive cognitive variables, Hilton (1994) reported that higher levels of uncertainty were associated with a reduced sense of coherence in women treated for breast cancer.

Further study has focused on the role of personality dispositions as mediators between uncertainty and negative outcomes. In such investigations, Mishel et al. (1984) proposed that a sense of optimism might weaken the impact of uncertainty on negative outcome variables. Mishel and Sorenson (1991) reported that, although uncertainty was related to lower mastery, mastery mediated the relationship between uncertainty and danger. With mastery considered, the relationship between uncertainty and danger was not significant. This finding was replicated with a second sample of women with gynecological cancer, and the mediation effect of mastery held. Mastery also strengthened the sense of opportunity for those with lower uncertainty levels, although the strength of the mediation effect differed across the two samples (Mishel, Padilla, Grant, & Sorenson, 1991).

The test of the mediation effect of mastery offers promise for learning how cognitive variables function. Although there is evidence that uncertainty is inversely related to positive cognitive states, these factors may still mediate between uncertainty and negative outcomes, but the mediation effect is rarely investigated.

MANAGEMENT OF UNCERTAINTY

Numerous investigators have studied the management of uncertainty in persons with acute illness and the findings from these investigations are very consistent. Congruent with the findings reviewed by Mast (1995), higher uncertainty was associated with emotion-focused coping strategies in the majority of studies that tested the direct relationship between uncertainty and coping. Across a variety of populations, the predominant strategies were less confrontive-oriented coping and more passive in nature, such as wishful thinking, cognitive avoidance, evasion, and fatalism (Christman, 1990; Hilton, 1989, 1994; Redeker, 1992; Webster & Christman, 1988).

Although the majority of findings were consistent, some inconsistencies emerged when subjects were followed over time. Redeker (1992) reported that at 6 weeks following coronary bypass surgery, patients exchanged passive strategies to manage uncertainty for the more active management strategy of seeking social support. In contrast, Christman et al. (1988) found that for patients with cardiac disease, uncertainty was not related to coping prior to hospital discharge but was associated with the use of less confrontive coping 1 week and 4 weeks after discharge. These were the few studies that tracked uncertainty and coping from the acute event into the rehabilitation phase. Although the findings on coping with uncertainty over time are sparse, this is a fruitful area for investigation, as coping strategies to manage uncertainty seem to change over time.

One limitation in the current work is the restricted view of coping as either problem- or emotion-focused based on the work of Lazarus and Folkman (1984). There are a few investigations in which coping has been broadened to include more diverse strategies. In a rare qualitative approach to the study of cancer patients receiving chemotherapy, Wiener and Dodd (1993) identified management strategies that they termed as ''uncertainty abatement work,'' which included pacing activities, being a professional patient, using ''worst'' case comparisons, constructing personal meaning for events, and finding supportive others. Molleman et al. (1984) attempted to devise a specific coping instrument for managing uncertainty, although the selected items were drawn from current literature, which heavily weighted them with avoidance and withdrawal items. Four strategies to manage uncertainty were self-instruction methods, which included withdrawal and avoidance, social means, which included using health care providers as resources, ego-defensive methods, and direct action. In a test of the effectiveness of these strategies in reducing uncertainty, no significant differences were found among subjects grouped by level of use of a strategy. In a secondary analysis of the use of social strategies, use of experts was found to be effective in reducing uncertainty (Molleman et al., 1984). Borgers et al. (1993) conceptualized information-seeking as a coping strategy among cancer patients. The investigators found that uncertainty was highly correlated with the intention to seek information about diagnostic tests, physical complaints, prognosis, and treatment.

Two studies were conducted to investigate compliance with treatment protocol as the behavioral management strategy. Whereas Richardson et al. (1987) found that uncertainty did not predict compliance in patients receiving cancer therapy, Di Iorio et al. (1991) found that unpredictability and ambiguity, two types of uncertainty, contributed significantly to discriminating compliant from noncompliant persons among those enrolled in a new test of an antiepileptic drug. Although the findings on compliance differ, they represent an attempt to investigate something different than the usual two categories of emotion- or problem-oriented coping. Compliance was selected because it was a management strategy appropriate for the population under study. Tying the study of coping to strategies specific to the population under study is a logical approach. Measures of coping that are relevant for the target population and the uncertainty being experienced are needed. The support found for the relationship between uncertainty and emotion-focused coping and lack of findings on uncertainty and problem-focused coping may be due to the coping measures used in these investigations. Qualitative studies have revealed a number of strategies that are used to manage uncertainty, but very few of these strategies are included in current instruments for measuring coping.

Some investigators have studied the indirect path between uncertainty and coping as proposed by Mishel (1988). Bennett (1993) found that uncertainty had an indirect effect on reducing problem-focused coping and reducing coping effectiveness by a path through negative emotion. Mishel and Sorenson (1991) and Mishel et al. (1991) found, in the original and replicated study, that uncertainty evaluated as a danger related to a higher level of emotion-focused coping, but when uncertainty was appraised as an opportunity, this strengthened the use of a problem-focused strategy.

Further study has been directed at the effectiveness of the coping strategies used to manage uncertainty during acute illness. Mishel and Sorenson (1991) and Mishel et al. (1991) tested mediating effects of coping in the relationship between uncertainty appraised as a danger and emotional distress in two different samples of women under treatment for cancer. If the coping strategies are effective in managing uncertainty, then the relationship between uncertainty appraised as a danger and emotional distress should be weakened by the addition of the coping methods. The emotion-focused coping strategy of wishful thinking did not function as an effective coping mechanism. The relationship between uncertainty appraised as a danger and emotional distress continued to be significant, although somewhat reduced by wishful thinking.

Christman et al. (1988) reported that prior to discharge and 4 weeks postdischarge, uncertainty was the major contributor to emotional distress in patients with a myocardial infarction. None of the coping strategies associated with uncertainty had a contributory effect on explaining emotional distress over time.

The ineffectiveness of coping strategies to mediate between uncertainty and emotional distress is likely due to the limited choice of coping strategies included on current coping scales. Developing new measures of coping should be of interest in future research in order to identify the strategies that will function to reduce the stressful nature of uncertainty. These strategies have been identified in qualitative investigations, and instruments need to be developed and tested that incorporate these management strategies (Mishel & Murdaugh, 1987; Molleman et al., 1986; Wiener & Dodd, 1993).

UNCERTAINTY AND ADJUSTMENT

A number of investigators have studied the relationship between uncertainty and a variety of psychosocial outcomes. As noted by Mast (1995), the most frequent finding is the positive relationship between uncertainty and emotional distress, anxiety, and depression across a variety of clinical populations (Bennett, 1993; Christman et al., 1988; L. L. Davis, 1990; Hawthorne & Hixon, 1994; Hilton, 1994; Mishel, 1981, 1984; Mishel et al., 1991; Mishel & Sorenson, 1991; Northouse, Jeffs, et al., 1995; Richardson et al., 1987; Webster & Christman, 1988; White & Frasure-Smith, 1995; Yates & Booton-Hiser, 1992). Yet, Northouse, Dorris, and Charron-More (1995) did not find uncertainty to be a predictor of either emotional distress or role adjustment in women with recurrent breast cancer or in their spouses. In that study, uncertainty was significantly associated with two of the three predictor variables and two dependent variables. It is likely that all of the variance in outcome measures attributable to uncertainty was accounted for by the relationship between uncertainty and the other predictor variables. The authors did not test for the prediction of the outcome variables by uncertainty alone.

Uncertainty has also been related to poorer psychosocial adjustment in the areas of less life satisfaction (Hilton, 1994), negative attitudes toward health care, family relationships, recreation, and employment (Mishel et al., 1984; Mishel & Braden, 1987), satisfaction with medical care and knowledge about the disease (Richardson et al., 1987), and perceived poor health of the caregiver (Stetz, 1989). Uncertainty also is associated with lower quality of life, particularly in the areas of family, spirituality, and physical and symptom distress (Hawthorne & Hixon, 1994; Padilla, Mishel, & Grant, 1992).

The relationship between uncertainty and psychosocial adjustment has been found to continue over time. Wong and Bramwell (1992) reported that the relationship between uncertainty and anxiety continued from hospitalization to home, and increased in strength over time among breast cancer patients. These results were supported by Christman (1990) who reported that uncertainty was a significant predictor of psychosocial adjustment problems 15 days into radiation therapy and at the last radiation treatment. In addition, uncertainty continued as the major variable influencing emotional distress in myocardial infarction patients in the transition from hospital to home and into the rehabilitation period (Christman et al., 1988). Among hysterectomy patients, Warrington and Gottlieb (1987) reported that women with higher uncertainty levels had no decrease in anxiety from surgery to 6 days postsurgery as compared with women with lower uncertainty levels. Mishel and Braden (1987) offered more support for the lasting relationship between uncertainty and adjustment problems, although they noted that the areas of adjustment effected by uncertainty change from diagnosis to 8 months posttreatment in women treated for gynecological cancer.

CAUSES OF UNCERTAINTY IN PARENTS OF ACUTELY ILL CHILDREN

There were seven studies identified in the literature on acutely ill children; four focused on the parents' experience during the child's hospitalization and three focused on the diagnosis phase of illness. These are included under acute illness, as the child is usually severely ill at the time of receiving a diagnosis. The diagnosis may be a chronic illness or an illness requiring severe lifesaving treatment or stabilization with the potential of recurrence and extension. There were no published studies on the child's experience of uncertainty in acute illness.

Diagnosis

Among parents of hospitalized children, lack of a diagnosis or receiving medical treatment created higher levels of uncertainty then being hospitalized for a specific surgical procedure (Mishel, 1983b). Using the Parent Perception of Uncertainty Scale, the perceived seriousness of the child's illness was significantly associated with higher uncertainty levels in the parents. Similar to the findings reported by Mishel (1983b), in grounded-theory studies of parents of children with cancer, investigators reported that undergoing diagnostic testing was a major cause of uncertainty (Clarke-Steffen, 1993; Cohen,

1995a; Cohen & Martinson, 1988). Many parents identified the waiting for results from diagnostic testing as the worst part of the experience, and that the distress from the uncertainty was relieved by diagnosis (Clarke-Steffen, 1993; Cohen, 1995a). Cohen described the process of considering multiple diagnoses and discarding some over time, thus narrowing the possibilities. This process involved waiting while the possible diagnoses were whittled down—an experience described as diffuse unbearable uncertainty by parents.

Further work is needed on the experience of receiving a diagnosis. Cohen's qualitative studies provide a direction that can be followed for further investigation and substantiation by other investigators. The limited publications in the area point to the need for further research.

Symptoms of Illness

Determining that symptoms are serious was described as a process that occurred over time and created uncertainty because the parents could not be sure what was significant and what could be disregarded. Prior to entering the health care system or prior to diagnostic testing, Cohen (1995a), Cohen and Martinson (1988), and Brett and Davies (1988) described a similar process for evaluating symptoms in the child. In all three studies, the investigators noted that parents went through a process of explaining away symptoms, trying to handle them in a number of ways until the problem was recognized as not normal, and the parents and child entered the health care system. Cohen (1995a) presented this process as three stages and offered exquisite detail about the components of each stage. Impaired confidence in the parents' ability to appraise health problems in the ill child and siblings resulted from their judgement or misdiagnosis of the ill child (Cohen & Martinson, 1988). Related findings addressed to illness changes due to treatment were reported by Turner, Tomlinson, and Harbaugh (1990) who found that parents lacked a cognitive map to interpret the relationship between treatment and expected changes in the child. Inability to classify treatments as common or unusual also generated uncertainty.

All of the work in this area is from a qualitative perspective. The excellent work on explaining the processes that parents experience is due to the sound qualitative investigations done by independent investigators with consistent findings and interpretations.

Health Care Providers

Health care providers were often described as not helpful in sharing information. Clarke-Steffen (1993) reported that families functioned under partial knowledge and believed that physicians withheld information. Turner et al. (1990), from the study of parents of a child hospitalized in a pediatric intensive care unit, reported that unfamiliarity with hospital routines and unfamiliarity with the roles of each staff member generated uncertainty about the environment of care. Inability to judge the competence of caregivers and the adequacy of response to emergencies led to uncertainty about caregivers. Similarly Cohen (1993b) gave the label of ''situational uncertainty'' to the experience of parents trying to navigate through an unfamiliar medical environment with unwritten expectations from the staff concerning expected parental behavior. Based on these studies, there was no evidence to support that caregivers functioned to reduce uncertainty among parents of acutely ill children, although the number of studies is quite small and the area has not been fully studied.

Family System

Changes in the family system were found to be sources of uncertainty in two studies (Clarke-Steffen, 1993; Turner et al., 1990). The illness of the child placed demands on the family that changed family roles, goals, family plans, and daily family life. The changes were unanticipated and still unknown resulting in uncertainty about the extent and duration of impact on the family system. Turner et al. (1990) labeled ''family system uncertainty'' as encompassing the issues and questions related to relationships within the child-rearing family.

Consequences of Uncertainty and Management of Uncertainty

In the only published study measuring parental uncertainty over time, Miles, Funk, and Kasper (1992) reported that parents of infants in a neonatal intensive care unit (NICU) experienced the greatest level of uncertainty in the area of unpredictability. Although uncertainty scores dropped over time, scores on the unpredictability factor decreased the least from the first week of the infant's admission to a week later. Unpredictability items refer to prognosis and outcome, and this may remain a constant issue during hospitalization. Turner et al. (1990) reported a number of negative consequences from uncertainty, including feelings of helplessness, anxiety, and overall lack of control over what happens to their hospitalized child. Uncertainty inhibited parents from naturally relating to their child and increased a sense of self-blame for the child's illness. Similarly, LaMontagne and Pawlak (1990), in a similar study of parents of children in a NICU, found that 40% of the parents identified uncertainty as a predominant stressor. In determining how these parents coped with uncertainty, the investigators reported that emotion-focused coping of escape and avoidance was more common than problem-focused coping. There was less use of social support in contrast to parents where uncertainty was not the major stressor. It is not surprising that emotion-focused coping strategies predominated in a situation where strong emotions may interfere with effective functioning (LaMontagne & Pawlak, 1990).

There is need for further research on the parental response to acute illness in the child and the role of uncertainty in that experience. A few studies have been done to investigate this topic, but further research is needed. Also, research is absent on the child's experience of uncertainty in illness. Nothing is known about when uncertainty occurs in ill children. The developmental issues surrounding the perception of uncertainty have not been studied, no instrument to address the child's uncertainty has been developed, and no qualitative studies have focused on the child's experience.

INTERVENTIONS TO MANAGE UNCERTAINTY

Although there has been extensive study of uncertainty in illness, only a few interventions to modify uncertainty and to promote health-related outcomes have been reported. Braden (1991, 1992) tested the efficacy of a series of 7-week community-based health promotion programs offered to 291 persons with systemic lupus erythematosus in reducing uncertainty and enhancing enabling skills, self-efficacy, and life quality. Using a one-group pre- posttest design, subjects were measured at the start of class, 7 weeks later, and 2 months postclass. Uncertainty decreased over time, while the other three variables increased over time. In a second report of the intervention, Braden (1992) divided the sample by scores on an investigator-devised 4-item measure of depression into high ($n = 37$) and low ($n = 35$) depression groups. Although both groups changed significantly over time on a number of variables, only those in the high depression group changed significantly in reducing uncertainty and increasing life quality. Using the same one-group pre- posttest design, Lemaire and Lenz (1995) reported the efficacy of an educational program on menopause in modifying uncertainty about menopausal changes. Using a convenience sample of women attending an educational program, 177 women were measured on the community form of the MUIS pre- and posteducational intervention. The decrease in uncertainty was statistically significant. Although both of these investigations found a significant decrease in uncertainty after educational intervention, the strength of the findings is weakened by designs that lack a control comparison. The study by Braden (1991) addressed the weakness of no comparison group by presenting offerings of the intervention over time to a sample of 291 subjects, and in each offering the findings for the decrease in uncertainty over time was significant.

In two other intervention trials, uncertainty was not affected. Andersson-Segesten (1991) reported that patients with cardiac disease who received two different models of nursing care did not differ in uncertainty levels. McCain, Zeller, Cella, Urbanski, and Novak (1996) found no effect for a 6-week stress management training program over standard care in reducing uncertainty in 45 men with human immunodeficiency virus (HIV), although changes were in the predicted direction of a decrease. Subjects were not randomly assigned to groups, so the intervention subjects were treated as a wait list control group with measures at baseline and 6 weeks prior to intervention. Intervention subjects differed significantly from controls on intrusive thinking. Increased frequency of practice of relaxation techniques was associated with less uncertainty.

Two recent reports of a longitudinal study testing the efficacy of two different interventions designed to enhance self-care and promote skill in managing uncertainty present encouraging results. Mishel, Braden, and Longman (1996) reported that women with breast cancer randomly assigned to an uncertainty management intervention differed from control subjects in problem solving and information seeking, two behaviors that are effective for managing uncertainty. Uncertainty levels significantly changed over time for all subjects. The intervention was specifically designed to teach women how to get information and how to manage uncertainty-related problems (McHenry, Allen, Mishel, & Braden, 1993). The two outcomes of problem solving and information-seeking were targeted by the intervention and significantly differed between experimental and control subjects. These two outcomes also were achieved among women being treated for breast cancer who participated in a combined uncertainty management intervention with a self-help class versus comparable women receiving standard care (Braden, Mishel, Longman, & Burns, 1996). From the evidence to date on interventions to manage uncertainty, the most supportive findings are from education-related interventions that provide information and build skills that are important in managing uncertainty.

SUMMARY AND FUTURE RESEARCH DIRECTIONS

Although conceptualizations of uncertainty have appeared in the past 10 years, much of the research continues to be atheoretical. There is a need for more theory-testing research to address the nursing perspectives of uncertainty in illness. Also, studies need to tie to existing theory through integration of findings into current literature and theory. Both qualitative and quantitative orientations can be used to test the nursing perspective on uncertainty. Substantive theory should be explored to see if it can be tied to existing conceptualizations of uncertainty, and in doing so, to build nursing knowledge.

In the study of uncertainty, most of the studies are cross-sectional and the findings are associative, although the analyses in many studies are considered predictive. Such designs are often selected in the building of information concerning a phenomenon. At this time, some consistent findings have emerged. Across all illnesses studied to date, uncertainty decreases over time and returns on illness recurrence or exacerbation, and uncertainty is highest or most distressing while awaiting a diagnosis. Current evidence is strong for the role of social support in reducing uncertainty among those with an acute illness. Due to consensus of the findings, if further research is done in this area, it should focus on building on what is known, instead of repeating similar findings.

Concerning the role of personality dispositions as antecedents of or modifiers of uncertainty, the evidence is not solid. In acute illness, there is some support for mastery in a mediating role, but the study of personality dispositions related to uncertainty has been limited to a small number of studies, all of cancer patients receiving treatment. Other acute illnesses require study in order to see which personality dispositions are associated with uncertainty and at which phase in the illness experience. Further research is necessary to determine if the acuity of illness immobilizes personality variables, and whether they come into play during the recovery phase or during the management of continual uncertainty in chronic illness.

The role of the expert health care provider in reducing uncertainty is substantiated for persons receiving treatment for cancer, yet few studies have been done to explore the role of the health care provider with other acute illness populations. Also, lack of support for the health care provider as a source for reducing uncertainty in parents of acutely ill children requires further exploration, since there are few studies in the area.

Studies of coping with uncertainty in persons with acute illness have resulted in consistent findings for the relationship between uncertainty and emotion-focused coping. In order to determine if a broader range of coping strategies exists, attention needs to be given to developing instruments that are related to the problem under study. If coping strategies were derived from the specific setting and population, results may differ from those consistently accrued from global measures of coping.

There is sufficient evidence that uncertainty has a negative impact on quality of life and psychosocial adjustment in acute illness populations. Because the evidence is consistent and strong, it provides direction for interventions to target outcome variables. There is some evidence for the effectiveness of supportive educational interventions in modifying the adverse outcomes from uncertainty. Repeated testing of these interventions and the development of other theory- and research-based interventions that build on the body of existing descriptive research should be the direction of future research.

REFERENCES

Andersson-Segesten, K. (1991). Patient's experience of uncertainty in illness in two intensive coronary care units. *Scandinavian Journal of Caring Sciences*, *5*, 43–47.

Bennett, S. J. (1993). Relationships among selected antecedent variables and coping effectiveness in postmyocardial infarction patients. *Research in Nursing & Health*, *16*, 131–139.

Borgers, R., Mullen, P. D., Meertens, R., Rijken, M., Eussen, G., Plagge, I., Visser, A. P., & Blijham, G. H. (1993). The information-seeking behavior of cancer outpatients: A description of the situation. *Patient Education & Counseling*, *22*, 35–46.

Braden, C. J. (1991). Patterns of change over time in learned response to chronic illness among participants in a systemic lupus erythematosus self-help course. *Arthritis Care and Research*, *4*, 158–167.

Braden, C. J. (1992). Description of learned response to chronic illness: Depressed versus nondepressed self-help class participants. *Public Health Nursing*, *9*, 103–108.

Braden, C. J., Mishel, M. H., Longman, A., & Burns, R. L. (1996). *Self-help intervention project efficacy*. Unpublished manuscript.

Brett, K. M., & Davies, E. M. B. (1988). What does it mean? Sibling and parental appraisals of childhood leukemia. *Cancer Nursing*, *11*, 329–338.

Christman, N. J. (1990). Uncertainty and adjustment during radiotherapy. *Nursing Research*, *39*, 17–20.

Christman, N. J., McConnell, E. A., Pfeiffer, C., Webster, K. K., Schmitt, M., & Ries, J. (1988). Uncertainty, coping, and distress following myocardial infarction: Transition from hospital to home. *Research in Nursing & Health*, *11*, 71–82.

Clarke-Steffen, L. (1993). Waiting and not knowing: The diagnosis of cancer in a child. *Journal of Pediatric Oncology Nursing*, *10*, 146–153.

Cohen, M. H. (1993a). Diagnostic closure and the spread of uncertainty. *Issues in Comprehensive Pediatric Nursing*, *16*, 135–146.

Cohen, M. H. (1993b). The unknown and the unknowable-managing sustained uncertainty. *Western Journal of Nursing Research*, *15*, 77–96.

Cohen, M. H. (1995a). The stages of the prediagnostic period in chronic, life-threatening childhood illness: A process analysis. *Research in Nursing & Health*, *18*, 39–48.

Cohen, M. H. (1995b). The triggers of heightened parental uncertainty in chronic, life-threatening childhood illness. *Qualitative Health Research*, *5*, 63–77.

Cohen, M. H., & Martinson, I. M. (1988). Chronic uncertainty: Its effect on parental appraisal of a child's health. *Journal of Pediatric Nursing*, *3*, 89–96.

Cooper, H. M. (1982). Scientific guidelines for conducting integrative research reviews. *Review of Educational Research, 52*, 291–302.

Corbin, J. M., & Strauss, A. (1991). A nursing model for chronic illness management based upon the trajectory framework. *Scholarly Inquiry for Nursing Practice: An International Journal, 5*, 155–174.

Davis, F. (1960). Uncertainty in medical prognosis clinical and functional. *American Journal of Sociology, 66*, 41–47.

Davis, L. L. (1990). Illness uncertainty, social support, and stress in recovering individuals and family caregivers. *Applied Nursing Research, 3*, 69–71.

Di Iorio, C., Faherty, B., & Manteuffel, B. (1991). Cognitive-perceptual factors associated with antiepileptic medication compliance. *Research in Nursing & Health, 14*, 329–338.

Dracup, K., Walden, J. A., Stevenson, L. W., & Brecht, M. L. (1992). Quality of life in patients with advanced heart failure. *Journal of Heart & Lung Transplantation, 11*, 273–279.

Galloway, S. C., & Graydon, J. E. (1996). Uncertainty, symptom distress, and information needs after surgery for cancer of the colon. *Cancer Nursing, 19*, 112–117.

Hallberg, L. R. M., & Erlandsson, S. I. M. (1991). Validation of a Swedish version of the Mishel Uncertainty in Illness Scale. *Scholarly Inquiry for Nursing Practice: An International Journal, 5*, 57–65.

Hawthorne, M. H., & Hixon, M. E. (1994). Functional status, mood disturbance and quality of life in patients with heart failure. *Progress in Cardiovascular Nursing, 9*(1), 22–32.

Hilton, B. A. (1989). The relationship of uncertainty, control, commitment, and threat of recurrence to coping strategies used by women diagnosed with breast cancer. *Journal of Behavioral Medicine, 12*, 39–54.

Hilton, B. A. (1992). Perceptions of uncertainty: Its relevance to life-threatening and chronic illness. *Critical Care Nurse, 12*(1), 70–73.

Hilton, B. A. (1993). Issues, problems, and challenges for families coping with breast cancer. *Seminars in Oncology Nursing, 9*, 88–100.

Hilton, B. A. (1994). The Uncertainty Stress Scale: Its development and psychometric properties. *Canadian Journal of Nursing Research, 26*(3), 15–30.

Koocher, G. P. (1985). Psychosocial care of the child cured of cancer. *Pediatric Nursing, 11*, 91–93.

LaMontagne, L. L., & Pawlak, R. (1990). Stress and coping of parents of children in a pediatric intensive care unit. *Heart & Lung: Journal of Critical Care, 19*, 416–421.

Lazarus, R. S., & Folkman, S. (1984). *Stress, appraisal, and coping.* New York: Springer Publishing Co.

Lemaire, G. S., & Lenz, E. R. (1995). Perceived uncertainty about menopause in women attending an educational program. *International Journal of Nursing Studies, 32*, 39–48.

Mast, M. E. (1995). Adult uncertainty in illness: A critical review of research. *Scholarly Inquiry for Nursing Practice: An International Journal, 9*, 3–24.

McCain, N. L., Zeller, J. M., Cella, D. F., Urbanski, P. A., & Novak, R. M. (1996). The influence of stress management training in HIV disease. *Nursing Research*, 45, 246–253.

McHenry, J., Allen, C., Mishel, M. H., & Braden, C. J. (1993). Uncertainty management for women receiving treatment for breast cancer. In S. G. Funk, E. M. Trornquist, M. T. Champagne, & R. A. Wiese (Eds.), *Key aspects of caring for the chronically ill: Hospital and home* (pp. 170–177). New York: Springer Publishing Co.

McIntosh, J. (1974). Processes of communication, information, seeking and control associated with cancer: A selective review of the literature. *Social Science & Medicine*, 8, 167–187.

McIntosh, J. (1976). Patients' awareness and desire for information about diagnosed but undisclosed malignant disease. *Lancet*, 2, 300–303.

Miles, M. S., Funk, S. G., & Kasper, M. A. (1992). The stress response of mothers and fathers of preterm infants. *Research in Nursing & Health*, 15, 261–269.

Mishel, M. H. (1981). The measurement of uncertainty in illness. *Nursing Research*, 30, 258–263.

Mishel, M. H. (1983a). Adjusting the fit: Development of uncertainty scales for specific clinical populations. *Western Journal of Nursing Research*, 5, 355–370.

Mishel, M. H. (1983b). Parents' perception of uncertainty concerning their hospitalized child. *Nursing Research*, 32, 324–330.

Mishel, M. H. (1984). Perceived uncertainty and stress in illness. *Research in Nursing & Health*, 7, 163–171.

Mishel, M. H. (1988). Uncertainty in illness. *Image: Journal of Nursing Scholarship*, 20, 225–231.

Mishel, M. H. (1990). Reconceptualization of the uncertainty in illness theory. *Image: Journal of Nursing Scholarship*, 22, 256–262.

Mishel, M. H. (1991). Response to "validation of the Swedish version of the Mishel Uncertainty in Illness Scale." *Scholarly Inquiry for Nursing Practice: An International Journal*, 5, 67–70.

Mishel, M. H., Belyea, M., Germino, B., Hamilton-Spruill, J., Harris, L. & Braden, C. J. (1996). Uncertainty and emotional distress in African-American cancer patients. Unpublished manuscript.

Mishel, M. H., & Braden, C. J. (1987). Uncertainty a mediator between support and adjustment. *Western Journal of Nursing Research*, 9, 43–57.

Mishel, M. H., & Braden, C. J. (1988). Finding meaning: Antecedents of uncertainty in illness. *Nursing Research*, 37, 98–127.

Mishel, M. H., Braden, C. J., & Longman, A. (1996). *Efficacy of the uncertainty management intervention for women receiving treatment for breast cancer*. Unpublished manuscript.

Mishel, M. H., Hostetter, T., King, B., & Graham, V. (1984). Predictors of psychosocial adjustment in patients newly diagnosed with gynecological cancer. *Cancer Nursing*, 7, 291–299.

Mishel, M. H., & Murdaugh, C. L. (1987). Family adjustment to heart transplantation: Redesigning the dream. *Nursing Research*, 36, 332–336.

Mishel, M. H., Padilla, G., Grant, M., & Sorenson, D. S. (1991). Uncertainty in illness theory: A replication of the mediating effects of mastery and coping. *Nursing Research*, 40, 236–240.

Mishel, M. H., & Sorenson, D. S. (1991). Uncertainty in gynecological cancer: A test of the mediating functions of mastery and coping. *Nursing Research*, 40, 167–171.

Molleman, E., Krabbendam, P. J., Annyas, A. A., Koops, H. S., Sleijfer, D. T., & Vermey, A. (1984). The significance of the doctor-patient relationship in coping with cancer. *Social Science & Medicine*, 18, 475–480.

Molleman, E., Pruyn, J., & Knippenberg, A. V. (1986). Social comparison processes among cancer patients. *British Journal of Social Psychology*, 25, 1–13.

Northouse, L. L., Dorris, G., & Charron-Moore, C. (1995). Factors affecting couples' adjustment to recurrent breast cancer. *Social Science & Medicine*, 41, 69–76.

Northouse, L. L., Jeffs, M., Cracchiolo-Caraway, A., Lampman, L., & Dorris, G. (1995). Emotional distress reported by women and husbands prior to a breast biopsy. *Nursing Research*, 44, 196–201.

Northouse, L. L., Laten, D., & Reddy, P. (1995). Adjustment of women and their husbands to recurrent breast cancer. *Research in Nursing & Health*, 18, 5-5–524.

Padilla, G. V., Mishel, M. H., & Grant, M. M. (1992). Uncertainty, appraisal and quality of life. *Quality of Life Research*, 1, 155–165.

Redeker, N. S. (1992). The relationship between uncertainty and coping after coronary bypass surgery. *Western Journal of Nursing Research*, 14, 48–68.

Richardson, J. L., Marks, G., Johnson, C. A., Graham, J. W., Chan, K. K., Selser, J. N., Kishbaugh, C., Barranday, Y., & Levine, A. M. (1987). Path model of multidimensional compliance with cancer therapy. *Health Psychology*, 6, 183–207.

Righter, B. M. (1995). Uncertainty and the role of the credible authority during an ostomy experience. *Wound, Ostomy, and Continence Nurses Society*, 22, 100–104.

Ronayne, R. (1985). Feelings and attitudes during early convalescence following vascular surgery. *Journal of Advanced Nursing*, 10, 435–441.

Selder, F. (1989). Life transition theory: The resolution of uncertainty. *Nursing & Health Care*, 10, 437–451.

Stetz, K. M. (1989). The relationship among background characteristics, purpose in life, and caregiving demands on perceived health of spouse caregivers. *Scholarly Inquiry for Nursing Practice: An International Journal*, 3, 133–159.

Turner, M. A., Tomlinson, P. S., & Harbaugh, B. L. (1990). Parental uncertainty in critical care hospitalization of children. *Maternal-Child Nursing Journal*, 19, 45–62.

Van Den Borne, H. W., Pruyn, J. F. A., & Van Den Heuvel, W. J. A. (1987). Effects of contacts between cancer patients on their psychosocial problems. *Patient Education & Counseling*, 9, 33–51.

Warrington, K., & Gottlieb, L. (1987). Uncertainty and anxiety of hysterectomy patients during hospitalization. *Nursing Papers*, 19(1), 59–73.

Webster, K. K., & Christman, N. J. (1988). Perceived uncertainty and coping post myocardial infarction. *Western Journal of Nursing Research*, 10, 384–400.

White, R. E., & Frasure-Smith, N. (1995). Uncertainty and psychologic stress after coronary angioplasty and coronary bypass surgery. *Heart & Lung: Journal of Critical Care, 24,* 19–27.

Wiener, C. L. (1975). The burden of rheumatoid arthritis: Tolerating the uncertainty. *Social Science & Medicine, 9,* 97–104.

Wiener, C. L., & Dodd, M. J. (1993). Coping amid uncertainty: An illness trajectory perspective. *Scholarly Inquiry for Nursing Practice: An International Journal, 7,* 17–31.

Wong, C. A., & Bramwell, L. (1992). Uncertainty and anxiety after mastectomy for breast cancer. *Cancer Nursing, 15,* 363–371.

Wurzbach, M. E. (1992). Assessment and intervention for certainty and uncertainty. *Nursing Forum, 27*(2), 29–35.

Wyler, A. R., Masuda, M., & Holmes, T. H. (1968). Seriousness of illness rating scale. *Journal of Psychosomatic Medicine, 11,* 363–374.

Yates, B. C., & Booton-Hiser, D. A. (1992). Comparison of psychologic stress responses in patients and spouses ten weeks after a cardiac illness event. *Progress in Cardiovascular Nursing, 7*(4), 25–33.

Chapter 4

Violence in the Workplace

JEANNE BEAUCHAMP HEWITT
SCHOOL OF NURSING
UNIVERSITY OF WISCONSIN—MILWAUKEE

PAMELA F. LEVIN
COLLEGE OF NURSING
UNIVERSITY OF ILLINOIS AT CHICAGO

ABSTRACT

This integrative review of research on workplace violence in Canada and the United States showed that risk factors for homicide and nonfatal assault injuries differed significantly. In 1993, there were 1,063 work-related homicides in the United States (Bureau of Labor Statistics, 1994). Workplace homicide was the second leading cause of fatal occupational injuries overall, but the primary cause for women. The highest risk for workplace homicide was observed among males, the self-employed, and those employed in grocery stores, eating and drinking establishments, gas service stations, taxicab services, and government service, including law enforcement. The majority of workplace homicides occurred during robberies. Unlike workplace homicide, the majority of nonfatal assaults that involved lost work time occurred to women, primarily employed in health care or other service sector work. The assault rates for residential care and nursing and personal care workers were more than ten times that of private non-health care industries. Minimal intervention research has been reported. In recent years, some governmental agencies and professional organizations have begun to address policy issues related to workplace violence.

Keywords: Workplace, Risk Factors, Homicide, Nonfatal Injury, Policy, Occupational, Violence, Physical Assault, Interventions

VIOLENCE IN THE WORKPLACE

In recent years, violence in the workplace has captured the attention of workers, employers, governmental bodies, and the news media (Bell & Jenkins, 1992; Burgess, Burgess, & Douglas, 1994; National Institute of Occupational Safety and Health [NIOSH], 1993; Northwestern National Life Insurance Company, 1993). Workplace violence has been conceptualized as occupational injuries due to violence (California Division Occupational Safety and Health Administration [CAL-OSHA], 1993). The CAL-OSHA uses the Occupational Safety and Health Administration's (OSHA) definition of occupational injury as being an injury which results in death, lost work days, loss of consciousness, restriction of work or motion, termination of employment, transfer to another job, or medical treatment other than first aid (Code of Federal Regulations [CFR], 1992). According to CAL-OSHA, injury is either "physical or emotional harm" with signs or symptoms that are "immediate or delayed" (CAL-OSHA, 1993, p. 38). Violence is defined in terms of assault which involves "any aggressive act of hitting, kicking, pushing, biting, scratching, sexual attack or any other such physical or verbal attacks directed to the worker . . . which arises during or as a result of the performance of duties and which results in death, physical injury or mental harm" (p. 38).

From a multidisciplinary perspective, violence in the workplace consists of behavior that involves a physical or psychological assault, threat, or harassment which occurs in the context of employment or work-related activities. Violence in the workplace broadly includes verbal abuse, sexual harassment, threat of harm, sexual assault, physical assault, homicide, suicide, and acts of terrorism (Alexander, Franklin, & Wolf, 1994; Bureau of Labor Statistics [BLS], 1994; CAL-OSHA, 1993; Emergency Nurses Association, 1994; Hales, Seligman, Newman, & Timbrook, 1988; Illinois Nurses Association, 1995; Lanza, 1988; New York Committee for Occupational Safety and Health [NY-COSH], 1995; Nurse Assault Project Team, 1992; Occupational Safety and Health Administration [OSHA], 1996; Simonowitz, 1995; Stultz, 1993). Researchers frequently used much more restrictive definitions (Lipscomb & Love, 1992; Simonowitz, 1995). A substantial proportion of the research on workplace violence has been focused on assaults. Although assaults do not invariably result in injury, when injury does occur, it may involve immediate or more delayed physical or psychological injury or trauma to the worker. In addition to the primary injury of the worker, those who witness workplace violence or are involved in the aftermath of violence—coworkers, supervisors, and safety, rescue, and health care personnel—may experience psychological trauma as well. Thus, violence in the workplace not only involves physical or psychological assault, threats, and harassment, but also broadly encompasses both short- and long-term effects, including injury, postincident trauma, and death. Such an expansive definition, however, makes violence in the workplace seem overwhelming to study.

To focus the issue of workplace violence on prevention, CAL-OSHA (1995) developed a classification scheme to assist employers and others to identify high-risk workplaces and situations and to design specific preventive measures. Type I workplace violence occurs in the context of interaction with the public and frequently involves the exchange of money, late night or early morning hours of operation, and working alone or with few workers. Examples of at-risk workers for Type I violence include taxicab drivers and convenience store personnel. Type II workplace violence occurs in the context of rendering service to the public, which includes health care and social service personnel, safety and correctional personnel, municipal bus and railway drivers, teachers, and sales personnel. Type III workplace violence occurs in the context of past or current employment relationships, such as coworkers, or past or current relationships of employees with a spouse, lover, relative, friend, or others with whom there is conflict. The criminal justice literature frequently refers to Type I workplace violence as ''instrumental'' in which assault or injury occurs secondarily to the commission of a crime such as robbery. Although Type III workplace violence receives the most attention from the news media (Burgess et al., 1994), it is least prevalent (CAL-OSHA, 1995).

The purpose of this chapter is to critically review and synthesize research on violence in the workplace, to highlight the implications for nursing practice and policymaking, and to make recommendations for further research. Specifically, the aims of the review of literature were (a) to describe the magnitude of workplace violence from a multidisciplinary perspective; (b) to identify risk factors for workplace homicide and assault and injury in high-risk occupations; and (c) to discuss the types of intervention studies conducted.

This integrative review used databased research reports of articles published in the English language and identified from online and manual searches of the medical, nursing, health, sociology, psychology, and criminal justice literature. Databases used for online searches consisted of MEDLINE (1975–1995), Cumulative Index of Nursing and Allied Health Literature (CINAHL, 1983–1995), Health Planning and Administration (1975–1995), Sociological Abstracts (1965–1995), PSYCHINFO (1967–1995), and the Criminal Justice Periodicals Index (1975–1995). Keywords used for online searches were: workplace, occupational, work-related, injury at work, abuse, physical assault, injury, homicide, and violence. Studies were limited to those conducted in the United States or Canada. There were 263 citations identified through the online search of the English language literature. Despite the attempt to provide a broad multidisciplinary review of literature, few citations outside the health-related literature qualified for inclusion. Additional studies and policy papers from professional organizations and governmental bodies were obtained through collegial networks and bibliographic ancestry. We limited this review to 60 databased articles and 12 policy-oriented articles that fit the aims of this chapter. Emphasis was placed on findings that address Type I and Type II workplace violence.

CONCEPTUAL FRAMEWORK

Data obtained from these published studies were analyzed using an epidemiological conceptual framework of person, place, and time to describe rates and risk factors for violence in the workplace (Levin, Hewitt, & Misner, 1992). Risk factors were examined in relation to the characteristics of the victims, occupation and industry of employment, nature of the crime, manner of death, and circumstances surrounding the event. Findings from intervention studies were described with respect to the implementation of environmental controls, training, and policy.

MAGNITUDE OF VIOLENCE IN THE WORKPLACE AND IDENTIFICATION OF GROUPS AT HIGH RISK

Violence in the workplace increasingly is being recognized as a formidable public health problem (Bell & Jenkins, 1992). From a public health perspective, homicide is the most easily recognizable endpoint of workplace violence, and as such, serves as a sentinel health event for workplace violence (Kraus, Peek, Silberman, & Anderson, 1995; Levin, Hewitt, & Misner, 1996). The National Census of Fatal Occupational Injuries (CFOI) is the most comprehensive study of workplace homicide ever conducted in the United States (U.S.) (BLS, 1993, 1994; Toscano & Windau, 1994). The CFOI showed that 1,063 work-related murders occurred in 1993 (BLS, 1994). Workplace homicide was the second leading cause of fatal occupational injuries overall (BLS, 1994; Toscano & Windau, 1993), compared to being the third leading cause in previous studies (Castillo & Jenkins, 1994; CDC, 1993; Jenkins, Layne, & Kisner, 1992) based on death certificates used by the National Traumatic Occupational Fatality (NTOF) database. Both the CFOI and studies based on NTOF data showed that workplace homicide was the leading cause of fatal injury at work for women (BLS, 1994; Levin et al., 1992; Toscano & Windau, 1993).

Disparities in workplace homicide risk were observed (BLS, 1994). Although men comprised 55% of the workforce, they were overwhelmingly the homicide victims (82%). The self-employed represented 12% of the workforce, but 22% of the homicides. High-risk industries identified were retail trade (49%), service (15%), transportation and public utilities (12%), and government (12%). Homicide in the retail trade division primarily involved grocery stores (17%), eating and drinking establishments (5%), and gas service stations (5%). The majority of homicides in the transportation and public utilities sector occurred to taxicab drivers. Seventy-five percent of all workplace homicides occurred during the commission of another crime, primarily robbery. Thus, homicide substantially fits the Type I profile of workplace violence.

In contrast to workplace homicides, 1993 figures for nonfatal events showed that although women comprised 45% of the national workforce, they experienced 55% of the work-related assaults that involved lost work time (BLS, 1995a). The majority of nonfatal assaults occurred in the health care service sector (38%) and in other services (29%) where females predominate. While the overall assault rate for private industry was 3/10,000 workers, the rates for the residential care industry and the nursing and personal care industry were 47/10,000 and 38/10,000, respectively. The BLS pointed out that a significant proportion of the 21,000 assault-related injuries in 1993 occurred to nursing personnel. These data suggest that workplace assaults fit the Type II profile and that nursing personnel are at greatest risk for nonfatal assaults.

LIMITATIONS OF STUDIES ON VIOLENCE IN THE WORKPLACE

The problems inherent with using existing data sources for surveillance of workplace violence have been discussed extensively (BLS, 1994; Davis, 1988; Kraus et al., 1995; Levin et al., 1992). Several limitations are highlighted here. On death certificates, the "usual" industry and occupation are recorded. It has been demonstrated that the usual industry and occupation frequently do not correspond to the employment at the time of the fatal injury. In one study that validated death certificate data using medical examiners' reports, among decedents whose industry was listed on death certificates as being either student, military, housewife, or other ($n = 28$), none accurately reflected their employment at the time of the homicide (Davis, 1988). The medical examiners' reports, however, indicated that at least 19 of these homicide victims worked in high-risk industries such as food and dairy stores, gasoline service stations, and eating and drinking establishments.

Other formidable challenges to the internal validity of studies result from the lack of standardized coding procedures for both occupation and industry, and determination as to where the fatal injury occurred and whether the injury occurred "at work." Although these factors result in random misclassification, it has been noted that considerably greater imprecision in coding occurred for women and older ($\geq$ 65) workers (Kraus et al., 1995). One of the advantages of medical examiners' and coroners' reports is that they provide much greater detail about the decedent and the prior events (Levin et al., 1996). However, a major limitation is that these data usually must be abstracted manually, which increases the cost and time of conducting large-scale studies that use these sources, and severely limits the feasibility of using them for routine surveillance.

Another limitation of death certificates, as well as workers' compensation claims and OSHA 200 logs, is that they have limited information that describes the injured worker or the events preceding the injury. Sometimes the limitations of various data sources can be offset by linking data from two or more data sources. However, in the United States, confidentiality issues preclude the linkage of datasets such as the NTOF data with Federal Bureau of Investigation (FBI) data, since by law, these datasets cannot contain identifiers.

Regardless of which data source is used to derive injury cases for the numerator, one of the major challenges is to identify appropriate denominator data for calculating rates (Levin et al., 1992). In particular, there is generally a lack of person–time data, which should be used to calculate rates based on full-time equivalents, which is particularly important when a notable proportion of the workforce is part time.

Despite the limitations associated with surveillance systems for studying workplace homicide, these systems do exist. In contrast, surveillance systems for nonfatal assaults and injuries are minimal. Although not designed for surveillance purposes, workers' compensation records have been used to estimate the magnitude of physical assaults and other forms of violence (Alexander et al., 1994; Barnett, Adelman, Bissell, Thomas, & Clower, 1994; Bensley, Nelson, Kaufman, Silverstein, & Kalat, 1993; Hales et al., 1988; Liss & McCaskell, 1994; NYCOSH, 1995; Sullivan & Yuan, 1995; Thomas, 1992). One of the major problems with using workers' compensation claims is that this system is designed to capture incidents that involve lost work days or medical treatment—a rather restrictive definition. Moreover, many workers never file a workers' compensation claim following assault (Levin et al., 1996). At present, workers' compensation systems differ from state to state (U.S.) and between provinces (Canada), and lack a centralized statistical analysis site. Thus, worker compensation records are limited in their usefulness for surveillance of nonfatal workplace injuries.

Besides workers' compensation claims, another potential source of surveillance data is agency-based incident reports. However, survey respondents frequently reported that they do not file an incident report following a physical assault at work (Lanza, 1988; Nurse Assault Project Team, 1992; Pane, Winiarski, & Salness, 1991). A similar problem exists with using police reports due to significant underreporting (56%) of violence-related crimes that occur in the workplace (Bachman, 1994).

The dearth of existing assault and injury surveillance data on nonfatal incidents has led some researchers to use survey research methods. However, the quality of most surveys identified for this review varied greatly. Many surveys had very low response rates (~25%), if reported at all. There was a lack of use of standard definitions and criteria (e.g., OSHA criteria for an injury case) and great variability in the analysis and reporting of findings. Consequently, we have largely excluded survey studies in this review.

RISK FACTORS FOR HOMICIDE IN THE WORKPLACE

Victim Characteristics

Across studies, workplace homicides occurred predominantly to males (~80%), to 25- to 44-year-olds (49%–55%), and to Whites (65%) (Bureau of Justice Statistics, 1995; BLS, 1996; Castillo & Jenkins, 1994; Centers for Disease Control [CDC], 1993; Fox & Levin, 1994; Hales et al., 1988; Jenkins, Layne, & Kisner, 1992; NYCOSH, 1995). Men also experienced the highest workplace homicide rates. During the 1980s, the average U.S. male workplace homicide rate was $1.0/10^5$ (CDC, 1993). Comparable national data are not available for Canada. Considerable variation was noted by states/provinces, ranging from a low of $0.26/10^5$ for Ontario men to highs of $2.1/10^5$ in Texas and $2.2/10^5$ in California (Davis, 1987; Kraus, 1987; Liss & Craig, 1990). Men experienced approximately a three- to fivefold greater risk of murder at work compared to women. The U.S. workplace homicide rate for women was $0.3/10^5$ (CDC, 1993). Similar to men, the highest homicide rates for women were found in Texas and California, and the lowest in Ontario, although state- and province-specific data are very incomplete. In Texas, North Carolina, and South Carolina, workplace homicide accounted for more than 50% of all injury deaths of women at work (Davis, Honchar, & Suarez, 1987; Sniezek & Horiagon, 1989; Stone, 1993), but approximately 40% nationwide. Although the workplace homicide rate is consistently lower for women than for men, homicide has been the leading cause of workplace injury fatalities among women since 1980 (BLS, 1994; Jenkins, 1994; Levin et al., 1992) and among health care workers (Stout, 1992).

Data on U.S. workplace homicides showed that victims' ages ranged between 16 and 93 years (Bell, 1991; CDC, 1987, 1990; Jenkins et al., 1992), with a mean age of 38 (CDC, 1987). In national studies that reported age-specific data, the greatest proportion of homicides occurred to workers between 25 and 54 years of age (Bachman, 1994; BLS, 1994; CDC, 1987, 1993; Fox & Levin, 1994), which is consistent with patterns of employment. However, the highest homicide rate occurred to workers 65 years of age or older (CDC, 1987, 1990, 1993; Davis et al., 1987; Jenkins et al., 1992). Rates varied between a low of $0.83/10^5$ for men in Ontario to a high of $6.7/10^5$ for men in Texas (Davis et al., 1987; Liss & Craig, 1990). Although the lowest homicide rates occurred to 16–17-year-olds (Castillo, Landen, & Layne, 1994), their deaths contribute heavily to years of life lost prematurely.

In studies that reported statistics by race, Blacks and other races (those excluding Whites and Blacks) experienced approximately a twofold higher workplace homicide rate than Whites (Bell, 1991; Castillo & Jenkins, 1994; CDC, 1987, 1993; Davis, 1987). In Texas, the workplace homicide rate for men of Hispanic origin was intermediate between that of Whites and Blacks (Davis, 1987).

Industry and Occupations

The most hazardous industries with respect to homicide were retail trade, service, transportation/utilities, and government/public administration (BLS, 1994; CDC, 1987, 1990, 1993; Davis, 1987; Davis et al., 1987; Hales et al., 1988; Jenkins et al., 1992; Liss & Craig, 1990; NYCOSH, 1995). Specific high-risk sectors included grocery stores, eating and drinking establishments, liquor stores, gasoline stations, jewelry stores, hotels/motels, and taxicab services. Not surprisingly, the high-risk occupations included cashiers, sales personnel, stock handlers/baggers, taxicab drivers, waiters and waitresses, bartenders, hotel clerks, and security guards. In addition, workers in government or public administration, which include police and detectives, were also at high risk for workplace homicide. During 1993, the CFOI showed that 67 police officers (6.3% of all workplace homicides in the United States) and 52 security guards (4.9%) were killed in the line of duty (Bureau of Justice Statistics, 1995).

Event Characteristics

When time-related factors were reported, the highest proportion of homicides at work occurred between 4 p.m. and 8 a.m., with the peak hour observed between 4–5 p.m. (CDC, 1987, 1990; Davis et al., 1987; Hales et al., 1988; Jenkins et al., 1992; Kraus, 1987). The majority of workplace homicides involved firearms (BLS, 1994; CDC, 1987, 1993; Davis, 1987; Davis et al.,

1987; Fox & Levin, 1994; Goodman, Jenkins, & Mercy, 1994; Hales et al., 1988; Jenkins et al., 1992; Kraus, 1987; Liss & Craig, 1990). Robberies or other crimes were involved in approximately three-fourths of all murders at work, whereas a much lower percentage was attributed to work associates (6%) or personal acquaintances (including current or ex-husbands, boyfriends, and others) (4%) (Bureau of Justice Statistics, 1995). Geographically, the Southern and Western regions of the U.S. accounted for 73% of all workplace homicides (Jenkins et al., 1992). In 1992–1993, New York City had only 3% of the U.S. workforce, yet experienced 12% of the nation's workplace homicides (NYCOSH, 1995).

RISK FACTORS FOR PHYSICAL ASSAULT AND INJURY IN HIGH-RISK OCCUPATIONS

Victim Characteristics

Bureau of Labor Statistics (1996) data indicate that females in general have experienced a disproportionate share of assault-related injuries (58%) based on their workforce participation. Nationally, nursing personnel, who are predominantly female, experienced the highest risk of assault-related injuries (BLS, 1995b, 1996). Findings based on workers' compensation and survey data, however, seem to suggest that men in the health care industry may be at greater risk for physical assault and injury (Liss & McCaskell, 1994; Nurse Assault Project Team, 1992). Unfortunately, the BLS does not report cause-specific rates by gender, age, or race/ethnicity, and the use of workers' compensation or survey data is problematic, as previously noted.

Industry and Occupations

The service industry, particularly the health care sector, clearly bears the highest risk of nonfatal assault injury (BLS, 1995a, 1995b, 1996; NYCOSH, 1995; "Workplace violence," 1995). The BLS (1995a, 1996) identified nursing personnel, including nursing aides, health aides, and registered nurses, as high-risk occupations. Rates based on workers' compensation claims suggest that workers in other occupations, including police, gasoline station attendants, and various service-related occupations, are at high risk for nonfatal injuries (Barnett et al., 1994; Hales et al., 1988; NYCOSH, 1995). Although nonfatal occupational assault and injuries fit the Type II profile of being service-related, nonfatal injuries identified through workers' compensation claims parallel the homicide risk profile.

Event Characteristics

Event characteristics associated with nonfatal assaults that involved lost work days were primarily due to hitting, kicking, or beating (43%) (BLS, 1996). Nursing aides and orderlies and other workers in health and residential care occupations were assaulted most commonly by patients or residents. In retail establishments, which accounted for 16% of the nonfatal assaults, perpetrators were likely to be customers or robbers. Survey data from the health care sector, however limited, suggest that risk of assault or physical injury may depend on the type of service provided (e.g., emergency care, mental health, long-term care) and the setting (inpatient or community-based) (Manitoba Association of Registered Nurses, 1989; Stultz, 1993; Williams, 1995; "Workplace violence," 1995). For example, in institutional health care settings, assaults seem to be correlated with understaffing and periods of high activity, such as mealtimes (Bensley et al., 1993; CAL-OSHA, 1993; Simonowitz, 1995).

INTERVENTIONS TO REDUCE VIOLENCE IN THE WORKPLACE

The three basic types of interventions consist of environmental controls, training, and policies, which, singly or in combination, are designed to reduce workplace violence and its sequelae. Guidelines and policies for reducing workplace violence have been developed (for example, CAL-OSHA, 1995; Illinois Nurses Association, 1995; Ministerial Committee on Abuse of Health Care Staff, 1991; Ontario Nurses Association, 1991; OSHA, 1996). However, relatively few intervention studies to reduce workplace violence were identified in the literature.

Environmental Controls

Despite the prevalence of Type I violence, there is a dearth of intervention research on reducing robberies and assaults or homicides, which frequently occur during the course of a robbery. Crow and Bull (1975) devised an intervention program to deter robbery based on making the convenience store less attractive to potential robbers. Efforts to assess the effectiveness of environmental controls to decrease violence-related injuries in retail establishments are being spearheaded by the NIOSH (Amandus et al., 1996).

Training

In an attempt to control the violence-related injury risk to late-night retail workers, Washington State enacted a rule that focuses on training employees in crime prevention (Brooker, 1993). This rule also stipulates that owners implement environmental controls, such as having the cash register be visible from the street, minimizing the amount of cash available, and having adequate lighting. Since implementing this rule, a 53% decrease in the violence-related workers compensation claims has occurred among food store workers ("Workplace violence," 1995).

In a forensic psychiatric hospital, Carmel and Hunter (1990) found that units that had at least 60% of its employees comply with mandatory training in the management of assaultive patient behavior significantly reduced assault-related worker injury. In another study, a Veterans' Medical Center instituted a behavioral emergency committee, whose function was to oversee incident reports of patient violence, which were used to assess high-risk patients (Drummond, Sparr, & Gordon, 1989). When patterns of serious behavioral problems were found for a given patient, the computerized scheduling system was "flagged" to alert admissions clerks and staff regarding the potential for violence and the need to initiate appropriate control measures, such as security standby and a search for weapons. In addition to using this warning system, many staff also participated in aggression management training. In the year following the implementation of the "flagging" system, the number of violent incidents were reduced by 91% ($p < .001$).

Policy

Health and human service community workers are at increased risk of assault at work (BLS, 1996; CAL-OSHA, 1993; OSHA, 1996). In response to 25 incidents of physical and verbal assault during a 1-year period, the New Jersey Division of Youth and Family Services implemented a number of policies and procedures to reduce violence directed at caseworkers (Scalera, 1995). These policies include a mandatory "team response" of two professionals for casework; the use of cellular telephones; a worker safety manual and mandatory safety training; the availability of postincident trauma counseling; and having the agency, on behalf of the worker, file charges against the perpetrator. Although others have discussed legal remedies, none have reported a procedure whereby the agency takes the responsibility—and the risk associated with angered patients/clients—to file charges (Hoge & Gutheil, 1987; Morrison, 1992; Phelan, Mills, & Ryan, 1985). However, some data indicate that patients who are prosecuted for assaulting workers may be less likely to repeat assaultive behavior (Hoge & Gutheil, 1987).

Although there is no OSHA regulation per se regarding violence in the workplace, in 1993, OSHA cited a Chicago psychiatric hospital for violating the "general duty clause" of the 1970 Occupational Safety and Health Act, which requires employers to provide a safe and healthful workplace (U.S.

Department of Labor, 1993). The plan outlined by OSHA required that this hospital train workers in the use of restraint and seclusion procedures, establish a written crisis prevention plan, provide multicultural sensitivity training, use critical-incident debriefing procedures, increase staffing, and control access to metal utensils, which can readily be used as weapons. This plan is consistent with the guidelines to protect health care and social service workers as set forth by OSHA (1996).

Patients, family members, and other visitors sometimes carry weapons into health care settings. One study evaluated the acceptance of a uniform weapons searching policy in a psychiatric emergency room (McCulloch, McNiel, Binder, & Hatcher, 1986). The researchers found that screening the contents of jackets, purses, and pockets yielded weapons in 8% of patients. According to staff, 97% of patients cooperated fully and both staff (93%) and patients (76%) reported feeling safer. In one Veterans' Medical Center, the policy is to mail confiscated weapons to the municipal police department near the patients' home, where the patients can retrieve their weapon (Sparr, Drummond, & Hamilton, 1988).

IMPLICATIONS FOR NURSING PRACTICE
AND POLICYMAKING

Violence in the workplace is a prevalent, but preventable, public health problem. All nurses can be involved in measures to reduce workplace violence and its sequelae. For example, one of the more recent thrusts of organized efforts by nurses has been to work with legislators to enact state laws to make the nonfatal assault of nursing personnel a felony.

Although all nurses have a role in reducing workplace violence, occupational health nurses in industry and businesses, including health care, and nurse administrators hold key positions for effecting violence prevention. Occupational health nurses, in particular, serve a vital function in the prevention of workplace violence and adverse sequelae in at least three ways: (a) by collaborating with administrators and employees to set policies; (b) by performing health surveillance activities (assess incidence and risk factors, implement changes based on the assessment data, and evaluate the effectiveness of prevention efforts); and (c) by doing follow-up and referrals (e.g., through employee assistance programs) for debriefing and counseling after critical incidents and for obtaining other services.

The role of nurse administrators in reducing workplace violence has received very little attention to date. However, nurse administrators can be instrumental in setting the organization's priorities and developing policies that take a ''zero tolerance of violence'' stand. In addition, nurse administrators can be invaluable by allocating necessary resources (e.g., adequate staffing, training, engineering controls) and by role-modeling a work environment that does not blame the victim for the violence. The CAL-OSHA (1995) model program and OSHA (1996) guidelines are excellent resources for workplace violence prevention for occupational health nurses and nurse administrators.

CONCLUSIONS AND FUTURE RESEARCH DIRECTIONS

The 1980s witnessed a growing awareness of violence in the workplace including assault, nonfatal injury, and homicide. The emerging science of workplace injury control has been focused largely on describing the magnitude of the problem of workplace violence and risk factors. Death certificate data has proven useful in describing homicide at work and some risk factors. Comparable data sources are not readily available for studying nonfatal injuries at work, so this area of research has progressed more slowly. Nonetheless, the data demonstrate that industries and occupations differ on their risk of assault, physical injury, and homicide.

Based on NTOF and CFOI data, certain sectors of retail trade (e.g., convenience stores and gasoline stations), service (e.g., taxicab), and public administration (e.g., police) were found to be at high risk for homicide. For nonfatal assault-related injuries, different patterns of high-risk industries were found, depending on which data source was used. The BLS data, based on OSHA 200 logs, indicate that the service-based health care industry has the highest risk of nonfatal assault-related injury. By contrast, workers' compensation data suggests that, as for homicide, the same retail trade and service sectors that are at high risk for homicide are also at high risk for nonfatal assault injuries. While significant progress has been made in defining the magnitude of the problem of workplace violence, there is a paucity of intervention research.

Directions for future research in the area of workplace injury control include: (a) continued surveillance of homicide at work; (b) development and use of state-of-the-science surveillance systems for nonfatal assaults and injuries; (c) in-depth studies of risk factors of Type I and Type II work-related violence; (d) improved surveillance methods for both fatal and nonfatal assault and injury; and (e) intervention studies. Here, some suggestions are provided as to how these research needs might be met.

The NTOF and CFOI data have proven invaluable for monitoring homicide at work. Because the NTOF database is a passive surveillance system based on death certificates, it is a cost-effective way to monitor progress at a national level, and should be continued indefinitely. It would also be cost-effective to use existing surveillance systems of injuries designed for purposes other than occupational health. For example, it may be feasible to use the active surveillance system for head injuries conducted by the Department of Public Health in Minnesota to examine patterns of and risk factors for occupational violence-related injuries. If industry and occupation are not currently obtained, it may be feasible to include these items with little added cost.

In addition to using existing surveillance systems, we suggest that a nationwide network of passive surveillance systems be implemented using selected emergency room, ambulatory care services, and police departments in urban, suburban, and rural locations that track both work-related and other violence-related injuries. Similarly, it would be important to develop an active surveillance system for selected health care agencies, including acute, ambulatory, long-term, mental health, and community health, to comprehensively examine trends and risk factors for work-related violence, including nonfatal injuries and homicide. This system could be based on incident reports if measures to assure complete ascertainment were undertaken.

Because most surveillance systems usually collect a limited amount of data on potential risk factors, there will be a continued need to conduct focused epidemiological studies of risk factors for workplace violence. Examples of data sources with more in-depth data include medical examiners' and coroners' reports, police records, and comprehensive surveys of worker populations, such as nursing personnel or police.

To facilitate studies of risk factors for workplace violence, it would be highly desirable to reexamine the issue of using identifying codes on state and federal databases, accessible only to state and federal agencies with assurances that confidentiality would be maintained. Identification codes would enable linkages between datasets such as death certificate files and Federal Bureau of Investigation files. Identifying codes then should be expunged from public use databases. Record linkages would enable more in-depth studies to be conducted in a very cost-effective manner.

To improve the quality of data, it is suggested that efforts to increase the standardization of procedures for collecting data on industry and occupation be undertaken. This type of effort would need to be directed toward funeral directors for death certificate data, physicians and nurses for medical records, and medical examiners and coroners for their reports. A similar program has been instituted by NIOSH for the coding "injury at work" item on death certificates (CDC, 1993). For data collection purposes, it would be advantageous to consider a "minimum dataset" (Health Information Policy Council, 1983) of items that should be included. When sample size is adequate, it is informative to do cause-specific analyses, and to analyze and report outcomes by specific characteristics of person, place, and time/event. Frequencies, such as the number of workplace homicides experienced by police during a certain time period, provide invaluable information on the magnitude of risk, while rates are used to determine risk factors; both should be reported when feasible.

Finally, there is an urgent need to do intervention studies, including the evaluation of the effectiveness of environment controls, training, and policy. For example, some cities have implemented policies whereby taxicab drivers can refuse to pick up passengers, and where they require bullet-proof barriers between the driver and passenger compartments. Yet, no studies were found that evaluated the effectiveness of these interventions on robbery or homicide of taxicab drivers. Importantly, a study on the effectiveness of Washington State's rule for retail trade workers was undertaken ("Workplace Violence," 1995), but needs to be continued to determine long-term outcomes. Intervention studies also are needed to evaluate which measures are most effective in reducing incidents of violence directed toward health care workers across work settings. For example, in long-term care and mental health settings, the evaluation should include the effectiveness of environmental controls, such as the design and layout of rooms and furniture, and administrative controls, such as staffing patterns and training in the recognition of impending violent behavior and de-escalation techniques. Because long waiting periods in emergency departments are thought to contribute to violent incidents, it would be worthwhile to measure the effect of innovative models of health care delivery. One example would be a system to triage persons with less serious injuries and illnesses to a nurse-managed advanced practice clinic adjacent to an emergency room, an approach that is designed to decrease waiting time and to provide more personalized care.

REFERENCES

Alexander, B. H., Franklin, G. M., & Wolf, M. E. (1994). The sexual assault of women at work in Washington State, 1980–1989. *American Journal of Public Health*, *84*, 640–642.

Amandus, H. E., Zahm, D., Friedmann, R., Ruback, R. B., Block, C., Weiss, J., Rogan, D., Holmes, W., Bynum, T., Hoffman, D., McManus, R., Malcan, J., Wellford, C., & Kessler, D. (1996). Employee injuries and convenience store robberies in selected metropolitan areas. *Journal of Occupational and Environmental Medicine*, *38*, 714–720.

Bachman, R. (1994). *National Crime Victimization Study: Violence and theft in the workplace* (NCJ–148199). Washington, DC: U.S. Department of Justice.

Barnett, K., Adelman, D., Bissell, E., Thomas, K., & Clower, R. I. (1994, September). *Violence in the workplace, Oregon, 1988–1992*. (Available from Department of

Consumer and Business Services, Information Management Division, 300 Labor & Industries Building, Salem, OR.)

Bell, C. A. (1991). Female homicides in United States workplaces. *American Journal of Public Health, 81,* 729–732.

Bell, C. A., & Jenkins, E. L. (1992, September). *Homicide in U.S. workplaces: A strategy for prevention and research* (DHHS [NIOSH] No. 92–103). Morgantown, WV: NIOSH.

Bensley, L., Nelson, N., Kaufman, J., Silverstein, B., & Kalat, J. (1993). *Study of assaults on staff in Washington state psychiatric hospitals.* (Available from Washington State Department of Labor and Industries, P.O. Box 44330, Olympia, WA 98504.)

Brooker, J. (1993). State of Washington acts to protect late-night workers. *Job Safety & Health Quarterly, 5,* 18–20.

Bureau of Justice Statistics. (1995). *Bureau of Justice Statistics Sourcebook of Criminal Justice Statistics—1994* (NCJ–154591). Washington, DC: U.S. Government Printing Office.

Bureau of Labor Statistics. (1993, October). *News: First national census of fatal occupational injuries reported by BLS* (USDL–93–406). Washington, DC: U.S. Department of Labor.

Bureau of Labor Statistics. (1994, August). *News: National census of fatal occupational injuries, 1993* (USDL–94–384). Washington, DC: U.S. Department of Labor.

Bureau of Labor Statistics. (1995a, April). *News: Work injuries and illnesses by selected characteristics, 1993* (USDL–95–142). Washington, DC: U.S. Department of Labor.

Bureau of Labor Statistics. (1995b, February). *Number of nonfatal occupational injuries and illnesses involving days away from work by selected injury or illness characteristics and industry, 1992.* Washington, DC: U.S. Department of Labor.

Bureau of Labor Statistics. (1996, May). *News: Characteristics of work injuries and illnesses resulting in absences from work, 1994.* Washington, DC: U.S. Department of Labor.

Burgess, A. W., Burgess, A. G., & Douglas, J. E. (1994). Examining violence in the workplace: A look at work-related fatalities. *Journal of Psychosocial Nursing, 32,* 11–18, 44–55, 53.

California Division of Occupational Safety & Health (CAL–OSHA). (1993). *CAL-OSHA guidelines for security and safety of health care and community service workers.* (Available from Department of Industrial Relations, Division of Occupational Safety and Health, 455 Golden Gate Avenue, Room 5202, San Francisco, CA 94192.)

California Division of Occupational Safety & Health (CAL-OSHA). (1995). *Model injury & illness prevention program for workplace security* (Available from Department of Industrial Relations, Division of Occupational Safety and Health, 455 Golden Gate Avenue, Room 5202, San Francisco, CA 94192.)

Carmel, H., & Hunter, M. (1990). Compliance with training in managing assaultive behavior and injuries from inpatient violence. *Hospital and Community Psychiatry, 41,* 558–560.

Castillo, D. N., & Jenkins, E. L. (1994). Industries and occupations at high risk for work-related homicide. *Journal of Occupational Medicine, 36,* 125–131.

Castillo, D. N., Landen, D. D., & Layne, L. A. (1994). Occupational injury deaths of 16- and 17–year olds in the United States. *American Journal of Public Health, 84,* 646–649.

Centers for Disease Control. (1987). Traumatic occupational fatalities—United States, 1980–1984. *Morbidity and Mortality Weekly Report, 36,* 461–464, 469–470.

Centers for Disease Control. (1990). Occupational homicides among women: United States, 1980–1985. *Morbidity and Mortality Weekly Report, 39,* 544–545, 551–552.

Centers for Disease Control. (1993). *Fatal injuries to workers in the United States. 1980–1989: A decade of surveillance (national and state profiles).* Washington, DC: U.S. Department of Health and Human Services.

Code of Federal Regulations. (1992). Recordkeeping and reporting occupational injuries and illnesses. 29CRF 1904: 12(c)(1)(2)(3). Washington, DC: U.S. Government Printing Office.

Crow, W. J., & Bull, J. L. (1975). *Robbery deterrence: An applied behavioral science demonstration.* La Jolla, CA: Western Behavioral Sciences Institute.

Davis, H. (1987). Workplace homicides of Texas males. *American Journal of Public Health, 77,* 1290–1293.

Davis, H. (1988). The accuracy of industry data from death certificates for workplace homicide victims. *American Journal of Public Health, 78,* 1579–1581.

Davis, H., Honchar, P. A., & Suarez, L. (1987). Fatal occupational injuries of women, Texas 1975–84. *American Journal of Public Health, 77,* 1524–1527.

Drummond, D. J., Sparr, L. F., & Gordon, G. H. (1989). Hospital violence reduction among high-risk patients. *Journal of the American Medical Association, 261,* 2531–2534.

Emergency Nurses Association. (1994). *Prevalence of violence in emergency departments.* Park Ridge, IL: Author.

Fox, J. A., & Levin, J. (1994). Firing back: The growing threat of workplace violence. In R. D. Lambert & A. W. Heston (Eds.), *The Annals of the American Academy of Political and Social Science, 536,* 16–30.

Goodman, R. A., Jenkins, E. L., & Mercy, J. A. (1994). Workplace-related homicide among health care workers in the United States, 1980 through 1990. *Journal of the American Medical Association, 272,* 1686–1688.

Hales, T., Seligman, P. J., Newman, S. C., & Timbrook, C. L. (1988). Occupational injuries due to violence. *Journal of Occupational Medicine, 30,* 483–487.

Health Information Policy Council. (1983). *Background paper: Uniform minimum data sets.* (Unpublished manuscript.)

Hoge, S. K., & Gutheil, T. G. (1987). The prosecution of psychiatric patients for assaults on staff: A preliminary empirical study. *Hospital and Community Psychiatry, 38,* 44–49.

Illinois Nurses Association. (1995). Guidelines for development of a personnel safety policy. *Chart, 92*(4), 3.

Jenkins, E. L. (1994). Occupational injury deaths among females in the US experience for the decade 1980 to 1989. *Annals of Epidemiology, 4,* 146–151.

Jenkins, E. L., Layne, L. A., & Kisner, S. M. (1992). Homicide in the workplace: The U.S. experience, 1980–88. *AAOHN Journal, 40,* 215–218.

Kraus, J. F. (1987). Homicide while at work: Persons, industries, and occupations at high risk. *American Journal of Public Health, 77,* 1285–1289.

Kraus, J. F., Peek, C., Silverman, T., & Anderson, C. (1995). The accuracy of death certificates in identifying work-related fatal injuries. *American Journal of Epidemiology, 141,* 973–979.

Lanza, M. L. (1988). Factors relevant to patient assault. *Issues in Mental Health Nursing, 9,* 239–257.

Levin, P. F., Hewitt, J. B., & Misner, S. T. (1992). Female workplace homicides: An integrative research review. *AAOHN Journal, 40,* 229–236.

Levin, P. F., Hewitt, J. B., & Misner, S. T. (1996). Workplace violence: Female occupational homicides in Metropolitan Chicago. *AAOHN Journal, 44,* 326–331.

Lipscomb, J. A., & Love, C. C. (1992). Violence towards health care workers: An emerging occupational hazard. *AAOHN Journal, 40,* 219–228.

Liss, G. M., & Craig, C. A. (1990). Homicide in the workplace in Ontario: Occupations at risk and limitations of existing data sources. *Canadian Journal of Public Health, 81,* 10–15.

Liss, G. M., & McCaskell, L. (1994). Injuries due to violence: Workers' compensation claims among nurses in Ontario. *AAOHN Journal, 42,* 384–390.

Manitoba Association of Registered Nurses. (1989, October). *Nurse Abuse Report.* (Available from Author, 647 Broadway, Winnipeg, Manitoba, Canada R3C0X2.)

McCulloch, E., McNiel, D. E., Binder, R. L., & Hatcher, C. (1986). Effects of a weapon screening procedure in a psychiatric emergency room. *Hospital and Community Psychiatry, 37,* 837–838.

Ministerial Committee on Abuse of Health Care Staff. (1991, October). *Protocol for the Prevention of Abuse of Health Care Staff.* (Available from Workplace Services Unit, Work Safety & Health Branch, Department of Labour, 1000-330 St. Mary Ave., Winnepeg, Manitoba, Canada R3C375.)

Morrison, E. F. (1992). What therapeutic and protective measures, as well as legal actions, can staff take when they are attacked by patients? *Journal of Psychosocial Nursing, 30,* 41–42.

National Institute of Occupational Safety and Health (NIOSH). (1993). *Fatal injuries to workers in the United States, 1980–1989: A decade of surveillance, national and state profiles* (DHHS [NIOSH] No. 93–108S). Cincinnati, OH: NIOSH.

New York Committee for Occupational Safety and Health. (NYCOSH). (1995). *Violence in the workplace: The New York State experience.* New York: Author.

Northwestern National Life Insurance Company. (1993). *Fear and violence in the workplace.* Minneapolis, MN: Author.

Nurse Assault Project Team. (1992, January). *Nurse assault survey.* (Available from Ontario Nurses' Association, 85 Grenville Street, Toronto, Ontario, Canada MSS 3A2.)

Occupational Safety and Health Administration (OSHA). (1996). *Guidelines for preventing workplace violence for health care and social workers.* (U.S. Department of Labor, OSHA 3148.) Washington, DC: Author.

Ontario Nurses Association. (1991). *Violence in the workplace: A guide for ONA members.* (Available from Author, 85 Grenville Street, Toronto, Ontario, Canada MSS 3A2.)

Pane, G. A, Winiarski, A. M., & Salness, K. A. (1991). Aggression directed toward emergency department staff at a university teaching hospital. *Annals of Emergency Medicine, 20,* 283–286.

Phelan, L. A., Mills, M. J., & Ryan, J. A. (1985). Prosecuting psychiatric patients for assault. *Hospital and Community Psychiatry, 36,* 581–582.

Scalera, N. R. (1995). The critical need for specialized health and safety measures for child welfare workers. *Child Welfare, 74,* 337–350.

Simonowitz, J. A. (1995). Violence in health care: A strategic approach. *Nurse Practitioner Forum, 6,* 120–129.

Sniezek, J. E., & Horiagon, T. M. (1989). Medical-examiner-reported fatal occupational injuries, North Carolina, 1978–1984. *American Journal of Industrial Medicine, 15,* 669–678.

Sparr, L. F., Drummond, D. J., & Hamilton, N. G. (1988). Managing violent patient incidents: The role of a behavioral emergency committee. *Quality Review Bulletin, 14,* 147–153.

Stone, P. W. (1993). Traumatic occupational fatalities in South Carolina, 1989–90. *Public Health Reports, 108,* 483–488.

Stout, N. A. (1992). Occupational injuries and fatalities among health care workers in the United States. *Scandinavian Journal of Work and Environmental Health, 18* (Suppl. 2), 88–89.

Stultz, M. S. (1993). Crime in hospitals 1986–1991: The latest IAHSS surveys. *Journal of Healthcare Protection Management, 9,* 1–25.

Sullivan, C., & Yuan, C. (1995). Workplace assaults on minority health and mental health care workers in Los Angeles. *American Journal of Public Health, 85,* 1011–1014.

Thomas, J. L. (1992). Occupational violent crime: Research on an emerging issue. *Journal of Safety Research, 23,* 55–62.

Toscano, G., & Windau, J. (1993). Fatal work injuries: Results from the 1992 national census. *Monthly Labor Review, 116*(10), 39–48.

U.S. Department of Labor. (1993). *Citation and notification of penalty (Inspection No: 102992021).* Des Plaines, IL: Occupational Safety and Health Administration. (Available from Occupational Safety & Health Administration, 2360 Devon Ave., Des Plaines, IL 60018.)

Washington Nurse. (1995). Workplace violence may be preventable. *Washington Nurse, 25*(4), 10–11.

Williams, M. F. (1995). The prevalence and impact of violence and sexual harassment of registered nurses in the workplace. *Chart, 92,* 5–6.

Workplace violence may be preventable. (1995). *Washington Nurse, 25,* 10–11.

Chapter 5

Interventions to Reduce the Impact of Chronic Disease: Community-Based Arthritis Patient Education

JEAN GOEPPINGER
SCHOOLS OF NURSING AND PUBLIC HEALTH
UNIVERSITY OF NORTH CAROLINA AT CHAPEL HILL

KATE LORIG
SCHOOL OF MEDICINE
STANFORD UNIVERSITY
SCHOOL OF NURSING
UNIVERSITY OF CALIFORNIA AT SAN FRANCISCO

ABSTRACT

Systematic development and testing of the efficacy of educational interventions to improve functioning, prevent disability, and reduce the impact of chronic disease has been limited, perhaps because many chronic diseases disable, do not kill, and because they are managed largely within home, work, and community environments and not within the medical care system. Until recently, these factors contributed to a paucity of arthritis educational interventions. But since the impetus provided by the establishment of the Multipurpose Arthritis Centers Program of the NIH (1977), a number of arthritis patient education programs have been established and evaluated. This chapter summarizes findings from community-based arthritis patient education studies conducted between 1980 and 1995, critiques the methods of these studies, and provides guidance for state-of-the-art community-based intervention research aimed at reducing the individual and social impact of arthritis and other chronic diseases.

Keywords: Arthritis, Patient Education, Intervention Research, Community, Chronic Disease Management

101

Systematic trials of educational interventions to improve functioning, prevent disability, and reduce the impact of chronic disease have been limited, perhaps because disability and "botheration" (Verbrugge, 1990, p. 741), not death, are the main effects of many chronic diseases. Chronic diseases such as arthritis are generally not fatal; they disable and bother individuals throughout a normal life span. They also are managed largely within home, work, and community environments and not within the medical care system. The impact of arthritis on the daily lives of persons with arthritis is not reflected in the frequency with which these persons are treated as arthritis patients by health professionals. And finally, strong links between health behaviors, disease incidence, and clinical outcomes, as exist in cardiovascular disease, diabetes, and asthma, have not been established. Most forms of arthritis are not preventable. Changes in health behavior are generally unrelated to the occurrence, remissions, and exacerbations of rheumatic disease. These factors have until recently contributed to the neglect of arthritis educational interventions by health care providers and researchers, although arthritis is clearly both a prevalent and disabling chronic disease with significant societal consequences (Yelin, 1992). The purpose of this chapter is to summarize findings from arthritis patient education studies, critique the methods of these studies, and provide guidance for state-of-the-art intervention research directed at reducing the personal and societal impact of arthritis and other chronic diseases.

There are over 100 recognized forms of arthritis; many of these are rare, but a few, such as osteoarthritis and rheumatoid arthritis, occur frequently (Schumacher, 1993). The most common symptoms of arthritis are musculoskeletal pain, loss of function, and the resultant disability, that is, the inability of the individual with arthritis to perform daily roles and tasks at home and on the job. The burden of these conditions is substantial.

In 1990, 37.9 million or approximately 15% of the people in the United States reported having arthritis (Centers for Disease Control and Prevention, [CDC], 1994a). Overall, arthritis is the second most common chronic condition; it is the single most prevalent chronic disease among women (Benson & Marano, 1994). A companion to these prevalence studies, conducted by the Centers for Disease Control and Prevention, established arthritis as the leading cause of disability in the United States (CDC, 1994b). The National Arthritis Data Work Group estimated that the cost of musculoskeletal conditions in the United States in 1992 was $149.4 billion; approximately 48% of these costs were due to medical care, that is, physician visits, drugs, and hospital inpatient and nursing home care, while 52% were estimated to be due to indirect costs resulting from restricted activity and wage losses (Yelin & Callahan, 1995). A few studies also have demonstrated the economic and emotional cost of disability in family work roles, unpaid roles generally assumed by women

(Katz, 1995; Reisine & Fifield, 1992). Early findings from a population-based prospective study of osteoarthritis suggested that the costs may disproportionately affect historically underserved populations (Jordan, Lindner, Renner, & Fryer, 1995). Jordan and her colleagues found that residents of rural communities have an increased prevalence of both arthritis and arthritis-related disability.

Arthritis is just as clearly a disease where medical and surgical interventions are of limited efficacy; most forms of arthritis are only somewhat responsive to physician treatment. Many other diseases (e.g., AIDS) that were life-threatening are now also becoming chronic. Consequently, the cumulative work establishing the importance of community-based arthritis patient education in decreasing the impact of arthritis and as a complement to medical and surgical interventions is both instructive and broadly applicable.

SCOPE OF THE REVIEW

The substance of the review was guided by three inclusion criteria. Each study reviewed examined the clinical outcomes of arthritis patient education, including indicators of disability and pain. The intervention was population-focused and community-based. The population sampled in each study reviewed included adult persons ages 18 and older with medically confirmed diagnoses of osteoarthritis, rheumatoid arthritis, systemic lupus erythematosus, fibromyalgia, or some combination of these diseases. The target of intervention and unit of analysis were aggregates, that is, populations of individual patients with arthritis. Studies reviewed were also community-based, i.e., the intervention strategy utilized community residents as leaders and was located in community settings such as churches, schools, homes, and meeting rooms in public libraries and shopping malls.

"Patient education" is here defined as a set of planned educational activities intended to improve patients' health behaviors and/or health status, or retard deterioration from disease (Lorig & Gonzalez, 1992), and more explicitly, as teaching the patient "what he or she should do . . . and how to approach situations and to make adjustments which are appropriate for each individual and his or her own needs" (Hirano, Laurent, & Lorig, 1994, p. 10). The individualized adjustments noted by Hirano et al. are necessitated by the long-term but not static consequences of arthritis on these persons' ability to participate in "typical and personally desired ways" (Verbrugge, 1990, p. 745) in their usual domestic, occupational, and recreational activities.

The search process for this chapter began with a computer search of literature published subsequent to that included in the review by Lambert

(1991). All computer searches included the MEDLINE database and the Cumu-lative Index of Nursing and Allied Health Literature (CINAHL). Author searches were conducted of nurse researchers who were listed as members of either the Association of Rheumatology Health Professionals or the Arthritis and Rheumatism Association in the 1995 membership directory. Abstracts of their publications were read to determine the subject of the research. Published abstracts of their presentations at the national meetings of the American College of Rheumatology and the Arthritis Health Professions Association between 1987 and 1995 were also reviewed. The outline for this chapter was then developed. From this outline keywords and phrases were identified and used to guide additional computer searches. Combination sets were identified with the key word ''arthritis'' included in each combination. The key words were patient education, community-based, self-care, intervention, pain, depression, secondary prevention, tertiary prevention, disability (function/dysfunction), cost-effectiveness, and health care utilization. The abstracts of all articles and presentations identified in the searches were screened using the three inclusion criteria outlined above. In addition, the following journals were hand-searched for the years 1987 through 1995: *Nursing Research, Research in Nursing and Health, Image, Applied Nursing Research, Public Health Nursing, Family and Community Health, American Journal of Public Health, Health Education Quarterly, Patient Education and Counseling, Journal of Rheumatology, Arthritis and Rheumatism*, and *Arthritis Care and Research*. Article titles and abstracts were reviewed for the identified keywords and phrases, and then screened for presence of the inclusion criteria. The work of nonnurse investiga-tors was included when needed to enrich and elaborate on the methods and findings of the studies examined.

    Several reviews of arthritis patient education studies published or pre-sented since 1983 were found. The series of reviews by Lorig and colleagues (Hirano et al., 1994; Lorig & Holman, 1993; Lorig, Konkol, & Gonzalez, 1987; and Lorig & Riggs, 1983) covers the development of arthritis patient education interventions subsequent to the funding impetus provided by the Multipurpose Arthritis Centers Program of the National Institutes of Health. These authors summarize the growing body of research findings documenting the effectiveness of arthritis patient education interventions in improving knowledge, behavior, and selected psychosocial and health status outcomes. A recent review chapter on rheumatoid arthritis patient education suggests ways the clinician can integrate patient education into practice (Lorig, 1994). The interested reader is referred to these reviews for historical perspective; study-specific detail about the research variables, design, instrumentation, sample, and analytic techniques; and practice guidelines.

    In this chapter, the earlier review (Lambert, 1991) of nurse researchers' investigations of psychosocial variables, nursing interventions, health care provider education, and instrumentation issues in the field of arthritis is both extended and focused. The present chapter is an integrative review of community-based arthritis patient education studies conducted by nurse researchers since the early 1980s; studies aimed at testing community-based, population-focused interventions to improve function, prevent disability, control pain and depression, and limit health care utilization. It describes chronologically what nurse researchers have learned about whether arthritis patient education works, how or why it works, and with whom it works. The theoretical work informing the research, particularly self-efficacy, learned helplessness, community development, and diffusion theory, is considered. Also reviewed are conditions under which arthritis patient education has been found to be effective: university-led and tightly controlled field experiments, and voluntary health organization-led national and international dissemination. The elements of successful educational programming, recently codified as arthritis patient education standards for the United States (Burckhardt, 1994), are presented, as is a synopsis of the international dissemination of one arthritis patient education program.

DOES COMMUNITY-BASED ARTHRITIS PATIENT EDUCATION WORK?

Historical Perspective: 1980–1987

By 1986 over 75 studies of the effectiveness of arthritis patient education had been reported in the published literature and at professional meetings (Lorig et al., 1987). Researchers had found that arthritis patient education increased knowledge and improved a wide range of arthritis self-care behaviors, selected psychosocial variables, and health status outcomes. One series of studies established the foundation for future effectiveness research in arthritis patient education by developing and beginning to test an intervention protocol, the Arthritis Self-Management Program (ASMP), that served as a model for much of the subsequent work. All studies highlighted the needs for future research to utilize more appropriate evaluation strategies and to work towards achieving stronger effects and a theoretically informed understanding of how and why arthritis patient education was effective.

Several studies in this period were conducted by nurse researchers (Goeppinger, Brunk, Arthur, & Riedesel, 1987a, 1987b; Goeppinger, Doyle, Brunk, Murdock, & Brunner, 1985; Holman & Lorig, 1987; Lorig, Cox, Cuevas, Kraines, & Britton, 1984; Lorig, Feigenbaum, Regan, Ung, & Holman, 1986; Lorig, Laurin, & Holman, 1984; Lorig, Lubeck, Kraines, Seleznick, & Holman, 1985). The goals of two of the earliest studies (Goeppinger et al., 1985; Cox et al., 1984) were to determine the expressed needs of arthritis patients for selected educational topics, and the congruence of patient and health professional perceptions of educational needs. The studies were conducted with convenience samples of Caucasian, Spanish-speaking, and rural persons with arthritis, as well as physicians, nurses, physical therapists, and chiropractors. The findings of the needs assessments directed these nurse interventionists to design arthritis patient education programs which included such topics as exercise and activity, energy conservation and joint protection, depression (''feeling low''), medicines, nutrition and diet, and sleep, and encouraged the active practice of self-care and thoughtful problem identification and management. Outcome evaluations conducted between 1984 and 1987 demonstrated the acceptability and effectiveness of arthritis patient education based on these needs assessments. Findings of improvements in clinical outcomes subsequent to community-based and population-focused patient education interventions substantiated the appropriateness of structuring a curriculum on the perceived needs of the target population.

Goeppinger et al. (1987a) conducted a randomized controlled assessment of the acceptability of two models (home study and small group) of a community-based intervention for arthritis self-care—Bone Up On Arthritis (BUOA)—among 450 residents of rural Virginia communities. Approximately 75% of the sample were adult and elder adult women and had medically verified diagnoses of osteoarthritis. Ninety percent were Caucasian; the average number of years of education was 12. Participation and retention rates were high and not significantly different between intervention groups, suggesting that both the content and format of BUOA were appropriate to the target populations. In a different study of the same sample (Goeppinger et al., 1987b), BUOA participants were found to demonstrate significant improvements over the delayed treatment control group in knowledge, performance of self-care behaviors, and helplessness at 4 months postintervention, but to make no changes in pain, depression, and function. Neither intervention model (home study or small group) was more effective than the other.

Concurrently, Lorig and her associates conducted several field trials of the efficacy of the ASMP. Findings were based on self-administered questionnaire data obtained from samples ranging in size from 100 persons with arthritis (Lorig et al., 1986) to 641 arthritis patients (Holman & Lorig, 1987). Longitudinal followup extended to 20 months posttest. As with Goeppinger's studies, the study samples were predominantly female, Caucasian, well-educated (the average number of years of formal education was 14), and had osteoarthritis; generally, ASMP participants had medically verified diagnoses of arthritis. Experimental subjects demonstrated significant initial and long-term increases in knowledge, practice of exercise, relaxation, and self-management activities, and perceived self-efficacy; they also had statistically significant and long-term decreases in pain and depression.

One study conducted during this same time period began the exploration of mediating variables, the intermediate processes that might explain the presence or absence of relationships between the educational interventions, changes in health behavior, and changes in health status (Lenker, Lorig, & Gallagher, 1984). Lenker and her colleagues utilized a guided interview to identify characteristics distinguishing ASMP participants with positive and negative health outcomes. The findings that personal control distinguished the two groups suggested to Lorig's team the utility of self-efficacy theory as a mechanism for explaining improvements in pain, disability, and depression.

Through 1987 the findings of nurse researchers' studies on the effectiveness of arthritis patient education were characterized by their orientation to patients, use of trained lay community members as interveners, and carefully designed experiments. First, the educational interventions, the Arthritis Self-Management Program [ASMP] and Bone Up On Arthritis [BUOA], were designed only after assessments of the educational needs perceived by members of the target populations were conducted (Goeppinger et al., 1985; Lorig, Cox, et al., 1984). Second, the interventions were led by trained volunteers who were respected community members and, to varying extents, recognized as community leaders. Third, the nurse researchers' studies utilized rigorous field experimentation with large samples. Individuals who volunteered to participate were randomly assigned to treatment and delayed treatment control conditions, and plans were made to examine the effects of the intervention longitudinally. Finally, differences between participants with positive and negative health outcomes began to be explored. The search for an explanatory theory began with interviews of ASMP participants; the approach to theory was inductive.

Despite these accomplishments, several limitations persisted. The study samples remained unrepresentative of persons with arthritis. Most participants were Caucasian and relatively well-educated. Another limitation was that outcome data were reported only for short-term intervals. Posttest effects at 4 and 8 months did not adequately reflect intervention impact on a long-term, that is, chronic, disease.

A meta-analysis of the effects of psychoeducational interventions among persons with arthritis was also reported in 1987 (Mullen, Laville, Biddle, & Lorig, 1987). It included 15 published studies that met stringent inclusion criteria. Each study assessed the impact of intervention on pain, depression, and/or disability; used a control or comparison group design; had > 10 subjects per experimental group; and reported sufficient information to calculate effect size. The meta-analysis concluded that arthritis patient education was not only effective in reducing pain, depression, and dysfunction but also improved the health status of patients with arthritis above and beyond the improvements obtained from clinical trials of nonsteroidal, anti-inflammatory drugs. Although these conclusions were based on 15 published studies, they included findings from only one of the studies by nurse researchers cited above (Lorig et al., 1985).

Historical Perspective: 1988–1991

In the most recent summary of arthritis patient education studies, Hirano et al. (1994) identified an additional 25 intervention studies measuring changes in knowledge, behavior, psychosocial status, and health status since 1987. Seven of these were conducted by nurse-researchers and met the review criteria (Arthur, Goeppinger, & Brunk, 1988; Burckhardt et al., 1991; Clark, Burckhardt, O'Reilly, Campbell, & Bennett, 1991; Goeppinger, Arthur, Baglioni, Brunk, & Brunner, 1989; Goeppinger, Arthur, Baglioni, Brunk, & Hawdon, 1988; Lorig & Holman, 1989; Lorig, Mazonson, & Holman, 1993). Two others (Braden, 1990, 1991) were identified in this review.

By the late 1980s most studies were reporting outcomes from longer posttest intervals. In 1988, for example, Goeppinger et al. reported on a 12-month followup of 259 BUOA participants who had been randomly assigned to small-group, home-study, and delayed-treatment control groups. Seventy-six percent of study subjects had osteoarthritis; 79% were female; all lived in rural areas. Intervention groups experienced statistically significant improvements in knowledge, behavior, helplessness, and pain at 4 months; these improvements were sustained at 8 and 12 months. Importantly, no significant differences in outcomes were found between participants in the home-study and small-group treatment conditions. These findings were replicated in a later study with 374 subjects by the same research team (Goeppinger et al., 1989). Once again, study subjects were followed for 12 months after intervention. The largest amount of explained variance in improvements in pain, that was the only clinical outcome to improve initially and show sustained improvements over time, was attributed to initial (4 months) and sustained (4–8 months) decreases in perceived helplessness. In neither study did function/ disability change. This finding was cautiously interpreted as positive given the length of followup (12 months) and the great likelihood of increased dysfunction with time among persons with osteoarthritis.

Holman, Lorig, and Mazonson (1989) reported findings from a longitudinal followup of ASMP participants who were initially randomized to treatment and delayed treatment control groups. They reported changes from baseline 4 years subsequent to participation in the ASMP course. The pain of study subjects decreased by 18%, physical disability increased by 9%, physician visits decreased by 34%, perceived self-efficacy for managing pain increased by 22% and for managing other symptoms by 9%, and increases in frequency of exercise and relaxation behaviors were statistically significant. The participants' levels and changes in perceived self-efficacy to cope with the consequences of arthritis correlated most strongly with improvements in clinical outcomes.

In addition to demonstrating the persistence of improvements over the long term, these studies continued to explore the theoretical explanations for the observed improvements. Two variables gained credence as mediators of the intervention effect: learned helplessness and self-efficacy. Both offered cognitive, not behavioral, explanations for change. The concept of learned helplessness suggests that given unpredictable and uncontrollable negative experiences, individuals learn to become helpless (Maier & Seligman, 1976). Developing a feeling of helplessness has been found linked to depression and decreased problem-solving behaviors among persons with arthritis (Stein, Wallston, Nicassio, & Castner, 1988). The concept of self-efficacy suggests that an individual's belief in his or her own ability to change a behavior or achieve a desired goal via behavior change is most important (Bandura, 1986). Still other studies demonstrated that the reasons for choosing a particular intervention mode had no effect on findings related to intervention effectiveness (Arthur et al., 1988), and that the persistence of improvement over the long term was unaffected by reinforcement (Lorig & Holman, 1989).

The findings regarding effectiveness were generally consistent with those of earlier studies. Only a few of the studies measured changes in knowledge alone. Exercise continued to be the most widely measured behavioral outcome, although self-care behaviors generally and specific pain relief and stress reduction behaviors were also studied. And, the trio of clinical outcomes termed the "gold standard" of arthritis outcomes research—pain, function/disability, and depression—were consistently measured and either found to be improved (pain and depression) or unchanged (function/disability). Importantly, given the temporal attribute of chronic diseases like arthritis, previously demonstrated short-term improvements were found to be maintained up to 4 years following intervention (Holman et al., 1989). And finally, for the first time, findings related to health care costs, that is, physician utilization, were reported (Holman et al., 1989).

The studies of Burckhardt and her colleagues (Burckhardt et al., 1991) and by Braden (1990, 1991) extended previous studies with osteoarthritis and rheumatoid arthritis patients to patients with fibromyalgia and systemic lupus erythematosus. (Sample demographics were, however, comparable.) These studies also extended the educational intervention with an aerobic conditioning and flexibility program (Burckhardt et al., 1991). Their findings added to the growing body of evidence substantiating the effectiveness of arthritis patient education interventions in increasing self-help and enabling skills (Braden, 1990, 1991), perceived helplessness (Goeppinger et al., 1989), and self-efficacy (Holman et al., 1989; Burckhardt et al., 1991).

By 1991 a positive answer to the question "Does community-based arthritis patient education work?" had been consistently reported in two major series of studies: those by Lorig and her colleagues on the West coast and by Goeppinger and her colleagues in the East. Although both urban and rural adults participated, study samples were predominantly composed of Caucasian and middle-aged-to-elderly women with osteoarthritis, and individuals with 12 or more years of schooling. Short- and long-term improvements in pain and depression, as well as in self-efficacy and helplessness, had been demonstrated.

Historical Perspective: 1992–1995

An occasional study using a sample comparable to those studied by Lorig and Goeppinger, investigating similar psychosocial variables, and conducted by a nurse-researcher new to the field had been reported subsequent to 1991 (e.g., Newman, 1993). The findings of these studies substantiated those reported earlier by Lorig and Goeppinger.

Studies of the effectiveness of arthritis patient education which made new contributions to the field after 1991 occurred in the area of health care costs and among new populations: persons with systemic lupus erythematosus (SLE) and fibromyalgia. Basic work in the assessment of fatigue, a symptom of rheumatic disease as common as pain, function, and depression, was also conducted.

Lorig and colleagues (1993) studied the relationship between participation in the ASMP and health care costs by comparing ASMP participants to individuals having arthritis, living in the same geographic region as ASMP participants, and serving as respondents in one of two observational studies of health system performance. They noted prolonged benefits in pain and medical service utilization among ASMP participants 4 years subsequent to intervention, estimated the costs of the ASMP and charges for physician visits, and extrapolated 4-year savings in medical costs of $648 for each ASMP participant with rheumatoid arthritis and $189 for each ASMP participant with osteoarthritis. No estimates were made of indirect cost savings.

Braden, in a series of studies of persons with SLE (1990, 1991, 1992; Braden, McGlone, & Pennington, 1993) found that SLE self-help course participants gained significantly in both enabling skill and self-efficacy; in addition, those who were depressed also improved in several of the variables indicating a learned response to chronic illness, the theoretical model underpinning Braden's work (1992). These variables were uncertainty, self-worth, and life quality. Findings from a 1993 study (Braden, 1993) were the first to suggest a treatment strength-outcome relationship. Treatment strength was indicated by the amount of time devoted to a particular activity or topic in the SLE self-help course; response or outcome was indicated by perception of limitations in ability to care for oneself, depression, enabling skill, and use of rest, relaxation, heat, and exercise activities.

Burckhardt, Clark, and Bennett (1991) and Burckhardt, Mannerkorpi, Hedenberg, and Bjelle (1994) conducted experimental studies of, respectively, 100 and 86 women with fibromyalgia. They demonstrated the effectiveness of self-management education and physical training in decreasing fibromyalgia symptoms and increasing physical and psychological well-being. They found that both experimental programs (1992, 1994) had significant positive effects on quality of life, self-efficacy, and fibromyalgia symptoms short-term. Only the physical training group showed significant long-term improvements. These programs are, however, among the first non-drug treatment strategies for persons with fibromyalgia, and a need exists for further research into who is helped by what strategies and the optimal program length (Burckhardt & Bjelle, 1994).

Research conducted by Belza (1994, 1995; Belza, Henke, Yelin, Epstein, & Gilliss, 1993) highlighted the importance of fatigue to individuals with many chronic diseases, including rheumatoid arthritis. The multiple problems resulting from a chronic physical condition require a significant amount of effort if successful disease adjustment and management are to occur. Adjustment and management require energy, not fatigue. Belza (1993) identified a constant high level of fatigue among persons with rheumatoid arthritis and found that the presence of fatigue was explained by pain, functional status, disease duration and comorbidity, and female gender. These findings were confirmed when persons with rheumatoid arthritis were compared to healthy controls (Belza, 1995). Belza (1994) suggested that fatigue improves with aerobic exercise of moderate intensity. Work in progress (B.L. Belza, personal communication, April 1996) is aimed at developing and testing biobehavioral strategies for fatigue modulation, work that will enrich future arthritis patient education studies.

During this same time period, the findings from a previous meta-analysis showing the efficacy of patient education above and beyond improvements obtained from standard clinical practice (Mullen et al., 1987) were substantiated by a meta-analytic comparison of the efficacy of patient education interventions and nonsteroidal anti-inflammatory drug treatment among persons with osteoarthritis and rheumatoid arthritis (Superio-Cabuslay, Ward, & Lorig, 1996). Superio-Cabuslay and her colleagues found that patient education interventions produced an additional, termed ''marginal,'' effect beyond the effects achieved by medication.

WHO BENEFITS FROM COMMUNITY-BASED ARTHRITIS PATIENT EDUCATION?

Research findings on the effectiveness of community-based arthritis patient education have provided convincing evidence that relatively well-educated, Caucasian, rural and urban adults and elders benefit. Individuals with diagnoses of osteoarthritis, rheumatoid arthritis, and to a growing extent, SLE and fibromyalgia also benefit. But arthritis patient education programs in the United States have not reached either racial and ethnic minorities (Native Americans, African Americans, Asian Americans, and Hispanics), those with less than a high school education, and inner-city residents. Successful programs require adaptation to reach these groups in culturally sensitive and cost-effective ways.

A Spanish version of the ASMP has been developed and is being systematically evaluated with Spanish-speaking residents of Northern California (Gonzalez, Stewart, Ritter, & Lorig, 1995). Another adaptation of the ASMP is occurring among First Nations populations of Canada, that is, indigenous or native Indian inhabitants (McGowan & Green, 1995). Preliminary results from this study suggest both the utility of participatory research strategies to the successful adaptation of health education programs in minority populations, and the effectiveness of the First Nations ASMP in decreasing arthritis pain and improving arthritis self-efficacy. Together the studies of Gonzalez et al. and McGowan and Green suggest ways the next decade of arthritis health education research might focus on testing theory-based interventions in new population groups and on implementing these interventions to better reach currently inaccessible populations in culturally sensitive and cost-effective ways. These suggestions are consistent with the recommendations of Daltroy and Liang (1993) and Marin et al. (1995) that successful programs be adapted to reach racial and ethnic minorities and inner-city communities.

Indirectly, clinicians have also benefited from arthritis patient education research, as many of their patients now have available at minimal cost in their own communities patient education programs that are both effective and complementary to the customary medical interventions for arthritis, medications, and joint replacement. Standards for structured arthritis patient education programs were established in 1990 (Burckhardt, 1994); they were later reviewed by the professional organizations who participated in their development (Arthritis Health Professions Association, American Physical Therapy Association, American Occupational Therapy Association, American College of

Rheumatology, and American Nurses Association) and finalized by the Arthritis Foundation. The arthritis patient education standards emphasize changes in behavior and health status, require patient participation in the development of interventions, recognize the ability of both health professionals and laypersons to become patient educators, and establish rigorous evaluation criteria for program approval (Lorig & Visser, 1994). These standards clearly show the influence of nurse researchers' work and encourage informed referral by the practicing clinician.

WHY IS COMMUNITY-BASED ARTHRITIS PATIENT EDUCATION EFFECTIVE?

Four concepts and theories—community development, self-efficacy, learned helplessness, and diffusion—have strongly influenced the development, testing, and dissemination of the major community-based arthritis patient education interventions designed by nurse-researchers. Common to both the ASMP and BUOA interventions is a firm foundation in community development theory. Both the ASMP and BUOA interventions are based on the findings of needs assessments of the target communities: patients with arthritis, and, secondarily, their professional health care providers. Relevance, or "starting where the people are," is a fundamental tenet of community development and health education practice. The design of the ASMP and BUOA interventions began with population-focused needs assessments. Both the ASMP and BUOA also initiate every program offering with needs assessments of participants. These questions are posed in the first lesson: What would you like to learn about your arthritis? What would you like to be able to do differently at the end of the program? When you think about arthritis, what do you think about? What things make your arthritis better? What things make your arthritis worse?

Second, both the ASMP and BUOA interventions conceive of program participants as active learners in problem-solving groups, as research *participants* and not as research *subjects*. Groups are led by trained volunteers. The roles of health professionals, like those of community developers, focus on "training the trainer," rather than on direct service. Project staff train local community members as lay leaders of small groups and as community coordinators and resource persons for home studies. They teach problem-identification and management techniques and group process skills to the volunteer leaders, as well as providing them with basic information about rheumatic disease. Project staff do not provide any direct participant instruction; they train the trainers.

Third, both the ASMP and BUOA conceive of small task and process-oriented groups as the medium of change. In the BUOA home study intervention model (Goeppinger et al., 1989; Goeppinger, Macnee, Anderson, Boutaugh, & Stewart, 1995) audiotapes include statements and testimonials from small group participants which are designed to create "virtual groups." Group work emphasizes self-contracting for selected changes, learning by doing, and role-modeling by group leaders, at least one of whom has arthritis.

And fourth, both the interventions conceptualize improved self-management (ASMP) or self-care (BUOA) as means to the desired clinical outcomes. Self-efficacy and learned helplessness, theoretical explanations for embracing self-help and self-care, gained credence as researchers reported counterintuitive results from early studies regarding the effects of behavior change on clinical outcomes. At this point, however, the theoretical orientations of the ASMP and BUOA research programs diverge.

The findings from Lorig's initial study, reported in the 1985 article by Lorig et al., provided the first evidence that healthful behavior changes were not strongly associated with improvements in health status. Participants in the ASMP did increase self-help behaviors and experience improved health status, but the changes in behavior and health status were not linked (Lorig et al., 1986). The next step (Lenker, Lorig et al., 1984) involved searching for the reasons.

Using a grounded-theory approach, researchers interviewed 54 persons who had participated in the ASMP. They asked questions about the participants' perceptions of the ASMP course; the effect of the course on their lives, health, and arthritis; and course benefits other than changes in pain, disability, and number of physician visits (Lenker, Lorig, et al., 1984). Participants were separated into two groups by their arthritis health outcomes (pain, disability, and number of physician visits), those with positive and those with negative outcomes.

The major dimension distinguishing the two groups was individuals' belief in their ability to control symptoms. This finding was of theoretical interest, because participants who believed themselves able to impact or control the disease process were thought most likely to adopt new self-help behaviors. The researchers' conceptualization of the link between control beliefs and self-management activities reflected the persistence of a belief in the efficacy of behavior change. (An alternative hypothesis suggesting that self-efficacy might directly affect health status was eventually explored [Lorig & Holman, 1993].)

A re-examination of the content and process of the ASMP revealed that several of Bandura's efficacy-enhancing mechanisms—skills mastery, modeling, reinterpretation of physiological symptoms, and persuasion—were already in place. This reinforced the explanatory promise of self-efficacy. Perceived self-efficacy was defined as people's beliefs in their abilities to effectively carry out the actions necessary to meet the demands of a particular situation (Bandura, 1986). An instrument to measure perceived self-efficacy in persons with arthritis was developed and piloted (Lorig, Chastain, Ung, Shoor, & Holman, 1989). The instrument was found to have acceptable psychometric properties; the study also found a correlation between improvements in self-efficacy and arthritis clinical outcomes subsequent to participation in the ASMP. Baseline self-efficacy predicted future health status, and changes in self-efficacy were associated with changes in health status. The question of whether changes in self-efficacy caused changes in health status remained unanswered.

A new ASMP was developed which deliberately emphasized efficacy-enhancing strategies (Lorig & Gonzalez, 1992). Course activities incorporated exercises to increase skills mastery, feedback about accomplishments, modeling by leaders and other participants, symptom reinterpretation, examples of how to change one's beliefs, and persuasion. Increases in health status improvements obtained with the self-efficacy enriched course ranged from 1.5 to 12 times that seen in the original course (Lorig & Gonzalez, 1992, p. 364).

In contrast, the BUOA intervention was neither designed nor redesigned within a theoretical rubric. Instead, learned helplessness was hypothesized as a mediating variable, and the Arthritis Helplessness Index (Stein et al., 1988) was used to reflect the effect of the intervention on helplessness. Learned helplessness is a state in which deficits in motivation, cognition, and affect cause individuals to expect that their efforts will be ineffective in producing desired changes (Abramson, Seligman, & Teasdale, 1978; Maier & Seligman, 1976; Seligman, 1975). This variable was chosen not because it directly suggests theory-driven interventions as does self-efficacy—it does not—but because it was thought to better explain responses to diseases like arthritis, where there is often a lack of relationship between self-care behaviors, symptoms, and clinical outcomes. Findings from the one intervention study which examined the explanatory power of learned helplessness (Goeppinger et al., 1989) suggest that decreases in feelings of helplessness, rather than changes in self-care behavior, are associated with improvements in clinical outcomes—in this case, pain.

Diffusion theory (Rogers, 1995) explains the success and failure of ASMP and BUOA dissemination activities across the United States and internationally. The dissemination of the ASMP and to a much lesser extent, BUOA, is the subject of the next section.

IN WHAT SETTINGS DOES ARTHRITIS PATIENT EDUCATION WORK?

In 1979 the ASMP was first offered in the United States in the San Francisco Bay Area. It was developed at Stanford University as intervention research aimed at determining the effectiveness of patient education in improving the health behaviors, health status, and health care utilization of persons with arthritis.

In 1982, before the findings of this study were widely known, the national Arthritis Foundation (AF) decided to sponsor a pilot dissemination. AF staff from 12 state chapters were trained at Stanford; they were taught how to teach the ASMP, how to train others to teach the ASMP, and how to manage the ASMP within their chapters. The trainees returned to their state chapters to pilot the course and train other ASMP leaders.

Within 18 months, the ASMP had spread to AF chapters across the country. Within 3 years, the national AF was sponsoring its own train-the-trainer workshops. Similarly rapid dissemination occurred in Australia, Canada, and Great Britain; it occurred more slowly in New Zealand, South Africa, and the Scandinavian countries (K. Lorig, personal communication, January, 1996).

Rogers (1995) describes diffusion as a process by which an innovation such as the ASMP is communicated through certain channels, like the AF, over time and among the members of a social system. Factors found associated with successful dissemination of the ASMP included: the growing body of evidence demonstrating the effectiveness of the ASMP; the detailed protocol used by leaders teaching the ASMP; and the minimal cost and low technology required by the ASMP, as course leaders are lay volunteers and require only meeting space and flip charts. These factors are all attributes of the innovative ASMP, attributes known to be linked to successful dissemination (Rogers, 1995). In addition, the acknowledged need of the AF and similar organizations internationally to better reach and serve their constituencies; enthusiasm among national organization program staff who were already skilled in training and supervising others; the presence of national and professional champions, charismatic leaders whose prestige and enthusiasm for the ASMP reflect the importance of venturesomeness and opinion leadership; early and active involvement of volunteers with arthritis; and national health care policies that encouraged adoption of low-cost health programs exemplify characteristics of diffusion networks highly supportive of innovation adoption (Rogers, 1995).

Slow adoption, such as occurred in New Zealand, South Africa, and Scandinavia, was attributed to the lack of adequate funding, especially for program management staff within the national organization; the necessity of offering programs in multiple languages; and political and health care reform occurring simultaneously at the national level. Even with these deterrents to innovation diffusion, however, the ASMP was offered sporadically, as resources allowed, in countries that Rogers would characterize as late adopters.

The history of the ASMP dissemination internationally, as well as the nationwide dissemination of BUOA by the AF (Goeppinger et al., 1995), suggest that these arthritis patient education interventions are effective in multiple, although not all, organizational and community environments. The only study (Oppewal, 1992) known to systematically examine the diffusion of a community-based, population-focused arthritis patient education intervention found that six processes are associated with successful implementation by a voluntary organization. They are: (a) "leaping," the process of adopting an innovation despite some risk, or what Rogers terms "venturesomeness" (Rogers, 1995); (b) "committing" the resources of the innovator supplier to support adoption; (c) "tailoring" the innovation to the disseminating organization and target community; (d) "attracting" volunteer leaders who will serve as the opinion leaders who recruit other participants; (e) "sharing" information between innovator suppliers, implementers, and volunteers; and (f) "nurturing" of both implementers and volunteers. These findings, especially those related to committing needed organizational resources and tailoring the intervention to the disseminating organization and target populations, are consistent with the outcomes observed in the international dissemination of the ASMP.

SUMMARY AND RESEARCH DIRECTIONS

The most compelling findings from 20 years of cumulative arthritis patient education research are threefold. The importance of interventions directed towards problems identified by patients, established as effective, and then further developed within theoretical frameworks was established. This is a marked difference from the deductive process used to develop many nursing interventions, despite the fact that patient-centered care has been a traditional focus of nursing practice. Patient-centered research and grounded theory are critical to the generation of new knowledge for practice.

Secondly, the effectiveness of population-focused, community-based interventions was documented among a wide variety of groups, although not with low-income and minority populations. Future investigations need to be designed with increased attention to the cultural appropriateness of the intervention, and funded for long enough periods for researchers to access the hard-to-reach populations representing Rogers' "late majority" and "laggards"

(1995). The work of McGowan and Green (1995) suggest the utility of participatory research methods in addressing issues of culture and timing.

Finally, systematic and detailed process evaluations of intervention implementation also need to occur, to specify the intervention component most responsible for observed improvements, and to describe the process of reinvention of innovative interventions which is associated with successful dissemination (Brunk & Goeppinger, 1990; Rogers, 1995).

ACKNOWLEDGMENTS

We gratefully acknowledge the assistance of Godfrey Hochbaum, Professor Emeritus, Health Behavior and Health Education, School of Public Health, University of North Carolina at Chapel Hill, for his thoughtful review and provocative comments, and of Barbara Speck, Graduate Research Assistant, for her skill in identifying articles and preparing the manuscript for publication.

REFERENCES

Abramson, L. Y., Seligman, M. E. P., & Teasdale, J. D. (1978). Learned helplessness in humans: Critique and reformulation. *Journal of Abnormal Psychology, 87*, 49–74.

Arthur, M. W., Goeppinger, J., & Brunk, S. E. (1988, May). *The impact of program choice on the effectiveness of two types of arthritis self-care education.* Paper presented at the 23rd Annual Meeting, Arthritis Health Profession Association, Houston, TX.

Bandura, A. (1986). *Social foundations of thought and action: A social cognitive theory.* Englewood, NJ: Prentice-Hall.

Belza, B. (1994). The impact of fatigue on exercise performance. *Arthritis Care and Research, 7*, 176–180.

Belza, B. L. (1995). Comparison of self-reported fatigue in rheumatoid arthritis and controls. *Journal of Rheumatology, 22*, 639–643.

Belza, B. L., Henke, C. J., Yelin, E. H., Epstein, W. V., & Gilliss, C. L. (1993). Correlates of fatigue in older adults with rheumatoid arthritis. *Nursing Research, 42*, 93–99.

Benson, V., & Marano, M. A. (1994). Current estimates from the National Health Interview Survey, 1993. *Vital Health Statistics, 10* (190).

Braden, C. J. (1990). A test of the self-help model: Learned response to chronic illness experience. *Nursing Research, 39*, 42–47.

Braden, C. J. (1991). Patterns of change over time in learned response to chronic illness among participants in a systemic lupus erythematosus self-help course. *Arthritis Care and Research, 4*, 158–167.

Braden, C. J. (1992). Description of learned response to chronic illness: Depressed versus nondepressed self-help class participants. *Public Health Nursing, 9,* 103–108.

Braden, C. J. (1993). Promoting a learned self-help response to chronic illness. In S. G. Funk, E. M. Tornquist, M. T. Champagne, & R. A. Wiese (Eds.), *Key aspects of caring for the chronically ill. Hospital and home* (pp. 158–169). New York: Springer Publishing Co.

Braden, C. J., McGlone, K., & Pennington, F. (1993). Specific psychosocial and behavioral outcomes from the Systemic Lupus Erythematosus Self-Help course. *Health Education Quarterly, 20,* 29–41.

Brunk, S. E., & Goeppinger, J. (1990). Process evaluation: Assessing re-invention of community-based interventions. *Evaluation and the Health Professions, 13,* 186–203.

Burckhardt, C. S. (1994). Arthritis and musculoskeletal patient education standards. *Arthritis Care and Research, 7,* 1–4.

Burckhardt, C. S., Clark, S. R., & Bennett, R. M. (1991). The fibromyalgia impact questionnaire: Development and validation. *Journal of Rheumatology, 18,* 728–733.

Burckhardt, C. S., & Bjelle, A. (1994). Education programmes for fibromyalgia patients: Description and evaluation. *Bailliere's Clinical Rheumatology, 8,* 935–955.

Burckhardt, C. S., Clark, S. R., Campbell, S. M., O'Reilly, C. A., Wiens, A., & Bennett, R. M. (1991, November). *Multidisciplinary treatment of fibromyalgia outcome assessment.* Paper presented at the 55th Annual Meeting, American College of Rheumatology, Boston, MA.

Burckhardt, C. S., Mannerkorpi, K., Hedenberg, L., & Bjelle, A. (1994). A randomized, controlled clinical trial of education and physical training for women with fibro-myalgia. *Journal of Rheumatology, 21,* 714–720.

Centers for Disease Control and Prevention. (1994a). Arthritis prevalence and activity limitations: United States, 1990. *Morbidity and Mortality Weekly Report, 43,* 433–438.

Centers for Disease Control and Prevention. (1994b). Prevalence of disabilities and associated health conditions: United States, 1991–1992. *Morbidity and Mortality Weekly Report, 43,* 730–739.

Clark, S. R., Burckhardt, C. S., O'Reilly, C. A., Campbell, S. M., & Bennett, R. M. (1991, November). *Exercise and patient outcome in fibromyalgia.* Paper presented at the 55th Annual Meeting, American College of Rheumatology, Boston, MA.

Daltroy, L. H., & Liang, M. H. (1993). Arthritis education: Opportunities and state of the art. *Health Education Quarterly, 20,* 3–16.

Goeppinger, J., Arthur, M. W., Baglioni, A. J., Brunk, S. E., & Brunner, C. M. (1989). A reexamination of the effectiveness of self-care education for persons with arthritis. *Arthritis & Rheumatism, 32,* 706–716.

Goeppinger, J., Arthur, M. W., Baglioni, A. J., Brunk, S. E., & Hawdon, J. E. (1988, May). *Effectiveness of arthritis self-care education: A longitudinal perspective.* Paper presented at the 23rd Annual Meeting, Arthritis Health Professions Association, Houston, TX.

Goeppinger, J., Brunk, S. E., Arthur, M. W., & Riedesel, S. (1987a). The effectiveness of community-based arthritis self-care programs. *Arthritis & Rheumatism, 30,* S194.

Goeppinger, J., Brunk, S. E., Arthur, M. W., & Riedesel, S. (1987b, October). *The impact of participant contracting on the outcomes of community-based arthritis self-care nursing intervention.* Paper presented at the 115th Annual Meeting of the American Public Health Association, New Orleans, LA.

Goeppinger, J., Doyle, M. A. T., Brunk, S. E., Murdock, M., & Brunner, C. M. (1985). Do you know what patients want? Lay and professional perceptions of the education needs of rural persons with arthritis (Abstract). *Arthritis & Rheumatism, 28* (Suppl. 4), S147.

Goeppinger, J., Macnee, C., Anderson, M. K., Boutaugh, M., & Stewart, K. (1995). From research to practice: The effects of a jointly sponsored dissemination of an arthritis self-care nursing intervention. *Applied Nursing Research, 8,* 106–113.

Gonzalez, V. M., Stewart, A., Ritter, P. L., & Lorig, K. (1995). Translation and validation of arthritis outcome measures into Spanish. *Arthritis & Rheumatism, 38,* 1429–1446.

Hirano, P. C., Laurent, D. D., & Lorig, K. (1994). Arthritis patient education studies, 1987–1991: A review of the literature. *Patient Education and Counseling, 24,* 9–54.

Holman, H. R., & Lorig, K. (1987). Patient education in the rheumatic diseases. *Bulletin on the Rheumatic Diseases, 37*(5), 1–8.

Jordan, J. M., Linder, G. F., Renner, J. B., & Fryer, J. G. (1995). The impact of arthritis in rural populations. *Arthritis Care and Research, 8,* 242–250.

Katz, P. P. (1995). The impact of rheumatoid arthritis on life activities. *Arthritis Care and Research, 8,* 272–278.

Lambert, V. A. (1991). Arthritis. In J. J. Fitzpatrick, R. L. Taunton, & A. K. Jacox (Eds.), *Annual review of nursing research* (Vol. 9, pp. 3–18). New York: Springer Publishing Co.

Lenker, S., Lorig, K., & Gallagher, D. (1984). Reasons for lack of association between changes in health behavior and improved health status: An exploratory study. *Patient Education and Counseling, 6,* 69–72.

Lorig, K. (1994). Arthritis patient education. In F. Wolfe & T. Pincus (Eds.), *Rheumatoid arthritis: Assessment, prognosis and therapy* (pp. 449–462). New York: Marcel Dekker.

Lorig, K., Chastain, R. L., Ung, E., Shoor, S., & Holman, H. R. (1989). Development and evaluation of a scale to measure perceived self-efficacy in people with arthritis. *Arthritis & Rheumatism, 32,* 37–44.

Lorig, K., Cox, T., Cuevas, Y., Kraines, R. G., & Britton, M. (1984). Converging and diverging beliefs about arthritis: Caucasian patients, Spanish-speaking patients, and physicians. *Journal of Rheumatology, 11,* 76–79.

Lorig, K., Feigenbaum, P., Regan, C., Ung, E., & Holman, H. R. (1986). A comparison of lay-taught and professional-taught arthritis self-management course. *Journal of Rheumatology, 13,* 763–767.

Lorig, K., & Gonzalez, V. (1992). The integration of theory with practice: A twelve year case study. *Health Education Quarterly, 19,* 355–368.

Lorig, K., & Holman, H. R. (1989). Long-term outcomes of an arthritis self-management study: Effects of reinforcement efforts. *Social Science and Medicine, 29*, 221–224.

Lorig, K., & Holman, H. R. (1993). Arthritis self-management studies: A twelve year review. *Health Education Quarterly, 20*, 17–28.

Lorig, K., Konkol, L., & Gonzalez, V. (1987). Arthritis patient education: A review of the literature. *Patient Education and Counseling, 10*, 207–252.

Lorig, K., Laurin, J., & Holman, H. R. (1984). Arthritis self-management: A study of the effectiveness of patient education for the elderly. *The Gerontologist, 24*, 455–457.

Lorig, K., Lubeck, D., Kraines, R. G., Seleznick, M., Holman, H. R. (1985). Outcomes of self-help education for patients with arthritis. *Arthritis & Rheumatism, 28*, 680–685.

Lorig, K., Mazonson, P., & Holman, H. R. (1993). Evidence suggesting that health education for self-management in patients with chronic arthritis has sustained health benefits while reducing health care costs. *Arthritis & Rheumatism, 36*, 439–446.

Lorig, K., & Riggs, G. (1983). *Arthritis patient education biblioprofile.* Arlington, VA: Arthritis Information Clearinghouse.

Lorig, K., & Visser, A. (1994). Arthritis patient education standards: A model for the future. *Patient Education and Counseling, 24*, 3–7.

Maier, S. F., & Seligman, M. E. P. (1976). Learned helplessness: Theory and evidence. *Journal of Experimental Psychology, 105*, 3–46.

Marin, G., Burhansstipanov, L., Connell, C. M., Gielen, A. C., Helitzer-Allen, D., Lorig, K., Morisky, D. E., Tenney, M., & Thomas, S. (1995). A research agenda for health education among underserved populations. *Health Education Quarterly, 22*, 346–363.

McGowan, P., & Green, L. W. (1995). Arthritis self-management in native populations of British Columbia: An application of health promotion and participatory research principles in chronic disease control. *The Canadian Journal on Aging, 14*, 201–212.

Mullen, P. D., Laville, E. A., Biddle, A. K., & Lorig, K. (1987). Efficacy of psychoeducational interventions on pain, depression, and disability in people with arthritis: A meta-analysis. *Journal of Rheumatology, 14*(Suppl. 15), 33–39.

Newman, A. M. (1993). Effect of a self-help course on adaptation in people with arthritis. In S. G. Funk, E. M. Tornquist, M. T. Champagne, & R. A. Wiese (Eds.), *Key aspects of caring for the chronically ill. Hospital and home* (pp. 150–157). New York: Springer Publishing Co.

Oppewal, S. R. (1992). Implementing a community-based innovation: Organizational challenges and strategies. *Family and Community Health, 15*, 70–79.

Reisine, S., & Fifield, J. (1992). Expanding the definition of disability: Implications for planning, policy, and research. *Milbank Quarterly, 70*, 491–508.

Rogers, E. M. (1995). *Diffusion of innovations* (4th ed.). New York: Free Press.

Schumacher, H. R. (Ed.). (1993). *Primer on the rheumatic diseases* (10th ed.). Atlanta, GA: Arthritis Foundation.

Seligman, M. E. P. (1975). *Helplessness: On depression, development and death.* San Francisco: Freeman.

Stein, M. J., Wallston, K. A., Nicassio, P. M., & Castner, N. M. (1988). Correlates of a clinical classification schema for the arthritis helplessness subscale. *Arthritis & Rheumatism, 31,* 876–881.

Superio-Cabuslay, E., Ward, M. M., & Lorig, K. (1996). Patient education interventions in osteoarthritis and rheumatoid arthritis: A meta-analytic comparison with nonsteroidal anti-inflammatory drug treatment. *Arthritis Care and Research, 9,* 292–301.

Verbrugge, L. M. (1990). Disability. *Rheumatic Diseases Clinics of North America, 16,* 741–761.

Yelin, E. (1992). Arthritis: The cumulative impact of a common chronic condition. *Arthritis & Rheumatism, 35,* 489–497.

Yelin, E., & Callahan, L. F. (1995). The economic cost and social and psychological impact of musculoskeletal conditions. *Arthritis & Rheumatism, 38,* 1351–1362.

Chapter 6

Parent–Adolescent Communication in Nondistressed Families

Susan K. Riesch
School of Nursing
University of Wisconsin—Madison

ABSTRACT

The focus of this chapter is parent and adolescent communication in nondistressed families. Communication is the assertive and unoffensive expression and accurate and attentive receipt of opinions, feelings, and ideas. Aspects of adolescent and adult development have been shown to influence as well as be influenced by perceptions of family communication. Though recently subject to extensive scrutiny and criticism, the paradigm of parent and adolescent conflict dominates this research area. Nurses and others have demonstrated strategies to enhance communication between parent and adolescents, with promising results. Issues of subject participation are reviewed and recommendations for future directions in research and practice are made.

Keywords: Parent, Child, or Adolescent Relations and Relationships; Communication

Communication is the cornerstone of all interpersonal relationships. One of the most important relationships between human beings is that of the parent and child. A challenging point in the parent and child relationship is the period of the child's adolescence. Communication between parent and adolescent has generated considerable attention among those conducting research with or caring for childrearing families.

The focus of this chapter is parent and adolescent communication within nondistressed families, the issues involved in studying it, and recommendations for future work. "Nondistressed families" refers to parents and adolescents who were not actively seeking treatment for a condition that may interfere with their relationship (Prinz, Foster, Kent, & O'Leary, 1979). These families often are referred to as "nonclinic" families, "typical" families, or families as they live in the community. This definition, then, excluded studies of communication among families of adolescents coping with acute or chronic biophysiological or socioemotional conditions.

An adolescent is a person aged 13 to 18 years. Though some studies define early adolescence to include 11- and 12-year-olds and late adolescence to include 19- to 21-year-olds, the focus of the research reviewed here was, by and large, 13- to 18-year-olds. The conceptual definition of communication guiding this review is the expression of ideas and feelings assertively but unoffensively and the receiving of ideas expressed by others attentively and accurately (Robin, 1979).

Nursing has not contributed in a significant manner to generating theory or knowledge of parent and adolescent communication, but the area is of importance to all professions who study and/or provide care to families. The recognition that an individual is born into a family that, in turn, is embedded in a society, necessitates a pluralistic approach to the study of family systems and interventions to promote healthy functioning. Building upon the integration of ideas and concepts from numerous disciplines (psychology, social work, medicine, and education), nursing is in a position to not only conduct research in this area, but also to apply research findings directly to the care of families. The study of parent and adolescent communication in nondistressed families illustrates the consistent orientation of nursing as a discipline to the provision of care that promotes well-being in the people served (American Nurses Association, 1995). There is a significant gap in knowledge about how to assist normally developing families at a potentially vulnerable point in their development.

The research reports included in this review were known to the author through continuing work in the field and through an online bibliographic search. For the online search of publications in English, the criterion of parent child relations (communication) in nondistressed families of adolescents aged 13 to 18 years was used. The search of CINAHL (Cumulative Index to Nursing and Allied Health Literature) for the years 1982 through 1995 yielded 11 papers; the search of Psychological Abstracts for the same years yielded 29 papers; and the search of MEDLINE for the years 1984 to 1995 yielded 2 papers. Master's-level or dissertation research was not reviewed.

THE IMPORTANCE OF COMMUNICATION
BETWEEN PARENT AND ADOLESCENT

Gibb (1961) described communication as a "people process" rather than a language process. According to Vangelisti (1992), when parents and their adolescents converse, problems emerge, making differences of opinion apparent. In other cases, problems may be problems because they are not discussed. Opinions are left unexpressed. Some topics, such as sex, drugs, or religion, may be avoided because of their potential to evoke conflict. Thus, communication between parent and adolescent may be perceived as challenging because the issues that emerge elicit differences of opinion or because of the implicit perceptions of certain issues. Two aspects critical to communication are that it is perceived as open (Barnes & Olson, 1985) and that it is able to facilitate the resolution of conflicts (Robin, 1979).

Communication between parent and adolescent has been deemed a "life skill" (Riesch, Jacobson, & Tosi, 1994) and considered a tool for negotiation; and it has also been described as a method to learn others' views, show interest, "keep tabs," and express affection (Lynam & Tenn, 1989). Communication has been linked to fostering decision making (Brown & Mann, 1990) and identity formation (Grotevant & Cooper, 1985); decreasing loneliness and depression (Brage & Meredith, 1994; Brage, Meredith, & Woodward, 1993); and promoting family strengths and self esteem (Demo, Small, & Savin-Williams, 1987). Communication has been found to be critical to adolescent autonomy achievement (Smollar & Youniss, 1985).

Communication between a parent and adolescent that is described as open or positive has been found to be associated with lower levels of substance use among teens (Kafka & London, 1991); increased beliefs and intentions regarding condom use (Strader, Beaman, & McSweeney, 1992); better school performance (Masselam, Marcus, & Stunkard, 1990); greater ability to resolve difficult life issues (Hops, Tildesley, Lichtenstein, Ary, & Sherman, 1990); sex education in the home (Baldwin & Baranoski, 1991); parental consultation on pregnancy and abortion issues (Resnick, Bearinger, Stark, & Blum, 1994; Zabin, Hirsch, Emerson, & Raymond, 1992); and increased knowledge of human immunodeficiency virus/acquired immunodeficiency syndrome (HIV/AIDS) (Crawford, Thomas, & Zoller, 1993). Adolescents who perceived the communication with their parents as open to topics of sexuality were not likely to be sexually experienced or pregnant, and were likely to have attempted avoiding HIV (Leland & Barth, 1993).

Communication between a parent and adolescent that is described as problematic or closed has been found to be associated with negative teen behavior, such as drug and alcohol use (Stoker & Swadi, 1990); delinquency (Patterson, 1986); premarital sex (Jaccard & Dittus, 1993) and pregnancy (Marcy, Brown, & Danielson, 1983); suicide (Stivers, 1988); and dropping out of school and running away (Engels & Lau, 1983). Tesser, Forehand, Brody, and Long (1989) demonstrated that better adjusted boys tended to perceive their interactions with their fathers as calm and more balanced than did the less well-adjusted boys. Strommen and Strommen (1985) documented that families were vulnerable to disengagement and chaos during the child's adolescence, and they recommended communication as a means to promote family functioning.

FACTORS INFLUENCING COMMUNICATION BETWEEN PARENT AND ADOLESCENT

Two major factors have been found to influence parent and adolescent communication—developmental tasks and family variables. After an extensive review of the developmental literature, Collins and Russell (1991) cautioned against viewing parent and child relationships as monolithic or a-developmental.

Developmental Tasks

Adolescent.   Enormous physical, cognitive, social, and emotional tasks face the adolescent. These challenges, when viewed from the perspective of a middle adult (an outsider view), may result in the appearance of a physically and verbally awkward individual (Manning, 1983) who is unpredictable, impulsive, moody, influenced by peers, and resistant to authority (Robin, 1985). Conger (1977) identified that independence from parents is the central issue of adolescence. Traditionally, independence has been perceived as achieved through a transitional period of "storm and stress" (Kenniston, 1970). This transitional period involves issues of power, sexuality, and personal identity (Elkind, 1984). The adolescent is expected to be resistive, belligerent, and hostile (Kett, 1977). There is little empirical evidence, however, to support the storm-and-stress view of adolescence.

Offer, Ostrov, and Howard (1981) emphasized development as continuous. They conceptualized adolescence as part of a larger developmental process that is not distinguished by any greater power struggles than any other developmental stage. Similarly, Hill (1987) pointed out that adolescents seek autonomy or self-governance. Subjectively, autonomy was associated with avowed closeness and positive feelings, participation in family activities, seeking parents out for advice and support, and wanting to be like one's parents. Freedom and autonomy during adolescence included continuing, harmonious relationships with parents.

A third perspective on adolescent development was proposed by Grotevant and Cooper (1986) and takes into account both the storm-and-stress and continuity perspectives. Parents and their adolescents were conceptualized as active relational partners who together negotiate and renegotiate new roles with regard to autonomy and individuation while remaining connected. Cockram and Beloff (1978) advanced the thesis that adolescence is a time of rehearsal for adulthood. They demonstrated that most adolescents hold the same values as their parents, do not go through a period of conflict, and have no collective conscious or unconscious.

When asked the major concerns of the teen years, adolescents cited appearance, scholastic competence, social acceptance, athletics, and behavioral conduct (Benson, Williams, & Johnson, 1987). Eme, Maisiak, and Goodale (1979) reported that the top concerns of adolescents were physical appearance, career preparation, grades, future school plans, present employment, and parents. Accommodation to pubertal changes, changes in ties to parents, mood changes, achieving a sense of self, acquisition of academic and work skills, and management of sexual arousal and opposite-sex relationships were cited by Brooks-Gunn and Peterson (1991).

When asked what is the major problem between teens and their parents, young adolescents expressed "not being listened to" (Benson & Elkind, 1990). In regard to communication, Vangelisti (1992) found that the most frequent complaint of older adolescents was their parents' personal criticism and that during middle adolescence it was their parents' behavioral restrictions. Barron and Yoest (1994) documented that the parent was the most frequently reported stressful relationship, followed by girlfriend, for a sample of adolescent boys.

Midlife adult.   Parents of teens are usually midlife adults, that is, between the ages of 40 to 60 years. Parents in this developmental stage deal with the highlights or disappointments associated with their own life situation, and often care for their own aging parents. In general, midlife adults possess a stable life pattern, though increasingly they may experience divorce, remarriage, and stepfamily formation (Vander Zanden, 1989). Two consistent findings in the literature addressing this stage are that persons identify themselves in their parents and in their children and that they continue to thrive on primarily occupational challenges (Neugarten, 1968).

Erikson (1963) characterized middle adulthood as that period when adults develop generativity versus stagnation. Peck (1968) expanded Erikson's ideas, juxtapositioning the values of wisdom versus physical powers, understanding and compassion versus sexuality, and emotional and mental flexibility versus rigidity. Middle adults tend toward androgyny (Sinnot, 1982) with women becoming forceful, managerial, and independent (Helson & Moane, 1987) and men becoming thoughtful, introspective, trusting, tolerant, and cooperative (Zubin, 1982).

Parents have reported fear and anxiety about parenting their children during adolescence (Ballenski & Cook, 1982). Much of this fear, however, may be the result of a generalizability gap. Many of the studies that reported teens as difficult to manage were based upon clinic samples and families with multiple problems. The view that the parent and child relationship is an evolving relationship, and not fraught with conflict, is gaining support in the literature (Koski & Steinberg, 1990; Ohashi, 1992; Weinmann & Newcombe, 1990).

Often overlooked in the application and interpretation of Erikson's work (1968) is the importance of relationships in the adolescent's identity formation. Achieving a stable sense of self allows greater closeness with others and potential for intimacy. Theoretically, communication that is perceived as open between a parent and adolescent contributes to discussion of issues essential to identity formation for adolescents.

Based upon the work to date, there is potential for adolescence to be viewed as a vulnerable time in family relationships. The developmental challenges of the adolescent and the parent could result in neither party's having the ability to take the other's perspective, and communication may be perceived as closed.

Family Variables

"Family variables," in this review, refers to the interparental relationship, parenting styles, and gender.

The interparental relationship.   The relationship between the parents may lay the foundation or directly influence the relationship between parents and children. In general, indicators of an amiable interparental relationship have been associated with beneficial child outcomes (Vuchinich, Vuchinich, & Wood, 1993). Upon an extensive review of the research on family communication, Doane (1978) concluded that the relationship between the parents significantly affected the other intrafamilial relationships. Montemayor, McKenry, and Julian (1993) found that the basic processes of the relationship between marital partners does not vary in other close relationships. The interparental relationship has been measured as marital satisfaction, quality, or conflict; spousal interaction style; interparental agreement; and parental coalitions.

Fitzpatrick and Ritchie (1994) established a clear relationship schemata for marital and parent-child communication. Based upon data from 169 family triads, they found that couple communication style and values dovetailed with parent-child communication style and values. These results are based upon a large knowledge base generated from two separate research programs focussing upon spousal communication and parent-child communication. McDonough, Carlson, and Cooper (1994) observed a series of family interaction tasks. They found that egalitarian spousal interaction was more functional in the completion of family tasks than other spousal interaction styles. An egalitarian style was characterized by mutual exchange and balance in the expression of individuality and connectedness.

Level of marital quality was found to be a significant variant in a sample of 54 two-child, intact, middle-class parents' and adolescents' ratings of themselves and each other of a videotaped interaction based on set topics (Callan & Noller, 1986). As the adolescent's perception of their parents' marital quality decreased, the adolescent's perceptions of anxiety and dominance increased and friendliness and involvement decreased. A strength of this study is its use of observational techniques in addition to self-report measures.

Vuchinich et al. (1993) defined "marital satisfaction" as the extent to which the parents agreed and supported each other in discussion of specific childrearing issues of concern to families. Though additional variables were evaluated, the relationship between the parents in this study of 68 lower middle-class, Caucasian mothers, fathers, and young adolescent sons indicated that parental agreement facilitated family problem solving as well as the child's ability to problem solve. Parental coalitions, however, served to limit problem solving, most likely because such a coalition inhibited the young adolescent's autonomy and ability to influence the solution. No assessment of the valence or emotionality of the problems discussed was provided.

The work of Amato and Keith (1991) on conflict between spouses in divorce is widely cited. They conducted a meta-analysis of 92 studies that was focused upon comparing measures of well-being among children living in divorced single-parent families with those of children living in continuously intact families. The samples were not limited to teens. Amato and Keith found that child well-being was compromised least in low-conflict, intact families, followed by divorced families. Children in high-conflict, intact families scored lowest on measures of self-concept, psychological adjustment, and conduct. Thus, interparental conflict was found to be disruptive on several measures of child development.

Smith and Forehand (1986) assessed the frequency of overt parental conflict that occurs in the child's presence using the 10-item O'Leary–Porter Scale (OPS) (Porter & O'Leary, 1980). The OPS was completed by a homogeneous sample of 36 female young adolescents and their parents who volunteered in response to announcements circulated in the community to complete the self-report measures. Findings indicated that adolescents' perceptions of interparental conflict closely matched their parents' ratings of marital discord. Marital discord emerged as a predictor of perceived conflict between parent and adolescent conflict for mothers and daughters, but not for fathers.

Neighbors, Forehand, and McVicar (1993) identified family and individual factors that may contribute to resilience among 55 young adolescents whose families were experiencing severe interparental conflict as measured by the OPS. "Resilient" adolescents were defined as those whose teachers rated them highly cognitively competent. Resilient adolescents were found to have better relationships with their mothers and higher levels of self-esteem than did the nonresilient adolescents. A critical recommendation of this study was that in the presence of high marital discord, parents should maintain a positive relationship with the adolescent, as this relationship may buffer the effects of stress. The temporal priority of self-esteem and cognitive competence was not established, and the sample size was too small to examine interaction effects among the stress and adjustment variables.

Based on the literature addressing the influence of the marital relationship on parent and adolescent communication, cumulative evidence indicates that the interparental relationship is reflected in the parent and adolescent relationship (Fitzpatrick & Ritchie, 1994). Across studies it was found that adolescents, using a number of different measures, generally were accurate in their assessment of their parents' relationship (Smith & Forehand, 1986). The adolescents' relationships with their mothers and fathers were found to be distinct (Vuchinich et al., 1993). Studies of conflict in families indicated that interparental discord can be detrimental to child development (Amato & Keith, 1991; Callan & Noller, 1986). Family and individual factors contribute to the adolescent's ability to cope with the effects of interparental conflict (Neighbors et al., 1993).

Parenting styles and characteristics of parents.   Baumrind (1978, 1991) identified four styles of parenting: authoritarian, permissive, authoritative, and rejecting–neglecting. A number of investigators have extended Baumrind's work and tested child developmental outcomes associated with each style of parenting. Steinberg (1990) proposed that parental acceptance (warmth), behavioral supervision and strictness (firmness), and psychological autonomy (democratic) constituted authoritativeness. He has developed a lengthy, valid, and reliable survey instrument to measure the construct, Authoritative Parenting (Steinberg, Elmen, & Mounts, 1989). With an ethnically and socioeconomically heterogeneous sample of 6,400 14- to 18-year olds from high schools in Wisconsin and California who lived in a variety of family structures, Steinberg, Lamborn, Dornbusch, and Darling (1992) found that those raised in authoritative homes performed better in school than their counterparts from nonauthoritative homes. Limitations of this work were that all measures, including academic outcomes, were self-reported by the sample, and characteristics of the adolescent that may influence the parenting style were not addressed.

In addition to the styles parents use, there is a growing body of literature to document that specific parental characteristics affect parent adolescent communication. Crawford et al. (1993) found in a sample of 130 African American mothers and their children (aged 8 to 14 years) that mothers who possessed more formal education were more knowledgeable about HIV/AIDS and sexuality and reported greater levels of parent and adolescent communication. Similarly, parents who possessed higher levels of self-esteem indicated they discussed sexual topics with their children more often than did parents with lower levels of self-esteem.

To determine characteristics of parents who talk with their adolescents about sexuality topics, Fisher (1986) studied the responses of 194 female and 88 male (31% return rate) college students and their parents to questionnaires designed to measure a number of psychological, sexual attitudes and knowledge, and demographic variables. The sample was of convenience and well educated. The adolescent, who was enrolled in a psychology class and under the age of 18 years, approached the parent to be surveyed. Fisher reported that mothers were more likely to have discussed sex if they perceived general family communication to be open, if the adolescent was a daughter, and if her own mother had discussed sexuality with her. For fathers, openness of general family communication, education, and the extent to which his father discussed sexuality with him predicted the likelihood of his discussing sexuality with his children.

To study problem-solving abilities among families of substance users, Hops et al. (1990) observed 128 single-parent and intact families of children aged 11 to 15 as they discussed three scenarios about the use of alcohol, cigarettes, and marijuana. In addition, the young adolescents completed self-report measures about their substance use. Data indicated that mothers' and fathers' alcohol use contributed to alcohol and cigarette use among their children, and fathers' smoking contributed to marijuana and hard drug use. Observations suggested poor parent–child communication, particularly in the area of problem solving. Adolescents' aversive affect during problem-solving tasks that were not related to substance use was a strong predictor of cigarette and marijuana use. Sophisticated discriminant function analyses were accomplished, though there were a large number of such analyses on many variables generated from a small sample. The nonindependence of the analyses was acknowledged as a limitation to the study.

"Sandwich generation" families is the term applied to families in which at least one parent is providing assistance to an aging grandparent. Hamill (1994) explored parent and adolescent communication in 62 three-generation predominantly Caucasian, stable, high-income, well-educated families with adolescents aged 14 to 19 years. Mothers reported poorer communication with their adolescent when the adolescent was less autonomous, had assumed more adult roles, and when the mothers were experiencing caregiver burden. Alternatively, adolescents reported poorer communication when they were less autonomous and when the grandparents were in better health.

The greater fathers' concerns were over midlife issues the poorer their perceptions of communication with the adolescent. Adolescents reported poorer communication with their fathers when the adolescent was less autonomous and the fathers were concerned with midlife issues. Thus, adolescents who exhibited greater psychological maturity, defined as autonomy, reported sharing more open communication with their parents than did less mature adolescents.

Hamill's (1994) work provides some evidence that mothers' relationships within their families of origin may permeate and have repercussions for their families of procreation. A perplexing finding—that when grandparents were in poorer health, adolescents perceived their communication as better with their mothers—may be attributed to how health status was measured—as a global index reported by the mother. A better indication of health status from the adolescent's perspective may shed additional light upon this finding. Assessment of the grandparent's assessments of communication, health status, and adolescent autonomy would strengthen work in this area.

Economic hardship has been found to affect parent and adolescent communication. Hawley, Shear, Stark, and Goodman (1984) examined a family medical practice of 79 low-income parents and their 121 teens to determine the prevalence and severity of adolescent behavioral problems, single parenting, coping, and family communication. They designed an 18-item scale to assess problem behavior and used the F–COPES (Family Coping Strategies) and Parent Adolescent Communication Inventory (PACI) to assess coping and communication.

Parents in the Hawley et al. (1984) study reported the major problems to be low school grades and attendance, and conflicts around chores and sibling relations. However, a small number of parents reported suicide ideation, running away, sexual activity, and gang membership among their adolescents to be severe. The single parents were found to report more of the severe behavioral problems and to use fewer community resources than the two-parent families. Contrary to expectations, the single parents were found to score highest on the PACI, indicating open communication. None of the problems were documented in the physicians' records, prompting the authors to recommend increased vigilance of adolescent behavioral problems by primary care providers. Adolescents were not asked to respond, thus, these data are from the parent's—chiefly the mother's—perspective.

In a series of studies to examine the effects of economic hardship upon family functioning and parent–adolescent communication, Conger's research team studied samples of rural Iowa families during the farm crises of the mid-1980s. The team developed a theoretically sound process model of family economic pressures and a number of adolescent behaviors. Conger et al. (1991) demonstrated that negative or aversive behaviors by parents were exacerbated by financial difficulties, which in turn increased adolescents' risk of developmental problems. The risks occurred in two ways: (a) parental modeling of inappropriate and coercive behaviors that could be emulated by the adolescent, such as alcohol use, and (b) disruption of the effectiveness of parents as socializing agents, through parental emotional distress, increased occurrence of hostile or irritable behaviors, and feelings of frustration, hopelessness, and depression.

In his research program, Conger has systematically tested the model and demonstrated that adverse financial circumstances affect parents' emotional state and the quality of family interactions. The direct and indirect effects on the adolescents have included increased alcohol use in girls and boys (Conger et al., 1993), reduced social and academic competence, diminished sense of self, and increased sensitivity among girls to changes in the moods and behaviors of their parents; both boys and girls experienced increases in emotional and behavioral problems (Ge, Conger, Lorenz, & Simons, 1994). The powerful group of studies conducted by Conger and colleagues over the past 20 years concluded that the consequences of economic hardship upon parent-child relationships and subsequently on child development can be described as devastating. To expand generalizability, Conger's theory and findings should be tested with other family structures, urban populations, and with children and adolescents of different ages.

Based on studies of parenting styles and characteristics of parents, it can be summarized that styles that promote adolescent expression and input into family decision making result in beneficial child outcomes (Steinberg et al., 1992). Parental self-esteem and education (Crawford et al., 1993), behavior (Hops et al., 1990), the type of communication parents experienced in their own upbringing (Fisher, 1986), economic status (Conger et al., 1993; Hawley et al., 1984), and extended family responsibilities (Hamill, 1994) contribute to parent and adolescent communication.

Gender.   Gender serves as an important variable in the research on parent–adolescent communication. In general, mothers take a larger and wider-ranging role than do fathers in communication with their adolescents (Fisher, 1986; Nolin & Petersen, 1992; Noller & Callan, 1990; Papini, Farmer, Clark, & Micka, 1990; Ritchie & Fitzpatrick, 1990; Tesser et al., 1989; Tucker, 1989; Werrbach, Grotevant, & Cooper, 1992). Bhushan (1993), in a study of 32 two-parent intact families with adolescents, found that mothers, as compared to fathers, reported more openness with male and female adolescents—a fact substantiated by the adolescents. Parents felt greater difficulty in communicating with sons than with daughters.

Communication with the mother more likely involves socioemotional topics (Nolin & Petersen, 1992), sexuality (Jaccard & Dittus, 1993), self-disclosure (Papini et al., 1990), and day-to-day problems of daily living (Flint, 1992). Communication with the father more likely involves problem solving (Werrbach et al., 1992) and politics (Noller & Bagi, 1985). Daughters have been found to initiate factual and moral discussion more regularly than sons (Nolin & Petersen, 1992). LeCroy (1988) examined the influence of parent–adolescent intimacy (defined as emotional closeness, affection, enjoyment, openness, respect, and solidarity) upon adolescent functioning (defined as self-esteem and problem behaviors). Intimacy was found to be greater with mothers than with fathers among both boys and girls, but intimacy with fathers was found to be a better predictor of adolescent functioning than was mother intimacy.

PARENT AND ADOLESCENT CONFLICT

Despite that fact that the storm-and-stress view of parent–adolescent relations has minimal empirical support (Gilligan, 1987; Ohashi, 1992) and that contentious interchange and systemic disorganization has been increasingly recognized as not characteristic of family relations during adolescence (Hill, 1987; Montemayor, 1983), a key aspect of communication that dominates the research on parent and adolescent communication is conflict and the ability to resolve conflict. As Hall (1987) indicated, families that work well communicate clearly and often in a noisy fashion! As a training ground for the adult world, conflict should be viewed as inevitable and manageable. Too much conflict, however, can lead to family violence or dissolution.

A conflict is a disagreement between two or more persons (Ohlson, 1979). Prinz (1976) defined conflict to include eight points: interruption, disagreement, tension, defensive and supportive communications, anxiety, antagonism, negative interpersonal expressiveness, and contradictory communications between verbal and nonverbal channels. When conflict occurs between adolescent and parent, emotion, hostility, and aggression may be involved because the conflict is interpersonal (Prinz, 1976). As Robin (1985) noted, the parent usually wants the adolescent to follow directions and not make the same mistakes the parent made as an adolescent. The adolescent, on the other hand, is striving for independence from the family, wishes to change the rules, and may test the limits of the rules.

Montemayor (1983) described the relationship between age and conflict as an inverted U with increases beginning in early adolescence, rising during middle adolescence, and declining in late adolescence. In a 1982 report, Montemayor reported a rate of 0.35 arguments with parents per day, with an average duration of 11 minutes, in nondistressed families.

Based on five descriptors, Novovo (1978) distinguished problematic conflicts that require therapeutic help from expected conflicts that can be managed using conflict resolution strategies. The descriptors include conflict that is too intense, too frequent, too long-lasting, leads to aggression, and disturbs work or relationships.

Topics Stimulating Conflict

Vangelisti (1992) asked 188 undergraduate students enrolled in an introductory communication course to describe, in detail, using a series of questionnaires, any communication problems they experienced when they were young teenagers and any problems they experienced at the time of the study. Using the steps of analytic induction, she developed a category system to describe the types of communication interactions respondents perceived as problematic. She used the same steps to develop a category system for the topics or issues most commonly perceived as problematic.

Interactions with the parent that were described as problematic by the adolescent included nine categories. The most frequently occurring topics of conflict included family relations, extracurricular activities, sex, romantic relationships, career/education, living circumstances, money/material items, and behavior problems. Extracurricular activities had been the most frequent topic in the past, whereas family relations, career/education, and living circumstances were the topics of current conflicts. Adolescents who had lived away from their parents for longer periods perceived fewer conflicts than those who had moved away relatively recently. The gender differences found were that males recalled more past interaction problems related to lack of disclosure than did females. Males also recalled more conflicts dealing with drinking, car accidents, and unlawful activities than did females.

This study contributed considerable new knowledge about adolescents' perceptions of conflicts with parents. The data analysis techniques, although reliable and valid, were unique and captured the adolescents' perspective. The past problems were limited to memory, prompting a recommendation that a similar technique be used to gather data from high school students.

Tesser et al. (1989) set out to document who argues with whom about what and to what extent various topics are discussed on a continuum from calm to angry. Using the Issues Checklist (IC) (Prinz et al., 1979), a widely used list of 44 topics commonly found to stimulate conflict, the most frequent issues were helping out around the house, cleaning up the bedroom, doing homework, time for going to bed, and fighting with siblings. These findings are congruent with previous literature documenting that conflicts typically involve mundane issues, not serious problems.

For each issue on the IC, the respondent is asked to identify how often it was discussed in the past month and at what intensity on a scale from 1 to 5, with 1 indicating "calm" and 5 indicating "angry." Girls tended to have calm discussions on the issues, while boys tended to be involved in angry discussions. Discussions with mothers tended to be calm for both boys and girls. The investigators also examined the relationship between intensity of discussion and adolescent adjustment—defined as teacher's judgement of actual competence, conduct disorder, socialized aggression, attention problems, anxiety-withdrawal, score on the Childhood Depression Inventory, and grade point average (GPA). Conflict accounted for over 30% of boys' variance in adjustment. A greater number of angry issues that boys discussed with mother but not father were associated with poorer adjustment. The relationship among girls was not nearly as strong. The authors concluded that a balance of calm and angry discussions provided the best form of emotional expression.

This study contributed knowledge about the frequency and intensity of parent and adolescent conflict and extended theory about internalizing and externalizing adjustment behavior among adolescents. The teacher ratings, GPA, and depression measures were creative, and most likely were valid measures of adjustment. The conclusion about balance, while intuitively appealing, is difficult to defend from the data.

Conflict-Resolution Processes

Skill at conflict resolution is the ability to resolve disputes or disagreements over issues of concern using self-disclosure, negotiation, or compromise, rather than exhibiting anger or using other strategies that erode self-concept (Robin, 1985). Assessment of parent–adolescent conflict through clinical interviews has produced mixed results with varying reliability (Robin & Koepke, 1990).

Self-report inventories, such as the Issues Checklist (Prinz et al., 1979), the Conflict Behavior Questionnaire (Prinz, 1976), the Family Environment Scale (Moos & Moos, 1981), and the Parent Adolescent Relationship Questionnaire (Robin & Koepke, 1990) meet minimum psychometric standards.

Parent–adolescent conflict can be assessed using direct observation. Measures include the Solving Problems in Family Interaction Coding System (SPI–FI) (Forgatch, Fetrow, & Lathrop, 1984); Living in Familial Environments (LIFE) system (Hops et al., 1990); Parent Adolescent Interaction Coding System (PAICS) (Robin & Foster, 1989); and the Interaction Behavior Coding Systems (IBCS) (Foster, Prinz, & O'Leary, 1983). The extent to which behavior observed is generalizable to the natural family environment depends on the interaction setting and task, reactions of the participants, and psychometric characteristics of the coding systems (Robin & Koepke, 1990). Grotevant and Cooper (1989) reported a thorough analysis of a number of observational coding systems. Coding systems are well suited to identifying relationship properties and indicators of patterns of interpersonal events that occur in a dyad or system.

Based on the review of the work addressing the conflict resolution process, it can be summarized that the topics and intensity of the conflicts differ among young, middle, and late adolescents (Vangelisti, 1992) and by gender (Tesser et al., 1989). Measures to assess the topics that stimulate the conflict and the processes used by parents and adolescents to resolve conflict include paper-and-pencil scales, interviews, and observation techniques with elaborate coding schemes. In choosing these measures for data collection, cost for implementation, training, and coding; convenience to the subject and researcher; and psychometric properties need consideration by the researcher.

PROMOTING PARENT AND ADOLESCENT COMMUNICATION

The importance of communication between parent and adolescent has spurred a number of investigators to develop theory-based interventions to promote communication between parent and child. Some investigators focused the interventions on school-aged children, others on young adolescents in anticipation of adolescence, and still others on older adolescents. The perspective of bidirectional influences or a dynamic interactional view of child and family development (Lerner & Spanier, 1978) is critical to the success of these interventions. According to this perspective, interventions should be aimed simultaneously at both parents and children due to the reciprocal nature of interaction (Cairns, 1979).

The literature on parent training, that is, assisting parents in the development of skills to apply to childrearing, indicates that significant outcomes can be expected across the life span and across topics. The methods, target, and outcomes of training, however, are diverse and usually do not consider the bidirectional perspective. An example of parent training is childbirth preparation, which—once considered novel but now a matter of routine—is associated with a cadre of outcomes to improve the families' participation in the birthing event.

Kagey, Vivace, and Lutz (1981) recommended that communication skills training be a ubiquitous primary prevention technique for families in the community. A few studies have demonstrated encouraging outcomes. Using a sample of families who already demonstrated high levels of interpersonal communication, Renz and Cohen (1977) obtained significant improvement in the skill of active listening. Graybill (1986) found that parents, after training, showed decreases in anxiety and concomitant increases in confidence, knowledge of how to respond to children's feelings, and active listening. Levant and Doyle (1983) found that fathers, after communication skill training, learned well what not to do, and the children's perceptions of their relationship with their fathers improved. Tebes, Grady, and Snow (1989) demonstrated improved decision making among school-aged children.

Communication skills training is not considered therapy, expensive, or intrusive. According to Robin and Koepke (1990), communication skills training is designed to identify and correct difficulties in the way parents and adolescents talk to each other. Communication skills training includes skill at conflict resolution.

Recent studies of communication skills training have demonstrated impressive outcomes. Robin and Koepke (1990) summarized over 25 years of research on the Problem Solving Communication Training (PSCT) intervention first developed by Robin (1979). In studies from 1977 to 1985, participating families improved significantly more than wait-list controls on measures of problem-solving ability and amelioration of parent and adolescent conflict, with stronger effects for parents than for adolescents (Foster et al., 1983; Robin, 1981). Social acceptability of the PSCT has been demonstrated (Finfrock-Mittl & Robin, 1987). However, the studies have lacked adequate control and attention groups, and the long-term effects of the intervention have not been examined.

Robin, Kent, O'Leary, Foster, and Prinz (1979) developed a behavioral approach to introduce conflict-resolution processes among parent and young adolescent dyads. Therapists delivered the treatment in five 1-hour sessions. They demonstrated significant increases posttherapy in problem-solving behavior, specifically, problem definition, option listing, and evaluation in the clinic situation. Their sample was small (12 mother-daughter and 12 mother-son pairings), without a comparison group, and findings were not generalized to the home situation.

Robin (1981) tested a treatment methodology, based on social learning theory, with 33 families. This included frequent explanations by parents of their rules of conduct and expectations, communication of one's own view of a problem in a nonthreatening manner, listening and understanding others' points of view, suggesting alternatives, projecting consequences of these alternatives, and negotiating solutions that meet everyone's needs. Problem-solving behaviors after participation in the treatment demonstrated a significant increase.

Noble, Adams, and Openshaw (1989) developed the Adolescent Social Skills Effectiveness Training (ASSET) program. Adolescent and parent participants were found to demonstrate improved social skills and reduced recidivism among delinquent adolescents (Hazel, Schumaker, Sherman, & Sheldon-Wildgen, 1981), greater use of reciprocal social skills (Serna, Schumaker, Sherman, & Sheldon, 1991), and decreased loneliness (Adams, Openshaw, Bennion, Mills, & Noble, 1988). Eight basic skills are taught: giving and accepting positive feedback, giving and accepting negative feedback, resisting peer pressure, problem solving, negotiation, following instructions, and conversation. The basis of the program is negotiation and problem-solving concepts.

Noble et al. (1989) found, on both self-reported and observational measures, that the ASSET program participants showed significant improvement in social skills, communication, and problem solving. The training effects were considerably greater for parents than for adolescents. The sample was small ($n = 43$) and restricted to families of Mormon faith. The design did not include a control group or measures of long-term effects.

Riesch et al. (1993) demonstrated that parents and young adolescents who participated in a 6-week communication training session were more satisfied with their family system, perceived communication between young adolescents and mothers as more open, and were better able to resolve conflicts than were parents and young adolescents who did not participate. One aspect of the training was a problem-solving process that emphasized the following steps: carefully defining the problem, brainstorming all possible solutions without judgment of feasibility, agreeing to a trial of a solution for a specified period of time, evaluation of the solution, and either continuing the solution or testing another. No change in perception of communication was attained with fathers and young adolescents. The findings were stable 6 months after participation. Though the sample size was adequate ($n = 459$ families) and the intervention standardized, the sample was nonrandom, urban, White, middle-class, and educated limiting generalizability of the findings.

Studies to test theory-based interventions designed to promote communication or reduce conflict have demonstrated significant outcomes. Step-by-step conflict resolution techniques have been developed, can be taught to parents and adolescents, and are effective in reducing negative behavior and promoting problem-solving behavior (Noble et al., 1989; Riesch et al., 1993; Robin, 1981; Robin et al., 1979). Investigators may target conflict-resolution techniques to specific parent–child dyads as in an individual client situation or to groups of parents and adolescents in the community.

RESEARCH ISSUES

Research addressing the communication between parent and adolescent has made significant strides, and caregivers and investigators can base their care and study upon the prior work in the field. Investigators are forthright in describing limitations of their work, which is categorized here in terms of design and methods, sample, measures, and procedures.

Design and Methods Issues

Other than Speicher (1992), who documented predictions 5 years after the initial study, most studies of parent and adolescent communication were cross-sectional. Issues surrounding parent–adolescent communication need confirmation using longitudinal designs. Additionally, many studies rely on retrospective data from college students or other easily accessible subject groups. Finally, nearly all studies, except for the notable exceptions of Lynam and Tenn (1989) and Vangelisti (1992), are based upon a neopositivist approach. Our knowledge would be significantly enriched if the adolescents' and parents' perspectives also were addressed directly through interpretive research approaches.

Often neglected in the research reports on studies of parent–adolescent communication is a sense of context. Parents and adolescents each live in multiple contexts—nuclear family, extended family, peer group, school, work, neighborhood, larger community—that exert influences upon behavior and development. Brooks-Gunn and Paikoff (1991), using teen pregnancy as an example, convincingly make a case for targeting research and programs to the teen perspective reinforcing the bidirectional influence perspective promoted by Lerner and Spanier (1978).

Sample Issues

To protect the rights of human subjects and the rights of children as a protected group, investigators must emphasize the confidentiality of participation. Randomization of individuals, dyads, and families requires creative approaches. Copeland and White (1991) suggested randomly assigning entire schools to study groups. The wait-list control strategy (Robin, 1981) is another approach if the study's aim is to evaluate an intervention.

In this body of research, the subject samples tended to be small and homogeneous, that is, confined to one ethnic group in one geographic locale. Contributing factors to the small sample sizes include the high cost of communication studies, the extensive commitment families are expected to make in such studies, and the need to include a variety of measures such as paper-and-pencil scales, observation and coding schemes, and interview techniques. Most samples were of convenience.

Descriptive characteristics of samples collected by investigators were extensive. The list of descriptive and intervening *family* variables included race, ethnicity, religion, and family structure; *adolescent* variables included age, gender, grade, academic performance, number of close friends, interests and hobbies, satisfaction with the family, self-esteem, previous traumatic experiences for the adolescent, such as parental loss or separation, quality of attachments to family members, and living arrangements; and *parent* variables included age, gender, income, occupation, education, marital status, quality of the marital relationship, quality of attachments to family members, and comfort with parenting. No standardized method for collecting these data was found in the literature.

Hill (1987) noted that the kinds of families studied often bear little resemblance to the kinds of families in which adolescents live. Research needs to be conducted in the domain of ethnic and family structure variations in adolescent family life.

Measures

Measures to document parent and adolescent communication abound. Most theorists have developed conceptually compatible instruments to test their tenets and demonstrated acceptable reliability and validity. In these studies, many measures were self-report instruments, sufficient for measures of perception. The target of the interaction should be addressed in the measure—for example, adolescent to father, mother to adolescent.

A thorough measure of parent and adolescent communication would include both self-report and observational methods. Observational methods may address micro or macro aspects of the communication. For example, microanalytic techniques measure sequences, base rates, and duration of behavior. Macro or molar techniques group a number of behaviors, such as hugging, teasing, and joking, and label it "warmth."

In setting up interaction to be observed, considerable controversy exists as to whether the situation should be structured or unstructured, hypothetical or salient, and located in the laboratory or in the home. Noller and Callan (1990) argued that a structured observation measures what a dyad or family *can* do, not what they typically do. Emotion, aggression, and hostility have been found to be more prevalent when salient, rather than hypothetical, issues are discussed (Reuter & Conger, 1995). Generalizability from the laboratory situation to the home has not been consistently demonstrated (Robin & Foster, 1989; Serna et al., 1991).

Procedures

Strategies to encourage parents and adolescents to participate in research revolve around the following issues: removing participation from the school setting, though schools are the optimal place to obtain study subjects; ensuring confidentiality of responses, particularly for the adolescent; providing an interactive component to participation; and providing minimal payment as incentive, but not to exceed the expectations of the community. In eliciting cooperation from adolescent subjects, it is best to explain the purpose of the study and their participation, stressing that the investigator is not merely "nosy" but sincerely interested in their response. Questions should begin with the least personal and progress to more sensitive topics. Providing positive feedback and praise frequently and appropriately is an effective strategy (Riesch & Forsyth, 1992).

Gaining the cooperation of agencies that provide access to adolescent and parent subjects, such as schools, frequently includes having to adjust the research protocol to very specific policies and procedures. Thus, establishing partnerships early in the study design may eliminate threats to the standardization of study procedures across sites.

Intervention studies to address the acquisition of particular communication skills share a number of methodological issues. Kazdin (1992), Tramontana, Sherrets, and Authier (1980) and Travormina (1974) summarized the issues to include: assessments of the effects of the programs on the child and the parent; random assignment of families to the treatment and control conditions; an adequate sample size based on power analyses; a direct observational sampling of parent and early adolescent behavior; a follow-up observational sampling of parent and child behavior to assess lag effects, but with enough time to allow the child to continue developmental progress; an attention group; an extensive description of the characteristics of children and parents; parent–child skill practice sessions; and step-by-step written protocols and interventions for the treatment application.

SUMMARY AND RECOMMENDATIONS

Based on developmental theory, families with adolescents may face challenges that result in neither the parents nor the adolescent having the ability to take the other's perspective, thereby inhibiting open communication. The interparental relationship has significant influences upon adolescent development and relationships. Parents who are authoritative, economically comfortable, educated, have high self-esteem, communicated openly with their own parents, and are not burdened with extensive extended family responsibilities are most successful in promoting adolescent expression. Mothers have been found to take a wider and larger role than fathers in communicating with the adolescent. Mothers are likely to be involved in interpersonal discussions with the teen, whereas fathers are more likely to be involved in problem solving. These findings are consistent, and most likely attributed to differences in male and female communication styles.

In nondistressed families, conflict between parents and adolescents is frequent, of varying intensity, and based on rather mundane issues. The interactions that are problematic and the topics of discussion differ from the early to late teen years, and boys tend to have more angry discussions with parents than do girls. A number of interventions based on social learning theory or behavioral therapy have been tested and found effective in promoting prosocial conflict-resolution techniques. Measures documenting skill in conflict resolution are evolving.

Programs to enhance communication skill have been developed and tested upon distressed and nondistressed families. Strategies and outcomes measured vary, but in general, effects are in the hypothesized direction.

The major function left to the postmodern family is the care and nurturance of its members, accomplished chiefly through the emotional climate of the family that is influenced significantly by communication among its members (Fitzpatrick & Ritchie, 1994). For a family to instill or pass on values, perspective, or information, they must communicate. The family serves as a training ground for teaching the child how to communicate with peers, coworkers, teachers, and, ultimately, a spouse. The greatest impact professionals could make is to give parents and adolescents the skills to engage in effective communication and problem-solving skills. LeCroy (1988) and Weinmann and Newcombe (1990) make convincing cases for the need for intimacy at all life stages, but particularly between the parent and the adolescent.

To diminish the discrepancies about perceptions of communication between parents and their adolescents and to further develop knowledge in the field, several important recommendations germane to the future of research in this area are (a) more should be done for fathers; (b) the reciprocal nature of communication should be addressed more fully; and (c) as suggested by Hill (1987), more studies of maternal and paternal role satisfaction are needed, as is more attention to the adolescent in situations of divorce, single-parent families, and reconstituted families, and finally to ethnic and structural variations.

More attention to fathers.   Noble et al. (1989), Riesch et al. (1993), and Smith and Forehand (1986) made little or no progress with fathers in training programs designed to improve communication skill. LeCroy (1988) found that father's intimacy with the adolescent was a better predictor of self-esteem and problem behavior than was mother's intimacy. Yet, adolescents describe communication with their fathers as judgmental and non-negotiable (Noller & Callan, 1990) or insufficient and insignificant (Stoker & Swadi, 1990). Therefore, it should be a priority to test methods to assist families to attain father and adolescent intimacy.

Reciprocal nature of communication.   Parent and adolescent perceptions of specific conflicts have been found to be generally congruent (Smith & Forehand, 1986; Tesser et al., 1989) but perceptions of the communication itself are weakly correlated (Barnes & Olson, 1985; Riesch et al., 1993). Perhaps this can be attributed to developmental differences. However, attention to the bidirectional influence of interactions and achieving a perception of openness and approachability about a range of subjects has been found to be associated with optimal family and child outcomes.

Parent–adolescent communication in structurally variant and ethnic families.   Congruent with Conger's work (Conger et al., 1991; Conger et al., 1993), parents' satisfaction with life work influences family and child outcomes. Opportunities for various roles are available to mothers and fathers—how does satisfaction with their parental, occupational, volunteer, or other roles influence communication and other aspects of the parent and adolescent relationship? Most studies of divorce, single parenting, and reconstituted families were conducted on families with younger children; the adolescent experience needs further investigation. Our knowledge is limited with respect to parent–adolescent communication among ethnic or rural families and those who have accessed the juvenile justice system.

Nursing research studies.   Other than the work of Brage et al. (1993, 1994) on depression, loneliness, and parent–adolescent communication, that of Riesch et al. (1993) on communication skills training, and that of Tucker (1989) on topics of sexuality, nurse investigators have contributed little to the study and enhancement of parent and adolescent communication, despite a history of significant research contributions toward families with infants and young children. Parent–adolescent communication is integral to parents' and adolescents' achieving developmental tasks, promoting health and preventing disease, and family decision making—all areas of interest to nursing as a discipline. A priority of the National Institute of Nursing Research continues to be "community-based prevention and intervention research" (Hardin, 1996), which may include research on family communication with an emphasis on adolescence.

REFERENCES

Adams, G. R., Openshaw, D. K., Bennion, L., Mills, T., & Noble, S. (1988). The effects of a social skills training program on lonely adolescents. *Journal of Adolescent Research, 3,* 81–96.

Amato, P. R., & Keith, B. (1991). Parental divorce and the well-being of children: A meta-analysis. *Psychological Bulletin, 110,* 26–46.

American Nurses Association. (1995). *Nursing's social policy statement.* (Available from American Nurses Publishing, 600 Maryland Avenue SW, Suite 100, Washington, DC 20024–2571.)

Baldwin, S. E., & Baranoski, W. (1991). Family interactions and sex education in the home. *Adolescence, 25,* 573–582.

Ballenski, C. B., & Cook, A. S. (1982). Mother's perceptions of their competence in managing selected parenting tasks. *Family Relations, 31,* 489–494.

Barnes, H. L., & Olson, D. H. (1985). Parent-adolescent communication and the Circumplex Model. *Child Development, 56,* 438–447.

Barron, C. R., & Yoest, P. (1994). Emotional distress and coping with a stressful relationship in adolescent boys. *Journal of Pediatric Nursing, 9,* 13–19.

Baumrind, D. (1978). Parental disciplinary patterns and social competence in children. *Youth and Society, 9,* 239–276.

Baumrind, D. (1991). Parenting styles and adolescent development. In R. M. Lerner, A. C. Peterson, & J. Brooks-Gunn (Eds.), *The encyclopedia of adolescence* (pp. 746–758). New York: Garland.

Benson, P., & Elkind, C. (1990). *Effective Christian education: A national study of Protestant congregations (Project Summary).* (Available from Search Institute, 700 S. Third St. Suite 210, Minneapolis, MN 55415.)

Benson, P., Williams, D., & Johnson, A. (1987). *The quicksilver years: The hopes and fears of early adolescents.* San Francisco: Harper & Row.

Bhushan, R. (1993). A study of patterns of family communication: Parents and their adolescent children. *Journal of Personality and Clinical Studies, 9,* 79–85.

Brage, D., & Meredith, W. (1994). A causal model of adolescent depression. *Journal of Psychology, 128,* 455–468.

Brage, D., Meredith, W., & Woodward, J. (1993). Correlates of loneliness among Midwestern adolescents. *Adolescence, 28,* 685–693.

Brooks-Gunn, J., & Paikoff, R. L. (1991). Promoting healthy behavior in adolescence: The case of sexuality and pregnancy. *Bulletin of the New York Academy of Medicine. 67,* 527–547.

Brooks-Gunn, J., & Peterson, A. C. (1991). Studying the emergence of depression and depressive symptoms during adolescence. *Journal of Youth and Adolescence, 20,* 115–119.

Brown, J. E., & Mann, L. (1990). The relationship between family structure and process variables and adolescent decision making. *Journal of Adolescence, 13,* 25–37.

Cairns, R. B. (1979). Social interaction methods: An introduction. In R. B. Cairns (Ed.), *The analysis of social interactions: Methods, issues, and illustrations* (pp. 1–9). New York: Wiley.

Callan, V. J., & Noller, P. (1986). Perceptions of communicative relationships in families with adolescents. *Journal of Marriage and Family, 48,* 813–820.

Cockram, L., & Beloff, H. (1978). *Rehearsing to be adults.* Leicester, England: National Youth Bureau.

Collins, W. A., & Russell, G. (1991). Mother-child and father-child relationships in middle childhood and adolescence: A developmental analysis. *Developmental Review, 11,* 99–136.

Copeland, A. P., & White, K. M. (1991). *Studying families.* Newbury Park, CA: Sage.

Conger, J. J. (1977). *Adolescence and youth* (2nd ed.). New York: Harper.

Conger, R. D., Conger, K. J., Elder, G. H., Lorenz, F. O., Simons, R. L., & Whitbeck, L. B. (1993). Family economic stress and adjustment of early adolescent girls. *Developmental Psychology, 29,* 206–219.

Conger, R. D., Lorenz, F. O., Elder, G. H., Melby, J. N., Simons, R. L., & Conger, K. J. (1991). A process model of family economic pressure and early adolescent alcohol use. *Journal of Early Adolescent Research, 11,* 430–449.

Crawford, I., Thomas, S., & Zoller, D. (1993). Communication and level of AIDS knowledge among homeless African-American mothers and their children. *Journal of Health and Social Policy, 4*(4), 37–53.

Demo, D. H., Small, S. A., & Savin-Williams, R. C. (1987). Family relations and the self-esteem of adolescents and their parents. *Journal of Marriage and the Family, 49,* 705–715.

Doane, J. A. (1978). Family interaction and communication deviance in disturbed and normal families: A review of the research. *Family Process, 17,* 357–376.

Elkind, D. (1984). *All grown up and no place to go.* Reading, MA: Addison-Wesley.

Eme, R., Maisiak, R., & Goodale, W. (1979). Seriousness of adolescent problems. *Adolescence, 14,* 93–99.

Engels, N. A., & Lau, A. D. (1983). Nursing care of the adolescent urban nomad. *MCN: American Journal of Maternal Child Nursing, 8,* 74–77.

Erikson, E. H. (1963). *Childhood and society (2nd ed.).* New York: Norton.

Erikson, E. H. (1968). *Identity: Youth and crisis.* New York: Norton.

Finfrock-Mittl, V., & Robin, A. L. (1987). Acceptability of alternative interventions for parent adolescent conflict. *Behavioral Assessment, 9,* 417–428.

Fisher, T. D. (1986). An exploratory study of parent-child communication about sex and sexual attitudes of early, middle, and late adolescents. *Journal of Genetic Psychology, 147*, 543–557.

Fitzpatrick, M. A., & Ritchie, L. D. (1994). Communication schemata within the family. *Human Communication Research, 20*, 275–301.

Flint, L. (1992). Adolescent parental affinity seeking: Age and gender mediated strategy use. *Adolescence, 27*, 417–434.

Forgatch, M. S., Fetrow, B., & Lathrop, M. (1984). *Solving problems in family interaction.* (Available from M. Lathrop, Oregon Social Learning Center, 207 E. Fifth St. Suite 202, Eugene, OR 97401.)

Foster, S. L., Prinz, R. J., & O'Leary, K. D. (1983). Impact of problem solving communication training and generalization procedures on family conflict. *Child and Family Behavior Therapy, 5*, 1–23.

Ge, X., Conger, R. D., Lorenz, F. O., & Simons, R. L. (1994). Parents' stressful life events and adolescent depressed mood. *Journal of Health and Social Behavior, 35*, 28–44.

Gibb, J. R. (1961). Defensive communication. *Journal of Communication, 3*, 141–148.

Gilligan, C. (1987). Adolescent development reconsidered. In C. E. Irwin, Jr. (Ed.), *Adolescent sexual behavior and health: New directions in child development* (pp. 63–92), *37*, San Francisco: Jossey-Bass.

Graybill, D. (1986). A multiple outcome evaluation of training parents in active listening. *Psychological Bulletin, 59*, 1179–1185.

Grotevant, M. D., & Cooper, C. R. (1985). Patterns of intervention in family relationships and the development of identity experience in the adolescent. *Child Development, 56*, 415–428.

Grotevant, M. D., & Cooper, C. R. (1986). Individuation in family relationships: A perspective on individual differences in the development of identity and role-taking skill in adolescence. *Human Development, 29*, 82–100.

Grotevant, M. D., & Cooper, C. R. (1989). Family interaction coding schemes. In M. D. Grotevant & C. R. Cooper (Eds.), *Family assessment: A guide to methods and measures* (pp. 17–40). New York: Guilford.

Hall, J. A. (1987). Parent-adolescent conflict: An empirical review. *Adolescence, 22*, 767–789.

Hamill, S. B. (1994). Parent-adolescent communication in sandwich generation families. *Journal of Adolescent Research, 9*, 458–482.

Hardin, J. T. (1996, April). *Federal update on nursing research.* Paper presented at the meeting of the Midwest Nursing Research Society, Detroit, MI.

Hawley, L. E., Shear, C. L., Stark, A. M., & Goodman, P. R. (1984). Resident and parental perceptions of adolescent problems and family communications in a low socioeconomic population. *Journal of Family Practice, 19*, 651–655.

Hazel, J. S., Schumaker, J. B., Sherman, J. A., & Sheldon-Wildgen, J. (1981). *ASSET: A social skills program for adolescence.* Champaign, IL: Research Press.

Helson, R., & Moane, G. (1987). Personality change in women from college to midlife. *Journal of Personality and Social Psychology, 53*, 176–186.

Hill, J. P. (1987). Research on adolescents and their families: Past and prospect. In C. E. Irwin, Jr. (Ed.), *Adolescent sexual behavior and health: New directions in child development* (pp. 13–31). San Francisco: Jossey-Bass.

Hops, H., Tildesley, E., Lichtenstein, E., Ary, D., & Sherman, L. (1990). Parent–adolescent problem-solving interactions and drug use. *American Journal of Drug & Alcohol Abuse, 16,* 239–258.

Jaccard, J., & Dittus, P. (1993). Parent-adolescent communication about premarital pregnancy. *Families in Society, 74,* 329–343.

Kafka, R. R., & London, P. (1991). Communication in relationships and adolescent substance use: The influence of parents and friends. *Adolescence, 26,* 587–598.

Kagey, J. R., Vivace, J., & Lutz, W. (1981). Mental health primary prevention: The role of parent mutual support groups. *American Psychologist, 71,* 166–167.

Kazdin, A. E. (1992). *Research decisions in clinical psychology (2nd ed.).* Boston: Allyn & Bacon.

Kenniston, K. (1970). Youth: A ''new'' stage of life. *American Scholar, 39,* 631–654.

Kett, J. F. (1977). *Rites of passage: Adolescence in America, 1790 to the present.* New York: Basic Books.

Koski, K. J., & Steinberg, L. (1990). Parenting satisfaction of mothers during midlife. *Journal of Youth and Adolescence, 19,* 465–474.

LeCroy, W. C. (1988). Parent-adolescent intimacy; Impact on adolescent functioning. *Adolescence, 23,* 137–147.

Leland, N. L., & Barth, R. P. (1993). Characteristics of adolescents who have attempted to avoid HIV and who have communicated with parents about sex. *Journal of Adolescent Research, 8,* 58–76.

Lerner, M. R., & Spanier, G. B. (1978). A dynamic and interactional view of child and family development. In M. R. Lerner & G. B. Spanier (Eds.), *Child influences on marital and family interaction: A life-span perspective* (pp. 1–22). New York: Academic Press.

Levant, R. F., & Doyle, G. F. (1983). An evaluation of a parent education program for fathers of school age children. *Family Relations, 32,* 29–37.

Lynam, M. J., & Tenn, L. (1989). Communication: A tool for the negotiation of independence in families with adolescents. *Journal of Advanced Nursing, 14,* 653–660.

Manning, M. L. (1983). Three myths concerning adolescence. *Adolescence, 18,* 823–829.

Marcy, S. A., Brown, J. S., & Danielson, E. (1983). Contraceptive use by adolescent females in relation to knowledge and to time and method of contraceptive counseling. *Research in Nursing & Health, 6,* 175–182.

Masselam, V. S., Marcus, R. F., & Stunkard, C. L. (1990). Parent adolescent communication, family functioning, and school performance. *Adolescence, 25,* 725–737.

McDonough, M. L., Carlson, C., & Cooper, C. R. (1994). Individuated marital relationships and the regulation of affect in families of early adolescents. *Journal of Adolescent Research, 9,* 67–87.

McMahon, R. J., Forehand, R., & Griest, D. L. (1981). Effects of knowledge of social learning principles on enhancing treatment outcome and generalization in a parent training program. *Journal of Consulting and Clinical Psychology, 49,* 526–532.

Montemayor, R. (1982). The relationship between parent adolescent conflict and the amount of time adolescents spend alone and with parents and peers. *Child Development*, *53*, 1512–1519.

Montemayor, R. (1983). Parents and adolescents in conflict: All families some of the time and some families most of the time. *Journal of Early Adolescence*, *3*, 83–103.

Montemayor, R., McKenry, P. C., & Julian, T. (1993). Men in midlife and the quality of father-adolescent communication. *New Directions in Child Development*, *62*, 59–72.

Moore, K. A., Peterson, J. L., & Furstenberg, E. F. (1986). Parental attitudes an the occurrence of early sexual activity. *Journal of Marriage and Family*, *48*, 777–782.

Moos, R. H., & Moos, B. S. (1981). *The Family Environment Scale*. Palo Alto, CA: Consulting Psychologists Press.

Neighbors, B., Forehand, R., & McVicar, D. (1993). Resilient adolescents and interparental conflict. *American Journal of Orthopsychiatry*, *63*, 462–471.

Neugarten, B. L. (1968). The awareness of middle age. In B. L. Neugarten (Ed.), *Middle age and aging* (pp. 93–98). Chicago: University of Chicago Press.

Noble, P., Adams, G., & Openshaw, D. (1989). Interpersonal communication in parent-adolescent dyads: A brief report on the effects of a social skills training program. *Journal of Family Psychology*, *2*, 483–494.

Nolin, M. J., & Petersen, K. K. (1992). Gender differences in parent-child communication about sexuality: An exploratory study. *Journal of Adolescent Research*, *7*, 59–79.

Noller, P., & Bagi, S. (1985). Parent-adolescent communication. *Journal of Adolescence*, *8*, 125–144.

Noller, P., & Callan, V. J. (1990). Adolescents' perceptions of the nature of their communication with their parents. *Journal of Youth and Adolescence*, *19*, 349–361.

Novovo, R. W. (1978). Anger and coping with stress: Cognitive behavioral interventions. In J. P. Foreyt & D. P. Rathjens (Eds.), *Cognitive behavioral therapy* (pp. 135–173). New York: Plenum.

Offer, D., Ostrov, E., & Howard, K. I. (1981). *The adolescent: A psychological profile*. New York: Basic.

Ohashi, J. P. (1992). Maternal role satisfaction: A new approach to assessing parenting. *Scholarly Inquiry for Nursing Practice: An International Journal*, *62*, 135–150.

Ohlson, M. M. (1979). *Marriage counseling in groups*. Champaign, IL: Research Press.

Papini, D. R., Farmer, F. F., Clark, S. M., & Micka, J. (1990). Early adolescent age and gender difference in patterns of emotional self-disclosure to parents and friends. *Adolescence*, *25*, 959–976.

Patterson, G. (1986). Performance models for antisocial boys. *American Psychologist*, *41*, 432–444.

Peck, R. L. (1968). Psychological developments in the second half of life. In B. L. Neugarten (Ed.), *Middle age and aging* (pp. 101–122) Chicago: University of Chicago Press.

Porter, B. P., & O'Leary, K. D. (1980). Marital discord and childhood behavior problems. *Journal of Abnormal Child Psychology*, *98*, 287–295.

Prinz, R. J. (1976). *The assessment of parent adolescent relations: Discriminating distressed from nondistressed dyads.* Unpublished doctoral dissertation, State University of New York at Stony Brook.

Prinz, R. J., Foster, S., Kent, R. N., & O'Leary, K. D. (1979). Multivariate assessment of conflict in distressed and nondistressed mother-adolescent dyads. *Journal of Applied Behavior Analysis, 12,* 691–700.

Renz, L., & Cohen, M. (1977). Interpersonal skill practice as a component in effective parent training. *Community Mental Health Journal, 13,* 54–57.

Resnick, M. D., Bearinger, L. H., Stark, P., & Blum, R. W. (1994). Patterns of consultation among adolescent minors obtaining an abortion. *American Journal of Orthopsychiatry, 64,* 310–316.

Reuter, M. A., & Conger, R. D. (1995). Interaction style, problem-solving behavior, and family problem-solving effectiveness. *Child Development, 66,* 98–115.

Riesch, S. K., & Forsyth, D. M. (1992). Preparing to parent the adolescent. *Journal of Child and Adolescent Psychiatric and Mental Health Nursing, 5,* 32–40.

Riesch, S. K., Jacobson, G. A., & Tosi, C. B. (1994). Young adolescents' identification of difficult life events. *Clinical Nursing Research, 3,* 393–413.

Riesch, S. K., Tosi, C. B., Thurston, C. A., Forsyth, D. M., Kuenning, T. S., & Kestly, J. (1993). Effects of communication training on parents and young adolescents. *Nursing Research, 42,* 10–16.

Ritchie, L. D., & Fitzpatrick, M. A. (1990). Family communication patterns: Measuring intrapersonal perceptions of interpersonal relationships. *Communications Research, 17,* 523–544.

Robin, A. L. (1979). Problem-solving communication training: A behavioral approach to the treatment of parent-adolescent conflict. *The American Journal of Family Therapy, 7,* 69–83.

Robin, A. L. (1981). A controlled evaluation of problem-solving communication training with parent-adolescent conflict. *Behavior Therapy, 12,* 593–609.

Robin, A. L. (1985). Parent-adolescent conflict: A developmental problem of families. In R. J. McMahon & R. D. Peters (Eds.), *Childhood disorders: Behavioral-developmental approaches* (pp. 244–265). New York: Brunner/Mazel.

Robin, A. L., & Foster, S. L. (1989). *Negotiating parent and adolescent conflict.* New York: Guilford.

Robin, A. L., Kent, R., O'Leary, K. D., Foster, S., & Prinz, R. (1979). An approach to teaching parents and adolescent problem solving communication skills. *Behavior Therapy, 8,* 639–643.

Robin, A. L., & Koepke, T. (1990). Behavioral assessment and treatment of parent-adolescent conflict. In M. Herson, R. M. Eisler, & P. M. Miller (Eds.), *Progress in behavior modification* (pp. 178–215). Newbury Park, CA: Sage.

Serna, L. A., Schumaker, J. B., Sherman, J. A., & Sheldon, J. B. (1991). In-home generalization of social interactions in families of adolescents with behavior problems. *Journal of Applied Behavior Analysis, 24,* 733–746.

Sinnot, J. D. (1982). Correlates of sex roles of older adults. *Journal of Gerontology, 37,* 587–594.

Smith, K. A., & Forehand, R. (1986). Parent-adolescent conflict: Comparison and prediction of the perceptions of mothers, fathers, and daughters. *Journal of Early Adolescence, 6,* 353–367.

Smollar, J., & Youniss, J. (1985). Parent-adolescent relations in adolescents whose parents are divorced. *Journal of Early Adolescence, 5,* 129–144.

Speicher, B. (1992). Adolescent moral judgment and perceptions of family interaction. *Journal of Family Psychology, 6,* 128–138.

Steinberg, L. (1990). Interdependency in the family: Autonomy, conflict, and harmony in the parent-adolescent relationship. In S. Feldman & G. Elliott (Eds.), *At the threshold: The developing adolescent* (pp. 11–32). Cambridge, MA: Harvard University Press.

Steinberg, L., Elmen, J. D., & Mounts, N. S. (1989). Authoritative parenting, psychosocial maturity, and academic success among adolescents. *Child Development, 60,* 1424–1436.

Steinberg, L., Lamborn, S. D., Dornbusch, S. M., & Darling, N. (1992). Impact of parenting practices on adolescent achievement: Authoritative parenting, school involvement, and encouragement to succeed. *Child Development, 63,* 1266–1281.

Stivers, C. (1988). Parent-adolescent communication and its relationship to adolescent depression and suicide proneness. *Adolescence, 23,* 291–295.

Stoker, A., & Swadi, H. (1990). Perceived family relationships in drug abusing adolescents. *Drug and Alcohol Dependence, 25,* 293–297.

Strader, M. K., Beaman, M. L., & McSweeney, M. (1992). Effects of communication with important social referents on beliefs and intentions to use condoms. *Journal of Advanced Nursing, 17,* 699–703.

Strommen, M. P., & Strommen, A. I. (1985). *Five cries of parents.* San Francisco: Harper & Row.

Tebes, J. K., Grady, K., & Snow, D. L. (1989). Parent training in decision making facilitation: Skill acquisition and relationship to gender. *Family Relations, 38,* 243–247.

Tesser, A., Forehand, R., Brody, G., & Long, N. (1989). Conflict: The role of calm and angry parent-child discussion in adolescent adjustment. *Journal of Social and Clinical Psychology, 8,* 317–330.

Tramontana, M. G., Sherrets, S. D., & Authier, K. J, (1980). Evaluation of parent education programs. *Journal of Clinical Child Psychology, 9,* 40–43.

Travormina, J. B. (1974). Basic models of parent counseling: A critical review. *Psychological Bulletin, 81,* 827–835.

Tucker, S. K. (1989). Adolescent patterns of communication about sexually related topics. *Adolescence, 24,* 269–278.

Vander Zanden, J. W. (1989). *Human development* (4th ed.). New York: Knopf.

Vangelisti, A. L. (1992). Older adolescents' perceptions of communication problems with their parents. *Journal of Adolescent Research, 7,* 382–402.

Vuchinich, S., Vuchinich, R., & Wood, B. (1993). The interparental relationship and family problem solving with preadolescent males. *Child Development, 64,* 1389–1400.

Weinmann, L. L., & Newcombe, N. (1990). Relational aspects of identity: Late adolescents' perceptions of their relationships with parents. *Journal of Experimental Child Psychology, 50,* 357–369.

Werrbach, G. B., Grotevant, H. D., & Cooper, C. R. (1992). Patterns of family interaction and adolescent sex role concepts. *Journal of Youth and Adolescence, 21,* 609–623.

Zabin, L. S., Hirsch, M. B., Emerson, M. R., & Raymond, E. (1992). To whom do inner-city minors talk about their pregnancies? Adolescents' communication with parents and parent surrogates. *Family Planning Perspectives, 24,* 148–154.

Zubin, M. (1982). Changing behavior and outlook of aging men and women: Implications for marriage in the middle and later years. *Family Relations, 31,* 147–156.

Chapter 7

Adherence to Therapy in Tuberculosis

Felissa L. Cohen
School of Nursing
Southern Illinois University at Edwardsville

ABSTRACT

Tuberculosis (TB) is a leading cause of morbidity and mortality worldwide. In the United States, TB has undergone a resurgence and the appearance of multidrug-resistant TB has caused new concerns. A critical part of TB treatment is adherence to the prescribed therapy for a considerable time period. Treatment "failure" is often due to nonadherence. Many factors influence adherence to therapy in TB. This chapter reviews research in the area of adherence to the TB treatment plan in the United States and worldwide. It discusses adherence as an outcome related to treatment regimens such as directly observed therapy, patient characteristics, life and family circumstances, motivation, education, incentives, and combination strategies. Themes across studies are compared and suggestions for successful future studies are identified.

Keywords: Adherence, Compliance, Therapy, Tuberculosis, Tuberculosis and Treatment

After a period of relative quiescence, tuberculosis (TB) has undergone a resurgence in the United States. The appearance of multidrug–resistant TB (MDR–TB) has caused new concerns and focus (Cohen & Durham, 1995). The incidence of TB in this country had been generally declining until 1986, when an increase in cases was seen (Bloom & Murray, 1992). In 1995, 22,813 cases of TB were reported in the United States (Centers for Disease Control and Prevention [CDCP], 1996). Worldwide, TB had continued to exact a toll and has been the leading cause of death among deaths from infectious diseases (Sudre, ten Dam, & Kochi, 1992). Various reasons have contributed to the rise in cases of TB in the United States. These include the human immunodeficiency virus (HIV) epidemic; social conditions such as poverty, crowding, poor nutrition, homelessness, drug use, and deinstitutionalization of the mentally ill; increased immigration from countries with high rates of TB; the previous apathy of both the public and health care workers to TB; high medication costs; treatment errors; nonadherence to therapy; decreased research about TB; and decreased funding to support TB control programs, resulting in inadequate surveillance and contact tracing (Brudney & Dobkin, 1991; Cohen, 1995; Joseph, 1993; Madsen & Cohen, 1995; Reichman, 1991).

In TB, distinction is made between tuberculous infection and tuberculosis. In those persons with tuberculous infection, living *Mycobacterium tuberculosis* may be present without clinically active disease. These individuals usually have a reactive tuberculin skin test, are not infectious to others, usually have negative sputum cultures and smears for tubercle bacilli, may be at risk for clinical disease if their immune systems are compromised, and may be candidates for preventive therapy. Those with active pulmonary tuberculosis are infected with *Mycobacterium tuberculosis*, usually have a reactive tuberculin skin test, usually have clinical symptoms, usually have positive sputum smears and/or cultures before therapy, and need adequate therapy over a relatively long period of time (CDCP, 1993). Persons at high risk for tuberculous infection or active disease include those who are of a racial minority, are poor, homeless, malnourished, immunologically compromised (including HIV infection), foreign-born from countries where TB is endemic, who are medically underserved, are alcoholics, are injecting drug users, are residents of or work in facilities such as jails, prisons, long-term care facilities, nursing homes and other institutions, and who live in crowded, unsanitary conditions.

ADHERENCE TO THERAPY IN TB

There can be many definitions for adherence (compliance). Sumartojo (1995) states that for TB, adherence "refers to patients taking medication as prescribed for the prevention of tuberculous infection or the treatment of active disease" (p. 122). Patients may take medication as part of preventive therapy if they have tuberculous infection or for treatment of active tuberculosis. In either case, a critical part of treatment is taking the prescribed medications properly for the appropriate period of time. Recommendations for the regimen vary depending on susceptibility of the organism, community TB rates, patient factors, and other considerations. However, the length of time for drug therapy is usually a minimum of 6 months, and can be 12 months or longer (CDCP, 1993). Over such a prolonged period of time, patients may simply stop taking medication, particularly if it is for preventive therapy and they do not really perceive that they are ill. Characteristics of the treatment regimen such as unpleasant side effects, treatment complexity, duration of treatment, packaging of the drug, route of administration, number of drugs taken, or the drug itself influence adherence (Madsen & Cohen, 1995). Beliefs about health and illness, understanding of disease-related information, and willingness and ability to carry out behavior related to health and illness are also important (Gentry, 1984; Janz & Becker, 1984). In addition, other factors influence adherence, such as cultural beliefs; language use; literacy; the patient's family and life circumstances; characteristics of the treatment site or clinic, such as availability of snacks, wait to be seen, hours, and so on; and the relationship with the health care provider (Cuneo & Snider, 1989; McDonald & Ma, 1987; Snider & Hutton, 1989; Sumartojo, 1993, 1995). Sbarbaro (1990) emphasized the need to treat the patient as a whole person; one who is part of a community and is cared about.

RESEARCH IN TUBERCULOSIS

Research in the field of tuberculosis has been concentrated on the areas of diagnosis, types of drug therapy, treatment regimens, detection and screening programs, and adherence to therapy. Strategies to impact on outcomes, particularly in regard to adherence, have been of special interest, and include the evaluation of patient characteristics, educational approaches and the use of incentives and enablers, and modifications of the treatment itself or the treatment environment.

Conducting research regarding adherence to the TB treatment plan is problematic and is compounded by the way in which adherence is measured. Both direct and indirect ways may be used in measurement. In TB, urine assays are one way to identify whether certain antituberculosis medication has been taken. Rifampin turns urine, feces, saliva, sweat, and tears a reddish orange. Isoniazid (INH) can be identified through using paper strips for urine testing. However, the urine assays only estimate adherence and may show a positive result even if the medication is only being taken intermittently (Sumartojo, 1995). Other methods are less direct and include patient self-report, pill counts, clinic or medical appointment records, and records of prescription filling or refilling (Sumartojo, 1995). Sometimes special microelectric devices have been used to record when and how often TB medications were removed from their container (Cheung et al., 1988; Moulding, Onstad, & Sbarbaro,

1970). However, the reliability of these devices is also in question, as patients may open medication containers simply out of curiosity, or for other reasons (Sumartojo, 1995).

Adherence has been a long-time nursing concern. Yet, health care providers are still relatively unaware of which patients will be adherent and which ones will not be. Among TB patients in one study, investigators found that physicians predicted nonadherence for 32% of nonadherent patients and for 8% of adherent patients (Wardman, Knox, Muers, & Page, 1988). In TB, the vast majority of nondrug efficacy studies have been focused on various factors that have influenced adherence and on methods for improving adherence.

Grateful Med's MEDLINE capability, the Cumulative Index of Nursing and Allied Health Literature (CINAHL), and the psychological literature (PsycLit) were used to identify articles for inclusion in this chapter. The searches were limited to the English language and human subjects. The keywords for searching were tuberculosis coupled with adherence (compliance), tuberculosis coupled with research, tuberculosis and nursing, tuberculosis and treatment and research. The years were limited to 1980 through January 1996. As articles were examined, their reference lists were used to identify further references within the same time period, and these articles were manually retrieved.

RESEARCH STUDIES RELATED TO TREATMENT STRUCTURE AND STRATEGIES

Research related to the way in which treatment is structured may refer to the drug dosage, the drug regimen or administration, the setting or environment in which treatment is delivered, and the treatment plan. A major focus of research has been on the mode of delivery of TB drugs, particularly directly observed therapy (DOT).

Directly Observed Therapy

Because of the potential seriousness of nonadherence to medications for tuberculosis, DOT has become increasingly popular (Iseman, Cohn, & Sbarbaro, 1993). Under DOT, another person (usually a health care worker) watches the patient take his/her medication in the home, the clinic, a school, shelter, or another agreed-upon facility. Patients on intermittent medication regimens are easier to manage under DOT than those on daily or more frequent treatment plans. However, patients can still avoid taking medication, even with DOT (Pozsik, 1993; Sumartojo, 1995), particularly if they view the plan as punitive

(Boutotte & Etkind, 1995). Some cities have used nontraditional providers, such as community workers, community-based organizations such as those concerned with substance use, or religious and social organizations to provide DOT (DeCock, 1996; Klein & Naizby, 1995).

In several studies researchers examined the effectiveness of DOT in patients with TB. Alwood and colleagues (1994) identified all patients with both TB and HIV from the medical records between January 1984 and June, 1992 in a chest clinic at the Baltimore Health Department. A total of 107 patients were located who were predominately African American (91%), male (78%), drug users (67%), alcohol users (48%), unemployed (73%), on Medicaid (88%), and had an incarceration history (18%). Due to the death of 29 patients, the remaining 78 patients received 8 or more weeks of therapy. They were either assigned to the DOT group, in which a nurse watched the patient swallow pills, or the indirect therapy group, in which medication was self-administered, partly supervised, or both. Completion of the 6 months of therapy was the measure of adherence, and survival after therapy also was examined. When the two groups were compared, no differences in sex were found between the two, but the DOT group had more African American patients than the indirect group (96% vs. 80%, $p = .02$). Patients in the DOT group were more likely to complete therapy than in the indirect treatment group (96% vs. 76%, $p = .02$). Overall survival was higher in the DOT group, with 85% of the patients alive versus 57% in the indirect group ($p = .01$), although some of the deaths at the time survival was measured were not TB-related. Although this study demonstrated the effectiveness of DOT for both adherence to therapy and survival, it was a retrospective review, not a controlled study, and the indirect group included mixed administration methods that included the DOT method used for the first group. The researchers did not report comparisons between the two groups in regard to other possibly significant variables such as CD4+ cell counts and laboratory and clinical parameters related to TB, such as sputum culture and cavitation. Therefore, it is not known if the findings could have been influenced by disease-related characteristics rather than therapeutic considerations. The time of survival measurement appeared to be at 6 months, but this is not clear. Finally, the use of multivariate data analysis might have been helpful in sorting out the multiple characteristics measured.

DOT was used in an intermittent preventive therapy program for homeless, predominately White (70.2%) men in a shelter in Seattle (Nazar-Stewart & Nolan, 1992). After purified protein derivative (PPD) testing, 47 of the eligible 64 men began preventive INH therapy and 23 (48.9%) completed the 6- to 12-month regimen. Reasons given for not completing therapy were adverse reactions to therapy, the loss of patients to followup, and refusal to comply.

The researchers also examined patient characteristics related to noncompliance and found that those men with contacts out of the state, those who used the shelter infrequently, and those who were born out of the country were less likely to complete therapy than were the others. Although the authors stated that alcoholics may have been slightly less likely to complete therapy than others, the difference was minimal. Men who did not complete therapy remained on the regimen for an average of 9 weeks. No control group was used in this study; therefore it is unknown to what extent results were due to using DOT as a method of compliance. The findings suggest the advantage of a medication regimen that is short-term in length for preventive TB therapy.

DOT was examined as a strategy for adherence for preventive therapy among Indians in Saskatchewan, Canada (Wobeser, To, & Hoeppner, 1989). DOT with education was compared to self-administered therapy alone and to self-administered therapy plus education. Additionally, self-administered therapy plus education was compared with self-administered therapy alone in the short and long term (1 year). Patients were randomly divided by household. The educational program included information about the disease and the importance of taking medication for a full year, personal and family counseling, and educational pamphlets. After 6 weeks, the compliance in the DOT plus education group was significantly greater than in the retrospective self-administered therapy alone group and the self-administered therapy with education group. The self-administered therapy with education group compliance rate was significantly greater than self-administration alone. Ten weeks after the DOT and education was discontinued, the compliance rates of the three groups were not significantly different. It was not clear why the DOT was not continued for a longer period or what the content and structure of the educational programs were. In addition, those in the self-administration group had to pick up their medications themselves, while those on daily observed therapy had drugs delivered to them. The use of the retrospective control group also raises questions of comparability. Further, division by household may have introduced bias.

Another study of DOT in Baltimore focused partly on clinic-based DOT versus community based DOT at sequential time periods (Chaulk, Moore-Rice, Rizzo, & Chaisson, 1995). The city of Baltimore has used clinic-based DOT since 1978 and community-based DOT since 1981. Most of the DOT is given at the home, workplace, school, drug treatment facility, jail, or nursing home; the remainder come to the clinic. Trained staff comprise an outreach team for those patients who miss clinic appointments. When comparisons were made both in absolute and relative terms with other major cities, Baltimore's annual TB case rates experienced the greatest drop. Further, from 1986 to 1992, the DOT-managed cases in Baltimore had the highest completion rates for anti-TB therapy, high bacteriologic evidence of cures, and rare incidence of drug resistance. Although cause and effect are difficult to demonstrate, these researchers attempted to compare variables (e.g., AIDS [acquired immunodeficiency syndrome] cases, unemployment, poverty and foreign-born TB patients) that could affect these rates in Baltimore and five comparison cities. The authors are appropriately conservative in their reporting of the results.

In Tarrant County, TX, from 1980 to 1986, TB therapy was unsupervised; after that time, DOT was instituted for the vast majority of patients (Weis et al., 1994). DOT was administered under a team of nurses, community-service aides, and public health investigators and was done at the site of patient preference (residence, clinic, place of work, or other). For the pre-DOT period, 407 patient episodes were compared with 581 episodes in the later time period. The groups were significantly different in regard to drug use, race, status as former prisoner or homeless, and other characteristics. However, in the DOT group, the proportion of cases with primary resistance declined; acquired resistance declined; rates of relapse decreased; and MDR-TB decreased significantly. DOT was judged to be effective and feasible. Differences in characteristics of the two groups and the use of different time periods inhibit the conclusions that can be drawn; however, results are consistent with other studies.

DOT with intermittent chemotherapy was used as a strategy to improve compliance in a rural area of China (Kan et al., 1985). The barefoot doctors of the village health cooperatives administered and supervised treatment. If a patient did not come to the treatment site, the barefoot doctor located the patient and administered the therapy on the same day. In this study of 229 patients over 1 year, the compliance rate was 99.4%, and the conversion of sputum from positive to negative was 95.2%. This study demonstrated the feasibility of treatment completion with DOT. Whether or not such a program could be implemented in other cultural settings because of cost and issues related to free choice remains to be tested. Interviews with 68 injecting drug users suggested that fear of involuntary detention was a major reason that they avoided services and treatment related to TB (Curtis et al., 1994).

Schluger, Ciotoli, Cohen, Johnson, and Rom (1995) described variance in the effectiveness of DOT in regard to adherence. Adherence was measured by completion of therapy. Patients who were being discharged from Bellevue Hospital in New York signed a contract for participation in the DOT program that included a series of incentives, including carfare and food at visits. After each successful week of therapy, an additional incentive of subway tokens was provided. If a dose of medication were missed, the outreach worker tried to telephone the patient; if not successful, they visited the patient's home. Patients were discussed at a weekly conference. One hundred and thirteen patients were discharged from the hospital and referred to the program during the study period. Of these, 90% completed therapy and 11 patients were lost to followup. The expected completion rate determined before implementation of DOT was 35%, and thus the difference was statistically significant ($p <$ .0001). The average cost for this program was approximately $2,082 per patient, as compared with self-medicated patients at $1,050. This study did not have a concurrent control group.

A community-based treatment program was developed to provide supervised intermittent ambulatory treatment (SIAT) for TB in Zululand (Wilkinson, 1994). Participating patients could chose a supervisor who observed the patient taking the medications; the supervisor signed a TB card. A TB health worker checked compliance with the supervisor monthly. The patients could choose sites such as a school, tribal authority, store, tea room, or a clinic. Of the 814 patients in the study, 89% completed treatment, as compared to an estimate of 18% in a retrospective time period. These results are muddied by the apparent combination of patients treated both on SIAT and on the ward in analyzing the results and by the "personal observation" estimate of the past 200 patients that led to the 18% retrospective compliance rate estimate. Nonetheless, the notions of the choice of the patients as to their supervisor and the selection of site of medication administration are interesting and need to be further explored.

During a 5-year period, 21 patients who were identified as TB treatment failures were given supervised therapy five times a week for the first 6 months on what the authors describe as a predominately ambulatory basis; however, 11 patients had some period of hospitalization during the study that ranged from 4 to 81 days with a mean of 27.2 (McDonald, Memon, & Reichman, 1982). Patients received daily refreshments or meals, transportation or carfare, and home visits when they could not attend clinic; in addition, the protocol minimized waiting in the clinic and provided medical care free of charge. After 6 months, oral medications were self-administered for another 18 months and evaluated monthly. Data reporting is somewhat confusing. It appears that there was an overall compliance rate of 80%, but it is not clear how this was determined. There were inconsistent numbers reported in various parts of the study. The authors also reported that past treatment failures appeared to be due not only to poor self-administration of TB medications but also to the lack of continuity of care. It is important to note that sputum conversion from positive to negative in individual patients did not necessarily occur more rapidly in those who were most compliant.

Elk and associates (1995) conducted a small study ($N = 5$) of drug-dependent women with TB requiring prophylactic treatment. Women could earn a monetary reinforcer related to the level of cocaine metabolites in their urine at the time of their daily visits. Patients received methadone, weekly counseling, and INH through DOT administration. One patient dropped out of treatment, presumably due to INH side effects, at week 12. The authors believed that the high rate of compliance with INH was due to the coordination of the drug and TB treatment programs at the same site and the effectiveness of methadone as a reinforcer. Although these investigators reported on a very small sample, the findings suggest a strategy that was effective in other adherence studies.

DOT was used as a strategy along with short-course drug therapy to treat patients in China (China Tuberculosis Control Collaboration, 1996). Between 1991 and 1994, patients with smear positives and smear negatives, for whom treatment was indicated, were registered into the TB program and received a TB treatment card and identity card. A copy of the card was sent to the village doctor, who observed every dose of the regimen and recorded witnessing the dose. Treatment was free. If the patients did not come in for treatments they were visited at home by the physician. Default rates were low, and treatment failures were attributed to a lack of drug susceptibility testing. This study was difficult to follow because the numbers in the summary do not coincide with the text and necessary methodological details were missing.

A fully supervised program was introduced in rural areas of Hong Kong, and those 15 years and older entered the 1-year study (Hong Kong Chest Service/British Medical Research Council, 1984). Drugs were given under DOT on weekly visits to the clinic after an initial hospitalization phase. Nearly half of the eligible patients did not participate because of refusing hospitalization. Of the 154 participating patients, 54% did not miss any doses; 18% missed one dose; 7%, two doses, 3%, four doses; 3%, five doses; 3% missed more than five doses; and 8% defaulted permanently. DOT appeared successful in this group, although no control group was available for comparison.

Characteristics of the Treatment

Characteristics of the medication itself, its administration, or the regimen have been found to influence adherence. Characteristics of the medication itself were found to be important in a study conducted in Hong Kong (Hong Kong Chest Service/British Medical Research Council, 1989). Adult Chinese patients ($N = 627$) received either combined ($n = 314$) or separate ($n = 313$) medication formulations during the 2-year study period. The separate group had three drugs to take. Medications were taken at the clinic. There were no significant differences between the two groups in regard to compliance, as measured by keeping clinic appointments and receiving medication at that visit. Patients were allowed to select their own drink to use when swallowing their medication. The combined medication was thought to be more acceptable to patients, but this did not affect either side effects or compliance.

Another study related to form of administration of medications as affecting adherence was conducted in Tanzania (Chum et al., 1995). Adherence was measured by comparison of actual numbers with the average number of patients expected in the clinic on a given day. Three regimens were compared: patients on a regimen containing injectable streptomycin; patients who received both the streptomycin-containing regimen and a completely oral regimen; and patients who received only oral medications. There were no significant differences among the three groups in terms of attendance. The authors believed that patients would perceive their need for medication as more important if the patients received injectable versus oral medication for TB. This belief was not supported. The adherence measurement may have influenced the results, and the actual numbers attending were not reported.

HIV-positive patients are at higher risk for TB than those who are HIV negative. Persons who were determined to be HIV positive after voluntary testing in Lusaka, Zambia were referred to a preventive therapy trial for TB treatment (Godfrey-Faussett et al., 1995). The purpose of the study was to compare efficacy of preventive therapy against TB in three groups: a 6-month intermittent INH group, a 3-month intermittent rifampin and pyrazinamide group, and a placebo group. Subjects were randomly assigned to one of the three groups. Of the 475 patients tested, 201 were HIV positive and returned for results of the HIV test. Of these 201 subjects, 181 were eligible, 156 accepted referral, and 77 (16.2% of those tested; 34.2% of those who were HIV positive) entered the trial. Reasons for not entering the trial were: not wanting to be in an experiment, confidentiality issues, reaction to being HIV positive, distance from center, and difficulty in getting off from work to come to the hospital. Of the 156 referred, 61 did not attend and were therefore nonadherent. Reasons given were ''no reason recorded,'' procrastination, adjusting to HIV result, family reasons, health provider attitudes and environment of the clinic, ambivalence, death of the subject, and other. This study was flawed in many ways. One problem is an ethical issue: that is, should there be a control group for TB prevention therapy, given what is known about TB and its treatment? Also, different numerical values were reported in the text of the report, the tables, and the abstract. Thus, interpretation of findings is problematic.

Valeza and McDougall (1990) reported on the use of blister calendar or bubble packs for TB treatment in the Philippines. In a 3-year period, the completion rates using these packs were over 80%, as compared with an approximate 41% before their introduction. Information is sparse in this report, and thus full interpretation is difficult.

An investigation ($N = 1062$) of the effectiveness, toxicity, and acceptability of a 6-month compared to a 9-month treatment regimen included assessment of noncompliance (Combs, O'Brien, & Geiter, 1990). Patients were defined as noncompliant if they missed more than 2 weeks of drugs, except for medical reasons. Patients on the shorter term therapy had significantly less noncompliance than those on the 9-month regimen (16.8% vs. 29.2%). Detailed information was lacking in this report.

Compliance was addressed in children with pulmonary and extrapulmonary TB in Papua, New Guinea (Biddulph, Mokela, & Sharma, 1987). The 321 children ranged in age from 1 year to 12 years. Methodological details such as sample selection are lacking. The authors reported that compliance with shorter term 6-month TB therapy was approximately 75% as compared with 25% on the 18-month regimen. However, as expected, the longer regimen was more expensive. The definition of compliance was not clear. In addition, children were followed by a special pediatric TB nurse and received education that included relatives. Because of the lack of details this study cannot be fully evaluated.

Investigators in Algeria examined a 28-week versus a 36-week course of chemotherapy in adults with pulmonary TB (Algerian Working Group/ British Medical Research Council Cooperative Study, 1991). Patients 15 years or older with previously untreated pulmonary TB were eligible; districts, rather than patients, were allocated to one of the two groups at random. The short-term therapy group enrolled 977 patients as compared with 1241 in the longer term group. Compliance was assessed through permanent default, treatment missed for at least 2 weeks during a 4-week period, and urine tests for isoniazid metabolites. Patients in the shorter term therapy had slightly less permanent default (9.3% vs. 6.7%). Presentation of data in this study was difficult to interpret. Significance tests were not reported. Many variables were identified that could have influenced the study, such as failure of personnel to enroll nearly 22% of those eligible to participate.

Research Relating to the Treatment Plan and Its Implementation

Tracing and direct contact were used to combat nonadherence to therapy in a rural district in southern Cambodia. Patients not returning for their medications after 10 days during initial therapy or 45 days after beginning continuation therapy were first contacted by letter. If this strategy did not work, then home visits were made by the district nurse via hospital motorbike on a weekly basis. One hundred seventy-one were admitted to treatment and 46 were considered "absconders." Of the 46 "absconders" or nonadherent persons, 57% were seen at home and 81% of these returned to treatment. The most frequent reasons given for not completing therapy were socioeconomic (work responsibilities and financial, 68%); drug toxicity (14%); feeling "too ill" (9%); feeling cured (9%); and "too poor" (2%). Distance from the treatment site was not a factor (Kimerling & Petri, 1995). The methods in this study were not precisely described. For example, the nurses attempted to trace absconders "depending on the season." This is not defined.

The use of a calendar to enhance medication-taking was used in an attempt to improve compliance in a study by Lange, Ulmer, and Weiss (1986). Participants attended a clinic at a community health center in East Los Angeles and included 28 subjects who were randomly assigned to either the experimental ($n = 18$) or control ($n = 10$) groups. All patients were diagnosed with inactive TB and were on daily INH. Patients in the experimental group received monthly calendars and were instructed by their physician to initial the calendar after taking their daily medication. In other respects, the groups were the same. Outcomes were measured in terms of short-term compliance (daily pill-taking) and long-term compliance (remaining in treatment from time of diagnosis until the study's end). Short-term compliance was calculated using a scoring algorithm based on daily pill-taking with adjustments for side effects and other factors. Pill-taking was measured by counting the pills remaining in the vial when the patient returned for the monthly visit. If the pills were not brought in, the patient's estimate was used. The number of dropouts was significant, and the authors believed this may have been due to the $10 visit fee. The authors concluded that the calendar intervention was not a benefit, and that preventing dropout, not taking medication daily, was the important compliance issue. Problems with this study include the small sample size, the various ways of measuring pill-taking, the use of the algorithm, and the lack of description of long-term compliance or its results.

A study conducted in Madras, India examined default in patients over 12-years of age (Krishnaswami et al., 1981). The 170 patients entering the study were assigned to either the routine or intensive group. One hundred and fifty subjects completed the study, 75 in each group. The intensive group received a home visit from a health visitor on the 4th day of default from their scheduled drug pickups at the clinic, a home visit on the 11th day, and home visits at 1 and 2 months. The routine group received a letter on the 4th day and a home visit on the 11th day. Default took place in both groups, 64 routine patients had 1 or more episodes as did 57 intensive patients. Patients in the intensive group were retrieved from default significantly more frequently with the first action than in the routine group ($p = .01$). The mean number of drug collections was higher in the intensive group than in the routine group. Data reporting was confusing. Further, the use of drug collection as an adherence variable is questionable, as collecting the drug is different than taking it.

In Barcelona, Spain, 318 children (mean age of 6.5 years) who were tuberculin positive assigned to INH preventative therapy were assigned randomly to one of 4 followup groups (Sanmarti et al., 1993). Those with active TB were excluded. The control group had no activity; treatment group I received a telephone call from the nurse every 3 months encouraging continuation with INH; treatment group II received home nursing visits every 3 months, with encouragement and urine testing for adherence; and treatment group III saw a physician at the TB center every 3 months, with urine testing for adherence. Adherence was measured by attendance at a clinic visit after 1 year of therapy and by a urine test showing adherence to INH. The urine test used detected INH if the drug was taken 3 days or less before the test. At the end of 1 year, treatment groups I and II had the highest adherence rates as measured by attendance (93.7% and 95%) and by positive urine test reaction (85% and 89.8%). The control group had attendance of 65% and positive urine tests of 55.8%, whereas treatment group III had attendance of 78% and urine tests of 74.5%. There was no significant difference between the group receiving nurses' phone calls (group I) and the group receiving nurses' visits (group II). The authors attributed the success of groups I and II to the mothers' perception that the attention from nurses was a separate act from the medical treatment, and thus they received additional attention. The lower rate of adherence in group III was speculated to be due to poor physician–patient relationship, inflexible appointment times, the center atmosphere, and the need to arrange work school schedules to see the physician when the child was not apparently ill. The study was basically well designed, with random assignment and appropriate data analysis. Gender of the health care provider was not included as a variable; this analysis might have provided interesting information.

Clinic Environment

A study conducted in Thailand included 160 patients attending a TB chest clinic (Buri, Vathesatogkit, Charoenpan, Kiatboonsri, & Buranaratchada, 1985). These patients attended a special TB clinic where they saw the same physician who repeated education self-care information, referred those in need to the social welfare department, diminished the waiting time, and monitored attendance, including reminders for those who missed appointments. After 3 months of no response, patients were classified as defaulters. Approximately 87% completed treatment. When comparing those who did not complete the course of treatment with those who did, those who did not complete the course of treatment were found to be significantly different from those who did complete the treatment in the following areas: irregular drug compliance, longer traveling time, presence of other illness, identified possible barriers to compliance, and regular use of alcohol. The clinic had a higher percentage of patients completing TB treatment (87%) than in another clinic at the same hospital (53%) and at an unnamed site. It was difficult to sort out the interaction of variables and the actual clinic program.

In a later study, Buri and Hathirat (1987) performed a retrospective analysis of 100 TB patients attending either the general medical outpatient department or the specialized TB clinic at a hospital in Bangkok. Sex and age were reported as similar; however, there was a higher proportion of extrapulmonary TB and other illnesses in the general medical clinic. There was a significantly higher degree of irregular drug compliance among the general medical clinic patients (25%) than the specialized TB clinic (11%; $p < .005$). Similar data were presented for treatment-compliance defaulters (25% in the general medical clinic vs. 13% in the specialized TB clinic; $p < .05$). Consistency of the physician made no apparent difference in compliance. The investigators did not report how the variables of drug compliance, treatment compliance, or physician consistency were defined or measured. Other information, such as details about sample selection and other parameters, was lacking.

RESEARCH RELATED TO PATIENT AND FAMILY CHARACTERISTICS AND CIRCUMSTANCES

Adherence research has demonstrated that certain demographic characteristics of patients such as age, sex, and occupation appear to influence adherence. The patients' living circumstances and the availability of family relationships also are important. In a survey of 68 local health authorities in one part of South Africa, investigators (Bell & Yach, 1988) examined patient characteristics in regard to compliance. All TB patients on a supervised short-course therapy attending outpatient clinics in the Western Cape were eligible. To be defined as compliant, patients had to receive 75% or greater of the number of doses they should have received. Analysis used compliance as a dichotomous variable: those with less than 75% compliance and those with 75% or higher compliance. Compliance was highest in those who were employed full-time regardless of sex; compliance between sexes was not significantly different. Compliance was lowest among children under 5 years of age (which raises a concern regarding their caregivers), and in teenagers. Compliance rates were lower in Blacks than in Whites. Recommendations were to increase education and access to health care and to target specific groups for compliance. It is hard to judge the results of this study, because the researchers did not define "supervised" therapy.

In a central African retrospective study (Harare City), 290 TB patients were assessed for compliance with therapy by demographic characteristics (Armstrong & Pringle, 1984). Fifty-eight percent completed therapy, and 24% of the total were traced and recalled to therapy. Eighteen percent were lost to followup after defaulting. The default rate was highest in housewives, laborers, the unemployed, and children. Better-educated and higher income patients were more likely to complete therapy. The authors believed that a major reason for default was due to social pressures and urban-rural migration. The authors noted that all patients with spinal TB defaulted, possibly due to transport difficulties. Interpreting the findings is problematic due to a lack of a clear definition of compliance.

Another study examining patient characteristics in regard to compliance was carried out in Malaysia (Chuah, 1991). Of 227 patients beginning therapy during the study, 146 completed therapy without default. "Defaulting" was defined as needing reminders for recall to treatment, regardless of the outcome of those reminders. When compliant and noncompliant groups were compared, no significant differences were found between defaulters and nondefaulters in terms of age, ethnic origin, area of residence, personal history of TB, treatment regimen, distance from the hospital, or month of presentation. Significant differences were found in regard to sex (females were less likely to default than males); occupation (professionals, nonmanual workers, and supervisory manual workers were more compliant); and source of referral (hospital referrals were more likely to default as were those who began initial therapy in the hospital). The compliance rate was high for housewives (91%). Patients were more likely to default in the initial 2 months of therapy than later. This latter fact may help with planning of followup for other populations and sites. The definition used for defaulting was somewhat problematic in interpreting the results of this study.

In a study in Canada in the Mistassini Cree territory, all patients ($n = 65$) on INH preventative therapy between 1988 and 1991 were eligible to participate, as was a random sample ($n = 40$) of patients between 1981 and 1987 (Rideout & Menzies, 1994). Subjects completed a questionnaire, and charts were reviewed. Overall, 33.7% were judged compliant. Gender, age, influence of family/friends, clinic convenience, and knowledge of TB were not significantly related to compliance. When the compliant versus the non-compliant groups were compared in regard to alcohol consumption, 54% of the noncompliant group reported drinking either frequently or sometimes, compared with only 30% of the compliant group ($p < .05$). It was thought that emphasizing the risk of liver damage from combining alcohol and INH caused patients to give up the INH rather than the alcohol. Noncompliant subjects spent more time in the bush than did the compliant subjects ($p = .06$). Attitudes regarding TB and treatment were significantly different ($p < .05$) between the two groups. For example, 49% of the noncompliant patients believed their risk of getting TB without medication was low as compared with 29% of the compliant patients. There was a startling difference in compliance rates between the time periods when treatment was started. Of those treated in 1981 to 1985, 79% were judged compliant compared to 16% of those in 1986 to 1991 ($p < .0001$). It was hypothesized that the change from native community health workers to nonnative nurses in regard to responsibility for the preventive TB program influenced the significant difference. This might relate to the importance of shared cultural traditions and language between the practitioner and patient. Such results might be tested in other settings.

In a study conducted at Leeds Chest Clinic in Britain, TB patients were profiled in regard to compliance (Wardman et al., 1988). One hundred and thirteen patients were entered into the study, and compliance was assessed by urine testing. The patient brought the urine specimens to certain visits; the number per patient varied. Noncompliance was defined by one negative urine test for rifampin during the course of the treatment. Noncompliant patients (17%) were said to be more likely to come from social classes IV and V (implying lower class status for the noncompliers) ($p < .01$), were more likely to be of Asian extraction, and to have defaulted from at least one clinic appointment without good reason. The authors speculated that despite the provision of an interpreter at the study site, poor comprehension and communication may have been factors in noncompliance. A problem with the interpretation of this study involved the measurement of compliance.

In Ghana, factors influencing adherence were examined in two parts (van der Werf, Dade, & van der Mark, 1990). In the first part, 569 patients in an unsupervised TB program were identified as defaulters or not. Males had a significantly higher default rate than females (52.3% vs. 39.9%, $p < .01$) and a lower cure rate (42.8% vs. 53.0%, $p < .025$). Younger persons had significantly higher cure rates and lower default rates than older persons; however, the age ranges were not clear in the report. In some of the regions, longer home-to-clinic distances were significantly associated with higher default rates, but this was not true in regions where followup occurred. In the second part of the study, 49 patients were interviewed. The defaulting patients were no different than the compliant patients in regard to marital status, socioeconomic circumstances, travel time, expense, or drug effects. However, the researchers noted that more males were defaulters than females. There was a lack of detail about the interviews.

In Addis Ababa, Ethiopia, all retreatment patients were entered into the study to examine reasons for noncompletion of therapy (Teklu, 1984). Patients received education regarding the importance of regularly taking medication, TB, safe sputum disposal, and the importance of a healthy diet. During the study, 7,466 patients were seen and 460 (6%) were classified as defaulters. According to data from the questionnaires, reasons for default were: clinical improvement, sickness or death of relative or friend, lack of transportation or guide, other illness or injury, lost treatment card, work inconvenience, moved away, and other reasons. The author discussed the social and cultural aspects of the reasons. For example, some jealous husbands would not allow their wives to travel to the clinic. However, many of the reasons transcend specific cultures and social customs. The author suggested using the Kebele, a political association whose members have identity cards, to track down defaulters, and even the use of punitive measures, such as reducing food rations, if the person did not attend the clinic. Such measures would be unacceptable in the majority of societies.

Cases of TB in a setting in Scotland were studied retrospectively and prospectively between 1978 and 1987 (Ormerod & Prescott, 1991). Patients were assessed for compliance by the physician and by monthly reports of the health visitor that included pill counts as well as clinic attendance. Compliance was defined as ''good'' if assessments were satisfactory and all clinic appointments were kept; ''fair'' if one or two assessments were unfavorable or clinic appointments were missed; and ''poor'' if three or more assessments were unfavorable or clinic appointments were missed. Over the study period, 1074 patients had TB, but some were lost due to death or other reasons. One thousand nine patients comprised the final sample. Compliance was reported as significantly lower for those in the years 1978 to 1980, but the authors did not speculate on the possible reasons. Compliance was reported as significantly worse for Indian Subcontinent ethnic origin patients than those of White ethnic origin ($p = .02$). Compliance was best in those over 60 years of age and worst in young adults 15 to 29 years of age. Relapse was most common in the later groups. The authors believed that liaisons with TB nurses or visitors were useful in monitoring compliance and in identifying those at higher risk for relapse. A problem with this study lies in the overlapping of the criteria for compliance, the lack of specificity of number of clinic appointments, and the mixing of retrospective and prospective data.

MEDICAL AND CLINICAL APPOINTMENTS AND ATTENDANCE

Automated telephone reminders were used to remind patients of upcoming appointments. Tanke and Leirer (1994) studied 2,008 patients with scheduled appointments in one TB control program over a 6-month period (858 in the reactor clinic; 536 in the preventative therapy clinic, and 615 in the case clinic). Males comprised 54% of the sample. Subjects spoke Spanish (39%), Vietnamese (28%), Tagalog (6%), and English (14%). A quasiexperimental design was used with message conditions of *No Message Control, Basic Reminder, Reminder plus Authority Endorsement, Basic Reminder plus Importance Statement,* and *Basic Reminder plus Importance Statement plus Authority Endorsement.* The evening before the scheduled appointment, the appropriate prerecorded message was delivered to the patient. The message identified the health department, called the patient by name, indicated that the patient had an appointment the next day, and gave the address and phone number of the clinic in the patient's primary language. Attendance on days that reminders were sent was greater, but there were no significant differences across the message variations. Effectiveness also did not differ by patient age, sex, or ethnicity. This study appeared well designed and suggests that voice messaging can be effective in decreasing appointment defaulters.

EDUCATION AND MOTIVATION

A variety of researchers have examined the use of motivation, including the use of incentives and enablers, as well as education of patients, families, and/ or health care providers in improving adherence to TB therapy. Motivation was examined in Bangalore, India among 250 eligible patients over 12 years old with newly diagnosed TB (Seetha, Srikantaramu, Aneja, & Singh, 1981). Patients were assigned to the motivation group ($n = 140$) or the control group ($n = 95$). Motivation consisted of four home visits with the patient and adult family members; these visits included education about TB and its treatment and time for questions. Controls received no home visits. At the end of 12 months, specimens were collected and treatment adherence was assessed. Drug "collection," apparently the medications obtained for treatment, was said to be significantly better in the motivation group than in the control group, particularly during the first 3 months. In the motivation group, 59.9% had made all three collections versus 27.8% in the control group. Varying time periods for comparisons, variance in subclassifications of patient visit times, failure to exclude drug reaction impact, and other problems made this study rather hard to interpret.

In the United States, compliance was assessed for inmates taking INH prophylaxis at Rikers Island, a prison facility in New York (Alcabes et al., 1989). The 63 subjects resided in two different facilities: one in which access to the pharmacy was relatively easy and one in which access was limited.

Knowledge about TB and its treatment was assessed, and an educational session with printed information was provided. Compliance was quantified by the number of doses taken divided by the number available. Predictors of greater compliance included the location of the inmate and certain knowledge about TB and its treatment. In one building, the inmates had to be willing to disrupt their evening activities to get their medications; this was found to decrease compliance. Surprisingly, compliance was lower for subjects who knew the difference between tuberculous infection and tuberculosis. The results in this study were compatible with the literature regarding knowledge and with the need to make taking medication as least disruptive to activities as possible.

In a retrospective chart review, researchers examined the records of all patients on TB therapy from 1987 to 1988 in the TB clinic at a hospital in Montreal for compliance and associated factors (Menzies, Rocher, & Vissandjee, 1993). Patients were defined as noncompliant if they failed to return to the clinic after at least three reminders and total duration of uninterrupted treatment was at least 1 month less than originally prescribed or if the physician discontinued therapy because the patient was not taking medication. Of the 352 patients, 207 (59%) completed therapy. Of the 145 who were noncompliant, 45% were lost to followup; 56 patients stated they did not believe treatment was necessary, 13 patients believed they could not tolerate the medication, 5 patients found the medication or clinic to be inconvenient, and 5 patients were advised by another health professional that treatment was not necessary. The variables of age, gender, immigration status, and spoken language were not associated with compliance. The interval from initiation of therapy to the first followup visit was important, that is, those seen earlier were significantly more likely to complete therapy ($p < .001$). Nurses assessed patient understanding, and only 57% of those who were judged to have fair or poor understanding completed treatment, compared to 73% of those whose understanding was good ($p < .05$). Shorter duration of therapy (6 to 9 months) also was associated with completion. The authors identified several limitations, such as a retrospective study design, small number of patients with disease, and the use of clinic attendance as the compliance measure.

A study using motivation to study defaulting in children with tuberculous meningitis was conducted in Madras, India (Ramachandran & Prabhakar, 1992). Children between 1 and 12 years of age were consecutively admitted to three drug study groups and hospitalized for 2 months for treatment; however, due to death and other reasons, only 32 of the original 180 patients participated in the study. These patients' "attendants" were educated in simple language about TB, its treatment, possible outcomes, and the need for regular therapy. As part of the education they saw patients of varying degrees of illness in the hospital and clinic. Subsequent motivation, tailored to individual patients, was done periodically. The authors concluded that there was a 90% rate of clinic punctuality and of compliance. This study suffers from small sample size, lack of a control group, lack of information about the type, frequency, and conditions of the intervention (motivation) provided, and lack of detail about the actual measurement of compliance.

In India, 60 patients with TB were divided into two groups, one who received verbal and written information about isoniazid toxicity and one who did not (control group) (Gupta, Gupta, Purohit, Sharma, & Bhatnagar, 1992). In the first 8 weeks of therapy, default was greater from the control group. After this time, default was similar. Statistical significance was not reported. A defaulter was someone who collected less than 80% of his/her drugs. Defaulting for drug toxicity was less in the educated group during the first 8 weeks (one patient vs. six patients). This study suffers from lack of detail related to methods and analysis.

Another plan to improve compliance was developed by Hill and Ramachandran (1992). Over a 13-month period, adults with pulmonary TB in a section of India were able to elect to participate in the study. This required a prepayment, refundable after the course of treatment was complete, and allowed the patients to purchase their medications at a 60% discount from the hospital pharmacy. Patients who did not attend within 1 week of the date of their appointment were contacted once and lost the deposit if they did not comply. Of the 82 patients who enrolled, 62% completed their treatment, as compared with a retrospective rate of 23%. However, these results need to be interpreted with caution, because of the selection bias inherent in the design and the lack of a concurrent control group.

RESEARCH IN ADHERENCE RELATED TO DETECTION AND SCREENING

Screening and detection of TB allows early diagnosis of active TB, tracing of contacts of those with TB, and the institution of preventive therapy for those who have tuberculous infection and would benefit (Harriman & Cohen, 1995). Major issues in screening and detection programs are means to ensure the return of subjects who have had tuberculin skin testing for the reading and interpretation of the tests.

Returning for the reading of a tuberculin test during a TB detection drive at a university was examined in regard to commitment (Wurtele, Galanos, & Roberts, 1980). Subjects were randomly assigned to a control group ($n = 653$), a verbal commitment group ($n = 629$), or a verbal and written commitment group ($n = 664$). Those in the verbal commitment group were asked to give a verbal commitment to return in 48 hours for a test reading, while those in the verbal and written commitment group gave the verbal assurance and endorsed a printed contractual agreement as well. No significant differences among the groups were found in regard to race, sex, or family history of TB and compliance with returning to have the test read. Differences were found among the three groups in relation to compliance. Compliance was 69.8% for controls, 76.9% for the verbal commitment group, and 78.2% for the verbal and written commitment group ($p = .001$). For those with a family history of TB, the most effective way to ensure compliance was to use both verbal and written commitment. For those without a history, there was little difference in the commitment condition among compliers. This study was basically well designed and well implemented.

Another effort to increase return compliance in a university TB skin test screening drive consisted of two experiments (Roberts, Wurtele, & Leeper, 1983). First, subjects were randomly assigned to one of eight groups which were a combination of two types of authorities (expert vs. nonexpert) with four types of return reminders (take-home card, postcard, phone call, and person-to-person reminders). The expert was identified as a District Health Officer and the nonexpert was a female undergraduate. The message was the same for all reminders. The person-to-person reminder was made by verbal statement by either the expert or nonexpert as they finished the detection test. The rates of return ranged from 81.2% for the postcard to 88.6% for the person-to-person contact. No significant differences appeared between the expert and nonexpert groups, nor was there significance on any interaction or combination.

A second experiment randomly assigned subjects to one of 12 groups. Factors included messages on importance of returning (enhanced vs. standard), two types of reminders (take-home card vs. no card), and three types of commitment to return (no commitment, verbal, or written and verbal). The lowest rate (63.6%) of return was for the no commitment, no reminder, enhanced message group; the verbal commitment, no reminder, enhanced message group had a rate of 82.6%. Using log-linear analysis for the 553 subjects in this experiment, neither the main effects nor interactions were statistically significant. The authors explained the differences between this study and that of Wurtele et al. (1980) as possibly due to setting and situation. It was well designed; however, the mixing of genders with the messages may have influenced the results in an unknown way.

Using combination strategies among the homeless in San Francisco, Pilote and colleagues (1996) investigated strategies to increase adherence to a follow-up appointment at the TB clinic following PPD screening. Of the subjects who were screened, 244 were eligible based on having a positive PPD and agreed to participate. Subjects were randomly assigned to one of three groups, a peer health adviser group ($n = 83$), a monetary incentive group ($n = 82$), and a usual care group ($n = 79$). All subjects received bus tokens and specific physician assignments. Both the monetary incentive and the peer health adviser groups demonstrated significantly higher rates of attendance at the first clinic visit than did the usual care group (84% vs. 75% vs. 53%, respectively). Patient characteristics of not using intravenous drugs and 50 years of age or older were statistically significant predictors of adherence. The authors stated that generalizability may be limited, because subjects had already demonstrated motivation by participating and returning for screening test results, and because there might have been an effect even in the usual care group. The authors hypothesized that stressing the importance of follow-up appointments could have had an intervention effect. Nonetheless, the basic design of this study allowed some differentiation of effects, and showed that financial incentives may be needed to maximize adherence in the homeless group.

At the American Indian Health Service, Inc. (HIS), the return rates for reading of TB tests were considered to be "below average" (Boskovich, 1994). This researcher decided to increase opportunities for test readings by training community workers to read and report the positive tests. From October to December 1992, 68 patients were screened, with a return rate of 68% as compared with previous rates of 61% and 49%. The researcher was unable to demonstrate how much the return rate was related to the worker intervention.

Rates of return of tine test cards were examined in a community health center in Massachusetts with a predominately Hispanic population (Wiecha & Lim, 1994). Eligibility criteria for the study were children whose mother received prenatal care from the center, delivered by the center, and attended clinic visits for a minimum of 12 months after delivery. Between 1985 and 1987, 152 mother/child pairs met eligibility criteria. A tine test was performed on 64.5% by 1 year of age, and 16.3% had a tine card returned. However, 71 infants had a written tine result, and of these 78.9% did not have a card. It was not known how the results were obtained and recorded. The usual procedure is that the tine test is done, the results are recorded by the parent, and are returned by mail or in person to the clinic. No stamp was provided. Those who had a Medicaid-financed delivery were less likely to return a tine card than were the others. The authors speculated that barriers to returning cards were related to cost of postage, in addition to other possible factors. The small sample size was a limiting factor in this study. Another potential source of error was that the cards could have been lost from the charts, rather than not returned, since the results were recorded.

During a 1-year period from 1980 to 1981, patients in Korea were recruited to the study and were divided into an intensive and routine service group (Jin, Kim, Mori, & Shiman, 1993). In the intensive group, special motivation or supervision was given to the workers in these areas, and patients were assessed in regard to their knowledge of TB. Drug collection was the measure of compliance. Those patients under intensive motivation were said to be more regular in drug collection than the other group ($p = .01$).

MULTIPLE STRATEGIES

Other approaches to increasing adherence to the medical regimen are by the combination of strategies, for example, patient education combined with techniques such as incentives, motivation, contracting, and individual contributions. Motivation to increase compliance with the treatment regimen was evaluated by Shukla, Singh, Jain, Agarwal, and Singh (1983) among 150 TB patients in one department. Two groups were matched for age and sex. One group received "extra" motivation for 15 to 20 minutes at their visit, while the other received "routine" motivation. Overall, 32% completed treatment without defaulting. Multivariate analysis was used to compare caste, literacy, and status and nature of family, and extra motivation. Motivation, caste, literacy status and nature of family explained about 34.5% of the total variability. The authors stated that motivation accounted for about two-thirds of the total variability. The description of how some of the variables were defined was not included in this study and makes interpretation difficult.

A TB treatment program was designed for residents of a refugee camp on the Thai-Cambodian border (Miles & Maat, 1984). Fifty-eight patients ranging in age from 10 to 64 years with pulmonary TB received therapy. Before treatment, education about TB, its treatment, and the need to complete therapy were discussed with the patient and family. After this, the patient signed a contract, and copies of the contract and a daily treatment calendar were given to the clinic and the patient. To enhance compliance, drugs were given under direct supervision of a bilingual provider in a separate special clinic to avoid long waiting times seen in other clinics, and streptomycin by injection was included because of cultural beliefs surrounding injection. After medications were received, the calendar was initialed, entitling the patient to an extra hot meal. Patients not coming in the morning were contacted in an unknown way. Fifty-one of 55 surviving patients completed full therapy, a high rate of compliance. Because of the multimodal approach to increasing compliance, it is not possible to tell if any one single intervention was more important than others. The researchers used cultural beliefs, contracting, incentives, a convenient, accessible environment with a provider who spoke their language, and coupled these with a short, free medication regimen administered in a clinic using DOT. This study is hard to fully evaluate because of a lack of information in regard to some of the methods.

In one California site, 205 subjects who were to receive either preventive therapy ($n = 117$) or treatment for active TB ($n = 88$) were randomized to a special intervention or usual care group over a 17-month period (Morisky et al., 1990). The usual care group who missed clinic appointments were contacted by telephone, postcard, or home visit; however, after two consecutive missed appointments they were not followed up. The special intervention group received behaviorally oriented, individually tailored health education, written instructions, verbal reinforcement, contingency contracting, and incentives which varied from bus tokens to food coupons, and from movie tickets to cash. Written materials also were given, and translators for Korean and Spanish were available. Counseling followed each clinic visit for 5 to 10 minutes. Both groups completed a questionnaire and were urine-tested for INH. Compliance was assessed in terms of appointment-keeping, medication-taking, and treatment completion. Although no significant differences in regard to appointment-keeping were seen between the usual care and special intervention groups who were receiving therapy for active TB, there was a significant difference between the usual care and special intervention groups receiving preventive therapy (65% vs. 47%, $p = .003$). In regard to medication-taking, there was no significant difference between usual care and special intervention subjects (90% vs. 93%, respectively). Patients receiving preventive care showed a significant difference between the usual care and special intervention groups (38% vs. 68%, respectively). For the active TB group, there was no significant difference found between the usual care and special intervention groups for completion of treatment (8.9% vs. 2.3%, respectively). In the preventive group, the special intervention group showed a significantly higher rate of completing treatment difference between the special intervention and usual care groups (36.2% vs. 72.9%, $p = .001$). Further, as the authors noted, followup efforts from the clinic were not consistent, although protocols had been formulated. This demonstrates the critical need for constant examination of the protocol and the monitoring of progress to insure that the protocol is being followed correctly when conducting a study.

In Taipei County, Taiwan, TB treatment outcomes were investigated in regard to "cognition" or knowledge about TB, adherence in regard to keeping appointments, taking medications as prescribed and on time, and family functioning (Lee et al., 1993). Family functioning was measured by the Family APGAR (Smilkstein, 1978; Smilkstein, Ashworth, & Montano, 1982) questionnaire. Three hundred and ninety-seven persons with active pulmonary TB were eligible. For analysis, subjects were considered in one of three groups:

complete or cured, incomplete, and other. A great number of individual statistical analyses were performed. The Family APGAR score and the compliance score were significantly associated with TB treatment outcomes. Those with higher Family APGAR scores (> 20), indicating higher satisfaction, had a chance to complete treatment as high as 72 times greater than those whose scores were 20 or below. Those with compliance scores of more than 12, indicating greater compliance, had a 2.7 greater chance to complete treatment than those whose scores were lower. Family APGAR scores were the best predictor of the outcome of treatment. Demographic variables such as sex, age, education, marital status, and occupation were not significantly associated with the TB treatment outcome. Cognition appeared more important in examining therapy completion in women than for men. The quantity of data made this study difficult to evaluate. Somewhat questionable is the decision to combine the categories of those who completed treatment with those who were cured without providing further information.

In the Wardha district of India, 52 compliant and 50 noncompliant (defined as failure to take drugs for more than 15 days) patients participated in a project on TB control (Barnhoorn & Adriaanse, 1992). A large number of variables were examined in regard to compliance including income, type of house, residence, occupation of patient and head of house, caste, religion, type of fuel, education, sex, age, marital status, family size, beliefs about TB, symptoms, self-rated health status, medication knowledge, social support, health beliefs, and health provider-patient interaction. Adherent people had significantly greater knowledge of their treatment and symptoms than the nonadherent. Adherent patients were more likely to report support in taking drugs than the nonadherent (67% vs. 32%, respectively; $p = 0.00$). Compliant people demonstrated more control of their own health, perceived benefits of treatment, and tended to care for themselves by eating good foods, whereas noncompliers tended to pray to God for a cure. Monthly income and type of house also differentiated the compliant and noncompliant groups. Satisfaction with the health care provider contributed to continuing to take medications. Those who complied perceived more symptoms at onset, whereas more noncompliers perceived a worsened health status at the conclusion of the study. Personal demographic characteristics such as age, sex, marital status, family type, and family size were not significantly different between compliers and noncompliers. This study has a wealth of information on individual variables too numerous to describe here. The authors presented a model of factors affecting compliance in terms of demographic, socioeconomic, reinforcing, predisposing, and enabling factors that influence health beliefs. It included barriers and supports that act with health beliefs to influence compliance with TB medication.

SUMMARY AND FUTURE RESEARCH DIRECTIONS

Tuberculosis is a disease that can be treated and/or prevented. Yet cases of TB continue to exact a worldwide toll, and multidrug-resistant cases are increasing. A major factor in treatment difficulty appears to be patient adherence to the treatment regimen, particularly over a period long enough to cure. Over the years, a vast body of literature on adherence in general, and some related to TB, has accumulated. In TB, directly observed therapy has seemed to hold the greatest promise for adherence to therapy, but can be costly to initiate in the short term. Studies described here also indicated that this approach is not a foolproof one, and in some cultures or societies, issues of personal freedom may arise.

Relatively few studies related to adherence to TB therapy are grounded in theory or have a conceptual basis. Many focus on aspects of the medication regimen, such as the type of drug or the length of time over which it has been given. In regard to this, researchers have found that shorter term chemotherapy tends to result in a greater degree of adherence than longer regimens. However, if the regimen is too short it will not be effective, and this is one of the challenges facing drug developers. Many of the studies report confusing information, are not well controlled, are subject to bias, have confounding elements (such as studying self-administration vs. DOT but adding another parameter besides DOT to that group), compare two groups that are significantly different in demographic characteristics without statistical control, do not specify the content of their intervention, or have other problems.

The research reported in this chapter includes many studies conducted throughout the world. Because cultural factors and social conditions influence adherence, results from these studies will need to be considered in the context of the population of interest.

The literature reports varying results on how and if patient characteristics influence adherence to therapy. Sumartojo (1993) stated that these characteristics tend to be surrogates for other causal factors. Certainly some demographic characteristics are not amenable to alteration but can be considered in some program designs. Other themes that appear relevant across studies are those that make the environment for taking medications easy, accessible, and pleasant. Education, incentives, and enablers including social support at home all contribute to adherence in TB. Education should be targeted to specific behaviors and information and not just be global (Sumartojo, 1993). Personal beliefs about health and risk continue to be important. Thus programs that are tailored for their local populations and incorporate multidimensional treatment elements will probably be the most successful.

Certainly there is room for more well-designed and well-controlled studies in TB. Such studies should be derived from existing theory, attempt to have concurrent control groups, minimize overlapping variables, give clear and unambiguous definitions of adherence, use randomized samples, and use appropriate data analysis. If indicators of adherence could be consistent over a group of nursing studies, some data comparisons might then be possible. It is notable, in examining this body of literature, that there is a dearth of research related to adherence to therapy in TB that has been carried out by nurse researchers. Yet nursing approaches are very important in the ultimate successful treatment of patients with TB and their families. Thus, this is an area that should be an attractive one for future nursing research.

REFERENCES

Alcabes, P., Vossenas, P., Cohen, R., Braslow, C., Michaels, D., & Zoloth, S. (1989) Compliance with isoniazid prophylaxis in jail. *American Review of Respiratory Disease, 140*, 1194–1197.

Algerian Working Group/British Medical Research Council Cooperative Study. (1991). Short-course chemotherapy for pulmonary tuberculosis under routine programme conditions: a comparison of regiments of 28 and 36 weeks duration in Algeria. *Tubercle, 72*, 88–100.

Alwood, K., Keruly, J., Moore-Rice, K., Stanton, D. L., Chaulk, C. P., & Chaisson, R. E. (1994). Effectiveness of supervised, intermittent therapy for tuberculosis in HIV-infected patients. *AIDS, 8*, 1103–1108.

Armstrong, R. H., & Pringle, D. (1984). Compliance with anti-tuberculous chemotherapy in Harare City. *The Central African Journal of Medicare, 30*, 144–148.

Barnhoorn, F., & Adriaanse, H. (1992). In search of factors responsible for noncompliance among tuberculosis patients in Wardha District, India. *Social Science and Medicine, 34*, 291–306.

Bell, J., & Yach, D. (1988). Tuberculosis patient compliance in the western Cape, 1984. *South African Medical Journal, 73*, 31–33.

Biddulph, J., Mokela, D., & Sharma, S. (1987). Compliance of children with tuberculosis treated by short-course intensive chemotherapy. *Papua New Guinea Medical Journal, 30*, 159–164.

Bloom, B. R., & Murray, C. J. L. (1992). Tuberculosis: Commentary on a reemergent killer. *Science, 257*, 1055–1064.

Boskovich, S. J. (1994). New concepts in nursing management of the TB patient: A community training program. *Journal of Community Health Nursing, 11*, 45–49.

Boutotte, J., & Etkind, S. (1995). Community based strategies for tuberculosis control. In F. L. Cohen & J. D. Durham (Eds.), *Tuberculosis: A sourcebook for nursing practice* (pp. 177– 196). New York: Springer Publishing Co.

Brudney, K., & Dobkin, J. (1991). Resurgent tuberculosis in New York City. *American Review of Respiratory Disease, 144*, 745–749.

Buri, P. S., & Hathirat, S. (1987). A simple way to enhance compliance and reduce default in tuberculosis treatment. *Journal of the Medical Association of Thailand, 70*, 317–320.

Buri, P. S., Vathesatogkit, P., Charoenpan, P., Kiatboonsri, S., & Buranaratchada, S. (1985). A clinic model for a better tuberculosis treatment outcome and factors influencing compliance. *Journal of the Medical Association of Thailand, 68,* 356–360.

Centers for Disease Control & Prevention. (1993). Initial therapy for tuberculosis in the era of multi drug resistance. *Morbidity and Mortality Weekly Report, 42* (No. RR–11), 61–71.

Centers for Disease Control & Prevention. (1996). Tuberculosis morbidity: United States, 1996. *Morbidity and Mortality Weekly Report, 45*, 365–370.

Chaulk, C. P., Moore-Rice, K., Rizzo, R., & Chaisson, R. E. (1995). Eleven years of community-based directly observed therapy for tuberculosis. *Journal of the American Medical Association, 274*, 945–951.

Cheung, R., Dickins, J., Nicholson, P. W., Thomas, A. S. C., Smith, H. H., Larson, H. E., Deshmukh, A. A., Dobbs, R. J., & Dobbs, S. M. (1988). Compliance with anti-tuberculous therapy: A field trial of a pill-box with a concealed electronic recording device. *European Journal of Clinical Pharmacology, 35*, 401–407.

China Tuberculosis Control Collaboration. (1996). Results of directly observed short-course chemotherapy in 112,842 Chinese patients with smear-positive tuberculosis. *Lancet, 347*, 358–362.

Chuah, S. Y. (1991). Factors associated with poor patient compliance with antituberculosis therapy in Northwest Perak, Malaysia. *Tubercle, 72*, 261–264.

Chum, H. J., Imolelian, G., Rieder, H. L., Msangi, J., Mwinyi, N., Zwahlen, M., Enarson, D. A., & Ipuge, Y. A. (1995). Impact of the change from an injectable to a fully oral regimen on patient adherence to ambulatory tuberculosis treatment in Dar es Salaam, Tanzania. *Tubercle and Lung Disease, 76*, 286–289.

Cohen, F. L. (1995). The epidemiology of tuberculosis. In F. L. Cohen & J. D. Durham (Eds.), *Tuberculosis: A sourcebook for nursing practice* (pp. 29–51). New York: Springer Publishing Co.

Cohen, F. L., & Durham, J. D. (1995). Tuberculosis: An introduction. In F. L. Cohen & J. D. Durham (Eds.), *Tuberculosis: A sourcebook for nursing practice* (pp. 3–14). New York: Springer Publishing Co.

Combs, D. L., O'Brien, R. J., & Geiter, L. J. (1990). USPHS tuberculosis short-course chemotherapy trial 21: Effectiveness, toxicity, and acceptability. The report of final results. *Annals of Internal Medicine, 112*, 397–406.

Cuneo, W., & Snider, D. E. (1989). Enhancing patient compliance with tuberculosis therapy. *Clinics in Chest Medicine, 10*, 375–380.

Curtis, R., Friedman, S. R., Neaigus, A., Jose, B., Goldstein, M., & Des Jarlais, D. C. (1994). Implications of directly observed therapy in tuberculosis control measures among IDUs. *Public Health Reports, 109*, 319–327.

DeCock, K. M. (1996). Editorial: Tuberculosis control in resource-poor settings with high rates of HIV infection. *American Journal of Public Health, 86,* 1071–1073.

Elk, R., Schmitz, J., Spiga, R., Rhoades, H., Andres, R., & Grabowski, J. (1995). Behavioral treatment of cocaine-dependent pregnant women and TB-exposed patients. *Addictive Behaviors, 20*, 533–542.

Gentry, W. D. (Ed). (1984). *Handbook of behavioral medicine.* New York: Guilford.

Godfrey-Faussett, P., Baggaley, R., Mwinga, A., Hosp, M., Porter, J., Luo, N., Kelly, M., Msiska, R., & McAdam, K. (1995). Recruitment to a trial of tuberculosis preventive therapy from a voluntary HIV testing centre in Lusaka: Relevance to implementation. *Transactions of the Royal Society of Tropical Medicine and Hygiene, 89*, 354–358.

Gupta, P. R., Gupta, M. L., Purohit, S. D., Sharma, T. N., & Bhatnagar, M. (1992). Influence of prior information of drug toxicity on patient compliance. *Journal of the Association of Physicians of India, 40*, 181–183.

Harriman, C., & Cohen, G. L. (1995). Screening for tuberculosis: An important prevention tool. In F. L. Cohen & J. D. Durham (Eds.), *Tuberculosis: A sourcebook for nursing practice* (pp. 139–156). New York: Springer Publishing Co.

Hill, J. P., & Ramachandran, G. (1992). A simple scheme to improve compliance in patients taking tuberculosis medication. *Tropical Doctor, 22*, 161–163.

Hong Kong Chest Service/British Medical Research Council. (1984). Study of a fully supervised programme of chemotherapy for pulmonary tuberculosis given once weekly in the continuation phase in the rural areas of Hong Kong. *Tubercle, 65*, 5–15.

Hong Kong Chest Service/British Medical Research Council. (1989). Acceptability, compliance, and adverse reactions when isoniazid, rifampin, and pyrazinamide are given as a combined formulation or separately during three-times-weekly antituberculosis chemotherapy. *American Review of Respiratory Disease, 140*, 1618–1622.

Iseman, M. D., Cohn, D. L., & Sbarbaro, J. A. (1993). Directly observed treatment of tuberculosis: We can't afford not to try it. *The New England Journal of Medicine, 328*, 576–578.

Janz, N. K., & Becker, M. H. (1984). The health belief model: A decade later. *Health Education Quarterly, 11*, 1–47.

Jin, B. W., Kim, S. C., Mori, T., & Shiman, T. (1993). The impact of intensified supervisory activities on tuberculosis treatment. *Tubercle and Lung Disease, 74*, 267–272.

Joseph, S. (1993). Editorial: Tuberculosis, again. *American Journal of Public Health, 83*, 647–648.

Kan, G., Zhang, L., Wu, J., Ma, Z., Liu, C., & Sun, F. (1985). Supervised intermittent chemotherapy for pulmonary tuberculosis in a rural area of China. *Tubercle, 66*, 1–7.

Kimerling, M. E., & Petri, L. (1995). Tracing as part of tuberculosis control in a rural Cambodian district during 1992. *Tubercle and Lung Disease, 76*, 156–159.

Klein, S. J., & Naizby, B. E. (1995). New linkages for tuberculosis prevention and control in New York City: Innovative use of non-traditional providers to enhance completion of therapy. *Journal of Community Health, 20*, 5–13.

Krishnaswami, K. V., Somasundaram, P. R., Tripathy, S. P., Vaidyanathan, B., Radhan-krishna, S., & Fox, W. (1981). A randomised study of two policies for managing default in out-patients collecting supplies of drugs for pulmonary tuberculosis in a large city in south India. *Tubercle, 61*, 103–112.

Lange, R. A., Ulmer, R. A., & Weiss, D. J. (1986). An intervention to improve compliance to year-long isoniazid (INH) therapy for tuberculosis. *The Journal of Compliance in Health Care, 1*, 47–54.

Lee, L.-T., Chen, C.-J., Suo, J., Chen, S.-C., Chen, C.-Y., & Lin, R.-S. (1993). Family factors affecting the outcome of tuberculosis treatment in Taiwan. *Journal of the Formosa Medical Association, 92*, 1049–1056.

Madsen, L., & Cohen, F. L. (1995). Medical treatment of tuberculosis. In F. L. Cohen & J. D. Durham (Eds.), *Tuberculosis: A sourcebook for nursing practice* (pp. 67–97). New York: Springer Publishing Co.

McDonald, S. J., & Ma, M. (1987). Identifying compliance incentives for screening and treatment of tuberculosis. *Journal of Community Health Nursing, 4*, 131–143.

McDonald, R. J., Memon, A. M., & Reichman, L. B. (1982). Successful supervised ambulatory management of tuberculosis treatment failures. *Annals of Internal Medicine, 96*, 297–302.

Menzies, R., Rocher, I., & Vissandjee, B. (1993). Factors associated with compliance in treatment of tuberculosis. *Tubercle and Lung Disease, 74*, 32–37.

Miles, S. H., & Maat, R. B. (1984). A successful supervised outpatient short-course tuberculosis treatment program in an open refugee camp on the Thai-Cambodian border. *American Review of Respiratory Disease, 130*, 827–830.

Morisky, D. E., Malotte, C. K., Choi, P., Davidson, P., Rigler, S., Sugland, B., & Langer, M. (1990). A patient education program to improve adherence rates with antituberculosis drug regimens. *Health Education Quarterly, 17*, 253–267.

Moulding, T., Onstad, G. D., & Sbarbaro, J. A. (1970). Supervision of outpatient drug therapy with the medication monitor. *Annals of Internal Medicine, 73*, 559–564.

Nazar-Stewart, V., & Nolan, C. M. (1992). Results of a directly observed intermittent isoniazid preventive therapy program in a shelter for homeless men. *American Review of Respiratory Disease, 146*, 57–60.

Ormerod, L. P., & Prescott, R. J. (1991). Inter-relations between relapses, drug regimens and compliance with treatment in tuberculosis. *Respiratory Medicine, 85*, 239–242.

Pilote, L., Tulsky, J. P., Zolopa, A. R., Hahn, J. A., Schecter, G. F., & Moss, A. R. (1996). Tuberculosis prophylaxis in the homeless: A trial to improve adherence to referral. *Archives of Internal Medicine, 156*, 161–165.

Pozsik, C. J. (1993). Compliance with tuberculosis therapy. *Medical Clinics of North America, 77*, 1289–1301.

Ramachandran, P., & Prabhakar, R. (1992). Defaults, defaulter action and retrieval of patients during studies on tuberculous meningitis in children. *Tubercle and Lung Disease, 73*, 170–173.

Reichman, L. B. (1991). The U-shaped curve of concern. *American Review of Respiratory Disease, 144*, 741–742.

Rideout, M., & Menzies, R. (1994). Factors affecting compliance with preventive treatment for tuberculosis at Mistassini Lake, Quebec, Canada. *Clinical Investigative Medicine, 17,* 31-36.

Roberts, M. C., Wurtele, S. K., & Leeper, J. D. (1983). Experiments to increase return in a medical screening drive: Two futile attempts to apply theory to practice. *Social Science and Medicine, 17,* 741–746.

Sanmarti, L. S., Megias, J. A., Gomez, M. N. A., Soler, J. C., Alcala, E. N., Puigbo, M. R. S., & Majem, L. S. (1993). Evaluation of the efficacy of health education on the compliance with antituberculosis chemoprophylaxis in school children: A randomized clinical trial. *Tubercle and Lung Disease, 74,* 28–31.

Sbarbaro, J. A. (1990). The patient-physician relationship: Compliance revisited. *Annals of Allergy, 64,* 325–330.

Schluger, N., Ciotoli, C., Cohen, D., Johnson, H., & Rom, W. N. (1995). Comprehensive tuberculosis control for patients at high risk for noncompliance. *American Journal of Respiratory and Critical Care Medicine, 151,* 1486–1490.

Seetha, M. A., Srikantaramu, N., Aneja, K. S., & Singh, H. (1981). Influence of motivation of patients and their family members on the drug collection by patients. *Indian Journal of Tuberculosis, 26,* 182–190.

Shukla, R., Singh, G., Jain, S. K., Agarwal, R. C., & Singh, M. (1983). Impact of extra motivation among tuberculosis patients on the duration of their unbroken drug continuity—A multivariate approach. *Indian Journal of Medical Sciences, 37*(2), 23–28.

Smilkstein, G. (1978). The Family APGAR: A proposal for a family function test and its use by physicians. *Journal of Family Practice, 6,* 1231–1239.

Smilkstein, G., Ashworth, C., & Montano, D. (1982). Validity and reliability of the Family APGAR as a test of family function. *Journal of Family Practice, 15,* 303–311.

Snider, D. E., Jr., & Hutton, M. D. (1989). *Improving patient compliance in tuberculosis treatment programs.* Atlanta: Centers for Disease Control.

Sudre, P., ten Dam, G., & Kochi, A. (1992). Tuberculosis: A global overview of the situation today. *Bulletin of the World Health Association, 70,* 149–159.

Sumartojo, E. (1993). When tuberculosis treatment fails: A social behavioral account of patient adherence. *American Review of Respiratory Diseases, 147,* 1311–1320.

Sumartojo, E. (1995). Adherence to the tuberculosis treatment plan. In F. L. Cohen & J. D. Durham (Eds.), *Tuberculosis: A sourcebook for nursing practice* (pp. 121–136). New York: Springer Publishing Co.

Tanke, E. D., & Leirer, V. O. (1994). Automated telephone reminders in tuberculosis care. *Medical Care, 32,* 380–389.

Teklu, B. (1984). Reasons for failure in treatment of pulmonary tuberculosis in Ethiopians. *Tubercle, 65,* 17–21.

Valeza, F. S., & McDougall, A. C. (1990). Blister calendar packs for treatment of tuberculosis. *The Lancet, 335,* 473.

van der Werf, T. S., Dade, G. K., & van der Mark, T. W. (1990). Patient compliance with tuberculosis treatment in Ghana: Factors influencing adherence to therapy in a rural service programme. *Tubercle, 71,* 247–252.

Wardman, A. G., Knox, A. J., Muers, M. F., & Page, R. L. (1988). Profiles of noncompliance with antituberculous therapy. *British Journal of Diseases of the Chest, 82,* 285–289.

Weis, S. E., Slocum, P. C., Blais, F. X., King, B., Nunn, M., Matney, G. B., Gomez, E., & Foreman, B. H. (1994). The effect of directly observed therapy on the rates of drug resistance and relapse in tuberculosis. *The New England Journal of Medicine, 330,* 1179–1184.

Wiecha, J. M., & Lim, M. (1994). Tine test cards for TB screening: Rates of return and associated factors. *Family Practice Research Journal, 14,* 51–57.

Wilkinson, D. (1994). High-compliance tuberculosis treatment programme in a rural community. *Lancet, 343,* 647–648.

Wobeser, W., To, T., & Hoeppner, V. H. (1989). The outcome of chemoprophylaxis on tuberculosis prevention in the Canadian Plains Indian. *Clinical and Investigative Medicine, 12,* 149–153.

Wurtele, S. K., Galanos, A. N., & Roberts, M. C. (1980). Increasing return compliance in a tuberculosis detection drive. *Journal of Behavioral Medicine, 3,* 311–318.

Research on Nursing Care Delivery

PART II

Research on Transitional
Care Delivery

Chapter 8

Health Promotion and Disease Prevention in the Worksite

SALLY LECHLITNER LUSK

SCHOOL OF NURSING

UNIVERSITY OF MICHIGAN

ABSTRACT

U.S. and Canadian research studies ($n = 73$) on health promotion/disease prevention programs in the worksite reported from 1990 through 1994 were reviewed
for this chapter. In those studies, diverse intervention foci were provided and
outcomes specific to the foci, as well as numerous additional outcomes, cost
and cost benefit being the most common, were measured. To aid future researchers, two appendices list reports by foci of intervention and by outcomes measured.
Deficiencies and inadequacies in reports and studies are described. Nearly all
(68 out of 73) of the published studies obtained positive results in terms of
benefiting health or reducing costs. The Johnson & Johnson LIVE FOR LIFE
Program® is presented as an exemplar of a comprehensive, multifaceted, worksite health promotion/disease prevention program whose effects were consistently assessed. Although health promotion and prevention of disease has always
been an important component of nursing practice, few reports included nurse
scientists as authors or coauthors. Potential explanations for the limited involvement by nurse scientists and recommendations regarding future research directions are presented. The worksite remains the best place to promote improved
health for adults and this area of research represents an opportunity for greater
involvement by nurse scientists.

Keywords: Health Promotion Interventions, Worksite Health Promotion:
Worksite Program Foci, Worksite Program Outcomes, Costs and Benefits
of Worksite Programs

This chapter includes a review of the research on health promotion/disease prevention programs in the worksite. The studies included are those conducted in the United States and Canada reported from 1990 through 1994 in which researchers measured the effect of an intervention delivered to workers to promote health or prevent disease, excluding interventions specific to occupational exposures or diseases. Analysis of studies on prevention of occupational illnesses or injuries requires a separate chapter. It was not a requirement that nurses were involved in the studies as investigators or authors, and in fact, very few of the reports identified nurses as authors or contributors. In addition to reporting on the desired effect of the program, many researchers also reported cost savings or cost-benefit analyses.

The review conducted for this chapter began with the studies ($n = 48$) identified by Pelletier (1991, 1993); the reader is referred to these two reports for details of the studies. In his previous review article, Pelletier (1991) stated that the studies selected for review were those of "comprehensive health promotion programs," but did not define this term (p. 311). His 1993 review, although purporting to be an update of the 1991 review, included studies of programs which would not logically be classified as worksite comprehensive health promotion programs because they dealt with narrowly focused interventions, e.g., an arthritis self-management program which was delivered to residents of five counties, not necessarily workers (Lorig, Mazonson, & Holman, 1993). In order to be more comprehensive, this review was expanded to include studies from 1990 to 1994. These were obtained through searches of a number of databases: MCAT (The University of Michigan Library Catalog, including medical, public health, and occupational health literature); Psychological Abstracts; CINAHL (Cumulative Index to Nursing and Allied Health Literature); MEDLINE; and Wilson's General Periodicals Database. The following keywords were used: health promotion studies, worksite prevention programs, wellness programs, disease prevention, risk reduction, health education, worksite health education, patient education interventions, occupational health programs, health care costs, and stress reduction. Manual review of several journals, *Journal of Occupational Medicine*, *American Journal of Public Health*, and *American Journal of Health Promotion* for 1994 yielded a number of articles that were not yet in the computer databases, and a few more were found through an ancestry approach. The ancestry approach yielded an additional 49 reports of studies of worksite health promotion or disease prevention interventions. These additional studies, including several published in nursing journals but not reported by Pelletier, and the studies included in Pelletier's articles (1991, 1993) that reported effects of an intervention and were published after 1989, comprised the body of literature for this review for a total of 73 studies. These are the studies classified according to foci of interventions and the outcomes measured (see Appendixes A and B).

The review conducted for this chapter had several limitations:

1. *Only published studies were included.* Many corporations offer health promotion/disease prevention programs and evaluate their effects, but their reports may be published only internally. Additionally, of those studies submitted for publication, those with positive results may be more likely to be accepted.

2. *The topic is broad.* Health promotion/disease prevention programs are designed to influence a large variety of behaviors, with the commonality being that the programs were offered to employees, or retirees. Thus, the conclusions will be based on a broad overview, resulting in general recommendations.

3. *All published studies may not have been included.* Even though a number of databases were searched, a few additional articles were identified through an ancestry approach, and even more were found through a manual search of the 1994 journals most likely to publish worksite health promotion studies.

This chapter includes five major parts. First, health promotion is defined and its history and application in the worksite are traced. Next, the foci of the interventions delivered in the worksite and of the outcome measures used to evaluate their effects, including cost data, are summarized for studies reported in the last 5 years. An exemplary worksite health promotion program is then described and critiqued. Next, major deficiencies in reports or studies and nursing's involvement in this area of research are reviewed. Finally, recommendations regarding future directions for research on worksite health promotion/disease prevention programs are made.

HEALTH PROMOTION

Definition of Health Promotion

Identifying health promotion studies is not a clear-cut task; no universally agreed-upon definition of health promotion programs exists. For the purposes of this review, health promotion programs are those designed to promote health or reduce illness-producing behavior. Thus, workplace health promotion and disease prevention encompass a large and diverse body of programs offered to retirees, employees, and employees' families.

History of Health Promotion

In the United States, the national emphasis on health promotion dates to the mid-1970s with the preparation of the *Healthy People: Surgeon General's Report on Health Promotion and Disease* (USDHEW, 1979). This was followed in 1980 (USDHHS) by the publication of the first national objectives, *Promoting Health/Preventing Disease: Objectives for the Nation*. This initiative grew out of the recognition that approximately one-half of premature deaths could be prevented by lifestyle changes. Previously, efforts to reduce deaths had been focused on community-wide efforts to improve sanitation and prevent infectious disease through immunizations. These efforts were very successful, but by the 1970s, offered little more margin for change. Thus, national attention shifted to changing individuals' behaviors; for adults, the logical place to offer programs to promote healthy behaviors and lifestyle changes was in the workplace.

Worksite Health Promotion

In 1985 and again in 1992, The Office of Disease Prevention and Health Promotion conducted a survey of worksite health promotion activities (United States Department of Health and Human Services [USDHHS], 1993). It was targeted to private worksites with 50 or more employees and was designed to measure progress toward the worksite objectives included in *Healthy People 2000*. The survey questionnaire classified activities in the worksite into four main types: policies, screening, information or activities, and facilities or services. Results indicated an increase in health promotion activities in the worksite. From 1985 to 1992, more worksite programs were offered on nutrition, weight control, physical fitness, high blood pressure, and stress management, and programs on back care and smoking cessation remained at about the same level. Of worksites with 50 or more employees, 81% offered at least one health promotion activity, in comparison with 66% in 1985. There were differences by size of worksite: 99% of those with 750 or more employees offered a program; 75% with 50 to 99 employees offered a program. However, it should be noted that a worksite offering one smoking cessation class was classified as offering a health promotion activity.

Although the large proportions are impressive, one should view these statistics with caution: (a) offering a single health promotion activity is of limited benefit; (b) no data were reported regarding programs for public employees or small worksites; and (c) there was no attempt to define essential components of comprehensive programs or activities, or to determine the percent of worksites with comprehensive programs. Based on experiential data, a small proportion of worksites offer comprehensive health promotion/disease prevention programs.

Interestingly, the 1992 survey was the first to obtain data on information or activities directed toward the prevention of job hazards and injuries, with 64% of worksites reporting information or activities in this area. A few occupational health specialists have recommended the integration of worksite health promotion/disease prevention programs with such prevention programs (Cohen, 1987; Lusk, 1992a, 1993); however, the federal goals are separate and distinct goals by disease category and by occupational disease and hazards. Lost in the second paragraph of narrative following goals 10–12 on worker health and safety programs are the benefits of offering health promotion programs in the workplace, but the integration of these programs with occupational health and safety programs is not suggested. To be most effective, health promotion and illness and injury prevention services should be combined in an integrated program, one that is coordinated with other community-based services (Lusk, 1992a, 1993). It is well documented that lifestyle factors account for 50% or more of premature deaths and that adopting healthier lifestyles will extend healthy years of life (USDHEW, 1979). Adults need facilitation to make these changes, and the worksite is the best place to access adults to provide health promotion. Adults spend the majority of their waking hours at work, and the worksite offers an opportunity to work with groups of adults. In addition, Cohen (1987) suggested that the approaches and objectives of health promotion programs can enhance occupational health and safety programs, offering three illustrations:

a. improvement of lifestyle can lower the risk of certain job hazards, e.g., smoking and occupational respiratory disorders, drinking and workplace accidents, and poor fitness and musculoskeletal stress in lifting;

b. emphasis on self-care in health promotion programs can translate to increased self-protection against workplace hazards; and

c. several of the 10 leading work-related disorders, namely, cancer, lung disease, traumatic injury, cardiovascular disease and psychological disorders, would probably be impacted by reducing behavioral risk factors through health promotion programs.

Changing lifestyles of the 110 million people in the workplace will have a significant impact on illness and its costs. For example, smoking-related illnesses cost more than $65 billion each year; avoiding one intervention, coronary bypass surgeries, would save approximately $9 billion each year (USDHHS, 1991).

Although there may be inconsistencies in defining health promotion, it is clear that such programs are increasingly offered in the worksite. Their goals typically include decreasing high-risk behavior and increasing health-promoting behavior. Those programs focusing on changing workers' lifestyles have generally not been integrated with occupational health and safety programs, even though a synergistic effect could accrue; no reports of effects of integrated programs were found. Thus, this review includes only those studies that reported the effect of an intervention delivered to employees to promote health or prevent nonoccupational disease.

STATUS OF RESEARCH

Pelletier (1991, 1993) summarized the research conducted in the worksite on health promotion/disease prevention programs. Pelletier indicated that 24 studies evaluating such programs were published from 1980 to 1991 and an additional 24 studies were published from 1991 and early 1993. However, he did not describe the process used for identifying the articles or the specific selection criteria for inclusion in his review; therefore, his work should be cautiously used as a source.

Foci of the Interventions

The foci of interventions and the studies addressing them are listed in Appendix A. In comparing the foci of these studies of health promotion programs with the worksite health promotion activities reported in the USDHHS survey (1993)—exercise/fitness and smoking cessation—the most frequently reported programs in the USDHHS survey were also among the most frequent research topics. However, although approximately one-third of the worksites in the USDHHS survey reported programs in stress management, alcohol/drugs, and back care, fewer research studies with those foci were found.

Some programs were referred to as comprehensive health promotion programs, but the components of each program varied slightly from one study to another. Therefore, rather than categorizing studies as comprehensive, the individual components included in those programs have been tallied separately in Appendix A. The foci most frequently occurring were those most likely to be included in a program identified as comprehensive.

In addition to the multiple and diverse content areas of the foci of the interventions, there were also studies that tested the method of delivery of health promotion programs, that is, mobile programs (Aldana, Jacobson, Harris, & Kelley, 1993; Aldana, Jacobson, Harris, Kelley, & Stone, 1993) and programs by mail (Bertera, Oehl, & Telepchak, 1990; Fries, Bloch, Harrington, Richardson, & Beck, 1993; Leigh et al., 1992). Further, a Health Risk Assessment or Appraisal (HRA), a structured assessment of risks, lifestyles, and behaviors, was identified as the intervention, or one of the interventions, in 13 studies. In these cases, the interventions reported to have been delivered as a result of the Health Risk Assessment were incorporated in Appendix A. One of the studies included in Pelletier's review (1993) measured the effect of a computerized medical claims record system (Burton, Hoy, & Stephens, 1991), but this study was excluded from this review because it did not measure the effect of an intervention delivered to persons.

Outcomes Measured

From considering the outcome measures used (Appendix B), it is apparent that these programs were intended to achieve multiple and diverse purposes. For example, in one study assessing a back injury program (Shi, 1993a) the investigator measured changes in health risk appraisal scores and employee satisfaction, as well as the prevalence of back injury or pain, workers' compensation and medical claims, and sick day costs related to back injuries. As can be noted by viewing Appendices A and B, outcomes specific to the foci were not necessarily measured in each study. Often foci would be included as part of a comprehensive health promotion program, but the outcome measured would be costs, absenteeism, or disability. Another example is stress management, which was often offered as part of comprehensive health promotion programs, but an outcome specific to stress was measured infrequently. It also should be noted these same studies measured the effect of an intervention and the mode of delivery of the intervention, for example, mailed information, or the participation rates in the program. To further complicate matters, one study's intervention (use of an HRA for counseling workers) was another's outcome measure (with the HRA used to contrast scores before and after an intervention). Worksite programs, more than those in any other setting, frequently measure program cost, cost-effectiveness, and medical care and claims costs. Other measures also have cost implications, such as absenteeism, injuries, disability, and turnover.

Cost-Benefit of Health Promotion Programs

A number of authors have expressed concern about reports of cost savings from offering health promotion programs in the worksite (O'Donnell, 1988; Pelletier, 1993; Warner, Wickizer, Wolfe, Schildroth, & Samuelson, 1988). Warner and colleagues (1988) carefully delineated the cost factors that are not usually included in any measurement of cost-benefit analysis of health promotion programs, such as increased costs due to the greater number of years of expenditures and greater demands for health care by the elderly resulting from increased participant longevity. Nonetheless, it is common for studies of worksite health promotion programs to report cost savings or a cost-benefit analysis. In fact, of the 24 studies analyzed in Pelletier's most recent review (1993), all but 4 reported on some aspects of costs. In this regard, although the economic analyses are likely flawed because they do not consider all potential cost factors (Lusk, 1992b) worksite studies are in the vanguard, as more researchers attempt to determine the costs and benefits of school, community, and hospital-based programs.

It is not difficult to understand the financial motivation of corporations in providing health promotion programs. According to *Business Week* (Flynn & Garland, 1993), the nation's health care costs were expected to exceed $889 billion for 1993, a 63% increase since 1988, with employers paying 51.7% of the total. Continued increases will absorb all corporate profits. Clearly, it is in the best interest of the employer to reduce health care costs. In *The Healthy Company: Eight Strategies to Develop People, Productivity and Profits* (Rosen, 1991), the author quotes Dick Wardrop of Alcoa Corporation: "If my employees are healthier than yours, I'm going to whip you. It's as simple as that" (p. 201).

Despite such clear corporate impetus to provide health promotion programs, it is interesting to note, as Pelletier (1993) reported in his review, that 47 of the 48 published studies included in his two reviews (Pelletier, 1991, 1993) attained positive results in terms of benefiting health, and when measured, attained positive cost-benefit analyses. In the additional 40 studies identified for the present review, only 4 failed to report positive results in terms of the outcomes measured. To sum, only 5 of the 73 studies included in this review did not obtain positive results. Although manuscript selection may be biased in favor of those with positive cost-benefit analyses, it is clear that a variety of behaviors were addressed, using diverse approaches to change behavior and to measure behavioral and economic outcomes of the programs. These results suggest that health promotion programs in the worksite are effective in changing behaviors that contribute to illness and premature death, and should be continued.

EXEMPLAR PROGRAM

A chapter could easily be, and probably should be, written for each of the many program foci of worksite health promotion/disease prevention programs.

Thus, this chapter will describe and critique one comprehensive worksite health promotion program: the Johnson & Johnson's LIVE FOR LIFE Program®, and critique two of the reports of its effects as exemplars of the research conducted on worksite programs.

LIVE FOR LIFE Program®

This early and comprehensive program, LIVE FOR LIFE® (LFL), is recognized as a leader; its effects have been reported in at least 10 publications. In 1979, the program was offered to 2,000 employees at three locations and, by 1982, had been extended to 16,000 employees at 22 locations (Wilbur, 1983). By 1987, the program had been implemented in so many of the Johnson & Johnson company sites that control sites were not generally available (Breslow, Fielding, Hermann, & Wilbur, 1990). Program goals were: (a) to provide the means for Johnson & Johnson employees to become among the healthiest in the world; and (b) to determine the degree to which LFL was cost-beneficial (Wilbur, 1983).

LFL has six main components:

1.   A health screening offered on company time, incorporating a lifestyle and attitudes questionnaire, measures of blood pressure, blood lipid levels, body fat, height, weight, and estimated oxygen uptake.

2.   A 3-hour Lifestyle Seminar, given on company time, to share results of testing, emphasize personal responsibility for health, and to make employees aware of the health enhancement programs offered by the company.

3.   LFL Action Programs include formal programs on smoking cessation, weight control, stress management, nutrition, exercise, and high blood pressure control. A variety of formats are used: groups, individual consultation, self-help kits, and telephone consultations or counseling.

4.   LFL shorter educational and health promoting programs encompass breast self-examination, biofeedback, nutrition, blood pressure, and, for smokers, carbon monoxide analysis.

5.   LFL efforts to sustain participation include company leaders promoting participation; incentives, feedback, and prizes; feedback to company leaders on the programs' performance; regular followup by phone or mail of program participants; a rotation of program leaders after 1 year; and a permanent program administrator.

6.   A healthful environment is created, including shower and exercise facilities; scales in restrooms; nutrition information where food is sold; nutritious food in cafeteria and vending machines; treatment and referral services for troubled employees; management training programs to improve supervisor-

employee relations; flextime; carpooling; self-administered blood pressure equipment; a clearly stated smoking policy and "thank you for not smoking" signs; LFL recruitment brochures; newsletters and bulletin boards; and a health fair (Wilbur, 1983).

A quasiexperimental design was used to evaluate the program. Epidemiological and economic datasets were created and merged. Outcomes measured include effects of the program on risk factors, health behaviors, cost savings, and morale (Breslow et al., 1990). Reports on results related to two of the outcomes will be described in more detail and critiqued.

Smoking cessation results.   Shipley, Orleans, and Wilbur (1988) reported the effect of LFL on employee smoking. Seven Johnson & Johnson companies in one geographic area participated, with four receiving the complete LFL program and three receiving only the health screening (HSO). The health screening received by both groups included a lifestyle questionnaire with questions on smoking status and history; lifestyle practices and attitudes; a measurement of blood pressure, blood lipid levels, body fat, height, weight, and estimated oxygen uptake; and provision of related health education by a registered nurse. In addition, those in the LFL program companies received the comprehensive 6-point program of services previously described. The activities specific to smoking were part of a multicomponent behavioral quit-smoking clinic with three phases: preparation for quitting (four sessions); quitting (five sessions); and maintenance (five sessions). Groups were led by "health professionals" (specific background was not identified) following detailed leader and participant manuals. Smoking behavior was measured by questions on the lifestyle questionnaire and by blood thiocyanate (SCN) at baseline and at a 2-year followup. At LFL companies, 22.6% of all smokers quit for a mean abstinence period of 14.8 months; 17.6% of smokers at HSO companies quit for a mean abstinence period of 12.3 months. In comparing results for smokers at high risk for cardiovascular disease, the LFL program was more successful than the HSO program (32% versus 12.9% quit rates).

Although there were serious limitations, specifically nonequivalent baseline comparability of the experimental and control groups, minimal participation in the smoking cessation clinic, and problems with the measurement of SCN, this study obtained very impressive quit rates. However, in looking at the smokers' behaviors, only 20.7% of the smokers did participate in at least one session of the smoking clinic, with heavy smokers participating at a higher rate (29.4%). Forty-one percent of smoking clinic enrollees (48% of those who quit smoking) also enrolled in other programs, such as stress management, exercise, and weight loss, but only 6% of the LFL smokers who did not participate in the smoking clinic enrolled in other programs. Thus, participation in other health promotion programs contributed to smoking cessation, and smokers who participated in the smoking clinic also participated in more health promotion programs. Although these results support a comprehensive approach that deals not only with the health/illness aspects of smoking, but also with other health promotion activities and environmental supports, it would have been useful to know in which of the other health promotion programs smokers enrolled.

In addition to the limitations previously described, this study's failure to analyze the effect of the amount of smoking clinic participation is of concern. An employee was defined as a participant if he or she attended at least one of the 14 sessions. Particularly in light of this corporation's interest in cost-benefit data, it would have been valuable to know more regarding the dose-response effect of clinic sessions. Further, there was insufficient information provided regarding the content and process used by health professionals in the smoking clinics. No mention was made of training for the health professionals, or of assessment of inter-intervenor reliability.

Morale results.   Although a few other studies have reported worker attitudes, the LFL program was unique in its early attention to effects of the health promotion program on morale. Holzbach et al. (1990) assessed the effect of the LFL program on work-related attitudes during the same time period and using the same methods previously described in the smoking study. Employees' attitudes in the participating sites (LFL) became significantly more favorable than those of employees at the HSO sites. Six scales assessed attitudes: organizational commitment, job involvement, growth opportunity, supervision, working conditions, and job competence. Four single items measured respect from family and friends, relations with coworkers, pay and fringe benefits, and job security. Baseline, year 1, and year 2 data were obtained from 63% of LFL ($n = 1019$) and 71% of HSO ($n = 586$) continuously employed workers. Three change scores were used in the analyses: change from baseline to year 1, change from baseline to year 2, and overall change from baseline to year 2 (year 2 plus year 1, divided by 2 minus baseline). At LFL sites, significant and positive change scores for all three time periods were seen for organizational commitment, supervision, working conditions, pay and fringe benefits, and job security, with improvement in job competence attitudes at year 1 and overall, and in relations with coworkers at year 1 only. (Baseline scores and demographic characteristics, gender, age, and job classification were used as control variables.) LFL sites showed significant positive effects on organizational commitment and working conditions among all employees, with significant effects on other attitude measures only in selected demographic groups. Among the sites for both the LFL and HSO programs there were significant differences in some attitude measure scores.

In this study, the authors also reported participation in three LFL activities—stress management, weight control, and smoking cessation—and its effect on attitude scores. In comparison with HSO sites, nonparticipants in LFL activities had significantly higher scores on organizational commitment and job competence. LFL participants and nonparticipants had significantly higher scores than HSO employees on working conditions and job security. Because there were significant positive changes in attitudes for nonparticipants in LFL activities, the authors postulate that these results indicate that the LFL program affected the underlying values and influenced the culture of participating sites. This conclusion may be correct, but the LFL program was in itself not sufficient to positively influence the climate at all four sites, as one of the sites actually had a decrease in employee attitudes at year 2 on four of the measures.

In contrast with the study of the effects of LFL's smoking cessation program (Shipley et al., 1988), where the participation in specific health promotion programs was not reported, these authors did identify the effect of participation in specific programs on attitude scores, which is a strength of this study. A major weakness of the study was the poor reliability of two of the measures of attitudes, that is, job involvement ($\alpha = .53$) and job competence ($\alpha = .49$), but this was not discussed in the report. Also, as noted, four of the attitudes were measured by single items.

Other LFL Programs

In addition to the two studies reviewed here, the LFL program has demonstrated a positive effect on exercise, physical fitness, weight reduction/control, blood pressure, absenteeism, seat-belt use, and reductions in health care costs and utilization (Breslow, 1990). Even though alcohol use, nutrition, and stress management were program components, these were not included in the summary of findings of the LFL program. No rationale for their exclusion was given.

Reports of studies of the LFL programs evidenced a number of strengths and weaknesses. The following section summarizes the deficiencies found in the 73 studies reported during 1990 through 1994.

CRITIQUE OF WORKSITE
HEALTH PROMOTION PROGRAMS

Deficiencies of Studies

In considering all of the studies identified for this review of worksite health promotion programs, it is apparent that there are a number of problems or inadequacies with the design, implementation, or reporting of the research studies. Control or comparison groups were often a problem, with a number of studies having no control groups and others reporting the use of nonequivalent comparison groups. Because treatment and control group assignment is often done by worksite and there are often differences between worksites, it is difficult to obtain equivalent comparison groups. For example, Johnson & Johnson discontinued their quasiexperimental evaluation of its LIVE FOR LIFE Program® because, once it was implemented in nearly all the corporation's worksites, there were no comparison groups available.

Only 2 of the 73 studies reviewed identified a theoretical model as a basis for their intervention: social learning theory (Shi, 1992) and transtheoretical model of change (Prochaska et al., 1992). But even in these, no information was provided regarding precisely how the theoretical model was translated into an intervention. In addition, one study used the PRECEDE model as a framework for planning and program development (Bertera, 1990a). Eight other reports made vague references regarding the philosophy underlying their approaches, such as behavior modification techniques: specifically, reinforcement (Anderson, Mavis, Robison, & Stoffelmayr, 1993), social engineering (Golaszewski et al., 1992), and "theory-based strategies" (Hunt et al., 1993).

Nearly all of the reports reviewed stated as their purpose the evaluation of program effectiveness in terms of changes in behavior, risk factors, or medical costs. Presented as rationale for the studies was the extent of the problem, such as the incidence and prevalence of heart disease for those dealing with preventing that condition, a few cited objectives in *Healthy People 2000* as the rationale.

Although some reports contained a fair amount of information about the process used to deliver the intervention and the specific content of the intervention, most of the information was inadequate to either understand how the intervention was accomplished or to replicate the studies. In most cases, however, there was a clear and appropriate relationship between the intervention and the outcome measures.

The evaluation period in the studies varied from a short 2 weeks to assess an incentive program (Jasheway & Sirota, 1993) to 8 years for a comprehensive health promotion program (Conrad et al., 1990). In the Indiana Blue Cross/Blue Shield "Alive and Well" program, which ran up to 8 years, there were significantly fewer absentee hours for participants than nonparticipants, demonstrating a sustained effect over a long time. The typical evaluation period for the studies was 1 to 2 years with a sizable number evaluating after a 4- or 5-year period.

Selection bias is operative in most of the studies which involved self-selection of subjects into health promotion programs. For example, the nonparticipant group in the Indiana Blue Cross/Blue Shield Study consisted of workers who had resisted participating in a single health promotion program over the 8 years of the program's existence. There may well have been other factors operating in the decision not to participate which would influence results. For example, are these "hard-core" nonparticipants those with physical disabilities or medical conditions that preclude or deter their participation while simultaneously contributing to greater absenteeism from work? Most studies have not attempted to try to obtain data regarding differences in the health status of comparison groups and intervention groups, or to consistently adjust for differences in health status that may have affected participation, level of participation, or continuation in health promotion programs. However, a number of studies reported adjustments in results of outcome measures by baseline measures, gender, and age groups.

The reports often do not contain enough information about the content of the intervention to be able to judge its appropriateness or replicate the study. For example, in the report of the smoking cessation program in Johnson & Johnson' s LFL, the developers of the intervention were identified and the number of sessions (14) and the general purpose of the sessions were stated; however, no information regarding the specific content, theoretical bases, or style of presentation of the individual sessions was given.

With the DuPont program (Bertera, 1990a) as a notable exception, only a few of the studies reported using an assessment of the needs of their employee group to design interventions to be offered in the worksite. While needs assessments are an essential prerequisite to program planning, these may well also influence the eventual effect found for the interventions. If an intervention is offered that is not related to the needs of the workers, there may be low participation and little effect.

Nursing's Involvement in Studies

A review of the research on worksite health promotion/disease prevention programs published since 1989 and Pelletier's work (1991, 1993) suggests there is room for a great deal of growth in the future of nursing research in this area. Since health education and prevention of disease has always been an important component of nursing practice, studies by nurse scientists would have been expected. Yet in Pelletier's reviews there were no articles whose first authors were identified as nurses, and only two where a nurse was a coauthor. It is possible, of course, that the RN designation could have been omitted from the listing and only the academic credentials used, but from reviewing the location of authors, that did not appear to be the case. Despite this absence from Pelletier's reviews, in the searches completed for this chapter five reports with nurses as first authors and three reports with nurses as coauthors were found.

There are a number of likely reasons for the dearth of representation of nurse scientists: (a) few nurses with doctoral degrees are practicing in the occupational setting; (b) few nurse scientists in academic settings are prepared in occupational health or focusing on worksite research; (c) although this is changing, the majority of corporations have not seen research as part of the role of occupational health nurses (Lusk, 1990; Lusk, Disch, & Barkauskas, 1988); (d) because most occupational health nurses have not been prepared for research, it is easy for the physicians and behavioral scientists to see worksite research as their province; (e) corporate programs are typically administered by physicians; and (f) some corporations contract with research firms for evaluation—for example, Johnson & Johnson contracted with Research Triangle Institute—and these firms may not employ nurse scientists. These factors are all amenable to change. Nurse scientists in academic settings would do well to align themselves with occupational health nurses in the worksite to collect data regarding programs they are implementing. Since many practicing occupational health nurses have not been prepared to conduct research, this arena is ripe for collaboration benefiting both the academician and the practitioner.

RECOMMENDATIONS REGARDING RESEARCH DIRECTIONS

Based on the critique of the studies for this chapter, several recommendations can be made for future research in this area. First, inasmuch as is possible, equivalent control groups should be used, or when they are not, greater efforts should be devoted to using statistical techniques to adjust for differential characteristics. Statistical treatment is recommended over instituting intervention and control treatments in the same worksite because it is very likely that diffusion of the intervention will occur. Further, due to the priority placed on production and profits, as opposed to research, random assignment to treatments is typically not possible (Lusk & Kerr, 1994).

Second, indication of a theoretical basis for design and selection of the intervention(s) would strengthen study design and facilitate synthesis of results, thereby contributing to more rapid building of a research base for interventions.

Third, reports of research need to provide more complete and detailed information regarding the content and process used in the intervention. No study reported assessing inter-intervenor reliability, and few described the preparation and training of intervenors.

Fourth, to achieve the most benefit, multiple-foci health promotion programs should be offered, as several studies reported carryover effects on change in a specific behavior from participation in programs directed toward changing another behavior. Further, although no studies of integrated health promotion and occupational health and safety programs were reported, there is rationale to support their synergistic effects, and they should be effected and evaluated.

Fifth, nurse scientists have a contribution to make to this area of research and could increase their involvement by linking with occupational health nurses practicing in the worksite to conduct studies of programs. Corporations, increasingly interested in documenting the effects of their programs, especially in regard to cost containment, may even provide limited financial support for such research.

Sixth, as previously noted, few programs determined their foci based upon an assessment of the needs of their employee group. Programs should be based on the characteristics and interests of the recipients, as the programs will be better received and achieve greater success.

Seventh, the evaluation period should be long enough to reasonably expect change in behavior or biological measures, with periodic measures to document effects and recidivism. Much more information is needed regarding interventions necessary to maintain the desired effects.

SUMMARY

A great deal of research has been reported on worksite health promotion, most commonly not conducted by nurses. Results of the studies supported offering programs in the worksite to reduce risk behaviors, encourage self-care, and promote health. In the instances where cost or cost-benefit analyses were done, positive results were obtained, but in most cases the calculations of the benefits probably did not include costs associated with long-term outcomes. Meeting the health goals expressed in *Healthy People 2000* (USDHHS, 1991) will require an expansion of workplace health promotion activities. The worksite remains the best place to access adults, and employers are motivated to improve the health of workers to obtain benefits in productivity and health care costs.

ACKNOWLEDGMENTS

The author gratefully acknowledges the assistance of Alice Horn with searches and manuscript preparation and of Leslie Martel Baer in reviewing the manuscript.

REFERENCES

Aldana, S. G., Jacobson, B. H., Harris, C. J., & Kelley, P. L. (1993a). Mobile work site health promotion programs can reduce selected employee health risks. *Journal of Occupational Medicine, 35,* 922–928.

Aldana, S. G., Jacobson, B. H., Harris, C. J., Kelley, P. L., & Stone, W. J. (1993b). Influence of a mobile worksite health promotion program on health care costs. *American Journal of Preventive Medicine, 9,* 378–383.

Aldana, S. G., Jacobson, B. H., Kelley, P. L., & Quirk, M. (1994). The effectiveness of a mobile worksite health promotion program in lowering employee health risk. *American Journal of Health Promotion, 8,* 254–256.

Anderson, J. V., Mavis, B. E., Robison, J. I., & Stoffelmayr, B. E. (1993). A worksite weight management program to reinforce behavior. *Journal of Occupational Medicine, 35,* 800–804.

Baer, J. T. (1993). Improved plasma cholesterol levels in men after a nutrition education program at the worksite. *Journal of the American Dietetic Association, 93,* 658–663.

Barr, J. K., & Warshaw, L. J. (1994). Worksite AIDS education: A case study of the New York City police. *AIDS Education and Prevention, 6,* 53–64.

Bertera, R. (1990a). Planning and implementing health promotion in the workplace: A case study of the DuPont company experience. *Health Education Quarterly, 17,* 307–327.

Bertera, R. (1990b). The effects of workplace health promotion on absenteeism and employment costs in a large industrial population. *American Journal of Health Promotion, 80,* 1101–1105.

Bertera, R. L. (1993). Behavioral risk factor and illness day changes with workplace health promotion: Two-year results. *American Journal of Health Promotion, 7,* 365–373.

Bertera, R., Oehl, L., & Telepchak, J. (1990). Self-help versus group approaches to smoking cessation in the workplace: Eighteen-month follow-up and cost analysis. *American Journal of Health Promotion, 4,* 187–192.

Breslow, L., Fielding, J., Herrmann, A. A., & Wilbur, C. S. (1990). Worksite health promotion: Its evolution and the Johnson & Johnson experience. *Preventive Medicine, 19,* 13–21.

Brigham, J., Gross, J., Stitzer, M. L., & Felch, L. J. (1994). Effects of a restricted work-site smoking policy on employees who smoke. *American Journal of Public Health, 84,* 773–778.

Briley, M. E., & Montgomery, D. H. (1992). Worksite nutrition education can lower total cholesterol levels and promote weight loss among police department employees. *Journal of the American Dietetic Association, 92,* 1382–1384.

Burton, W., Erickson, D., & Briones, J. (1991). Women's health programs at the workplace. *Journal of Occupational Medicine, 33,* 349–350.

Burton, W., Hoy, D., & Stephens, M. (1991). A computer-assisted health care cost management system. *Journal of Occupational Medicine, 33,* 268–271.

Burton, W. D., & Conti, D. J. (1991). Value-managed mental health benefits. *Journal of Occupational Medicine, 33*, 311–313.

Cohen, A. (1987). Perspectives on self-protective behaviors and work place hazards. In N. D. Weinstein (Ed.), *In taking care: Understanding and encouraging self-protective behavior* (pp. 298–322). Cambridge, England: Cambridge University Press.

Cohen, R., & Mrtek, M. B. (1994). The impact of two corporate lactation programs on the incidence and duration of breast-feeding by employed mothers. *American Journal of Health Promotion, 8*, 436–441.

Conrad, K. M., Riedel, J. E., & Gibbs, J. O. (1990). Effect of worksite health promotion programs on employee absenteeism. *American Association of Occupational Health Nurses Journal, 38*, 573–580.

Ellis, E., Koblin, W., Irvine, M. J., Legare, J., & Logan, A. G. (1994). Small, blue collar work site hypertension screening: A cost-effectiveness study. *Journal of Occupational Medicine, 36*, 346–355.

Erfurt, J., Foote, A., & Heirich, M. (1991a). The cost-effectiveness of work-site wellness programs for hypertension control, weight loss, and smoking cessation. *Journal of Occupational Medicine, 33*, 962–970.

Erfurt, J., Foote, A., & Heirich, M. (1991b). Worksite wellness programs: Incremental comparison of screening and referral alone, health education, follow-up counseling, and plant organization. *American Journal of Health Promotion, 5*, 438–448.

Erfurt, J., Foote, A., Heirich, M., & Gregg, W. (1990). Improving participation in worksite wellness programs: Comparing health education classes, a menu approach, and follow-up counseling. *American Journal of Health Promotion, 4*, 270–278.

Falvo, D. R., & Tippy, P. K. (1993). Comparison of interventions to increase asymptomatic women's use of mammography screening. *Health Values: The Journal of Health Behavior Education and Promotion, 17*, 12–17.

Fielding, J. E., Knight, K., Mason, T., Klesges, R. C., & Pelletier, K. R. (1994). Evaluation of the IMPACT blood pressure program. *Journal of Occupational Medicine, 36*, 743–746.

Fisher, E. B., Bishop, D. B., Levitt-Gilmour, T., Cappello, M. T., Ashenberg, Z. S., & Newman, E. (1994). Social support in worksite smoking cessation: Qualitative analysis of the EASE project. *American Journal of Health Promotion, 9*, 39–47, 75.

Flynn, J., & Garland, S. (1993, January 11). The final option: Radical surgery. *Business Week*, p. 95.

Foote, A., & Erfurt, J. (1991). The benefit to cost ratio of work-site blood pressure control programs. *Journal of the American Medical Association, 265*, 1283–1286.

Fries, J. F., Bloch, D. A., Harrington, H., Richardson, N., & Beck, R. (1993). Two-year results of a randomized controlled trial of a health promotion program in a retiree population: The Bank of America. *The American Journal of Medicine, 94*, 455–462.

Fries, J., Fries, S., Parcell, C., & Harrington, H. (1992). Health risk changes with a low-cost individualized health promotion program: Effects at up to 30 months. *American Journal of Health Promotion, 6*, 364–371.

Fries, J. F., Harrington, H., Edwards, R., Kent, L. A., & Richardson, N. (1994). Randomized control trial of cost reductions from a health education program: The California public employees' retirement system (PERS) study. *The American Journal of Medicine, 8,* 216–223.

Gleason-Comstock, J., Lando, H. A., McGovern, P., Pirie, P., & Rooney, B. (1994). Promotion of worksite smoking policy in two Minnesota communities. *American Journal of Health Promotion, 9,* 24–27.

Goetzel, R., Sepulveda, M., Knight, K., Eisen, M., Wade, S., Wong, J., & Fielding, J. (1994). Association of IBM's "A Plan For Life" health promotion program with changes in employees' health risk status. *Journal of Occupational Medicine, 36,* 1005–1009.

Golaszewski, T., Snow, D., Lynch, W., Yen, L., & Solomita, D. (1992). A benefit-to-cost analysis of a worksite health promotion program. *Journal of Occupational Medicine, 34,* 1164–1172.

Gomel, M., Oldenburg, B., Simpson, J. M., & Owen, N. (1993). Work-site risk reduction: A randomized trial of health risk assessment, education, counseling, and incentives. *American Journal of Public Health, 83,* 1231–1238.

Harrell, J. S., Cornetto, A. D., & Stutts, W. C. (1992). Cardiovascular risk factors in textile workers. *American Association of Occupational Health Nurses Journal, 40,* 581–589.

Hartman, T. J., McCarthy, P. R., & Himes, J. H. (1993). Use of eating-pattern messages to evaluate changes in eating behaviors in a worksite cholesterol education program. *Journal of The American Dietetic Association, 93,* 1119–1123.

Harvey, M., Whitmer, R., Hilyer, J., & Brown, K. (1993). The impact of a comprehensive medical benefits cost management program for the city of Birmingham: Results at five years. *American Journal of Health Promotion, 7,* 296–304.

Heirich, M. A., Foote, A., Erfurt, J. C., & Konopka, B. (1993). Work-site physical fitness programs. *Journal of Occupational Medicine, 35,* 510–517.

Henritze, J., Brammell, H., & McGloin, J. (1992). LIFECHECK: A successful, low touch, low tech, in-plant, cardiovascular disease risk identification and modification program. *American Journal of Health Promotion, 7,* 129–136.

Herbert, J., Harris., D., Sorensen, G., Stoddard, A., Hunt, M., & Morris, D. (1993). A worksite nutrition intervention: Its effects on the consumption of cancer-related nutrients. *American Journal of Public Health, 83,* 391–394.

Holzbach, R., Piserchia, P. V., McFadden, D. W., Hartwell, T. D., Herrmann, A., & Fielding, J. E. (1990). Effect of a comprehensive health promotion program on employee attitudes. *Journal of Occupational Medicine, 32,* 973–978.

Hunt, M. K., Herbert, J. R., Sorensen, G., Harris, D. R., Hsieh, J., Morris, D. H., & Stoddard, A. M. (1993). Impact of worksite cancer prevention program on eating patterns of workers. *Journal of Nutrition Education, 25,* 236–243.

Jasheway, L. A., & Sirota, H. (1993). Challenging employees to health: An incentive contest approach. *American Journal of Health Promotion, 7,* 165–166.

Jeffery, R., Forster, J., French, S., Kelder, S., Lando, H., McGovern, P., Jacobs, D., & Baxter, J. (1993a). The healthy worker project: A work-site intervention for weight control and smoking cessation. *American Journal of Public Health, 83,* 395–401.

Jeffery, R. W., Forster, J. L., Dunn, B. V., French, S. A., McGovern, P. G., & Lando, H. A. (1993b). Effects of work-site health promotion on illness-related absenteeism. *Journal of Occupational Medicine, 35,* 1142–1146.

Jeffery, R. W., Kelder, S. H., Forster, J. L., French, S. A., Lando, H. A., & Baxter, J. E. (1994). Restrictive smoking policies in the workplace: Effects on smoking prevalence and cigarette consumption. *Preventive Medicine, 23,* 78–82.

Jones, R. C., Bly, J. L., & Richardson, J. E. (1990). A study of a work site health promotion program and absenteeism. *Journal of Occupational Medicine, 32,* 95–99.

Kingery, P. M., Ellsworth, C. G., Corbett, B. S., Bowden, R. G., & Brizzolara, J. A. (1994). A closer look at the case for work-site health promotion. *Journal of Occupational Medicine, 36,* 1341–1347.

Kishchuk, N., Peter, C., Towers, A. M., Sylvestre, M., Bourgault, C., & Richard, L. (1994). Formative and effectiveness evaluation of a worksite program promoting health alcohol consumption. *American Journal of Health Promotion, 8,* 353–362.

Knight, K. K., Goetzel, R. Z., Fielding, J. E., Eisen, M., Jackson, G. W., Kahr, T. Y., Kenny, G. M., Wade, S. W., & Duann, S. (1994). An evaluation of Duke University's LIVE FOR LIVE® health promotion program on changes in worker absenteeism. *Journal of Occupational Medicine, 36,* 533–536.

Kurtz, M. E., Kurtz, J. C., Given, B., & Given, C. C. (1994). Promotion of breast cancer screening in a work site population. *Health Care for Women International, 15,* 31–42.

Larsen, P., & Simons, N. (1993). Evaluating a federal health and fitness program. *American Association of Occupational Health Nurses Journal, 41,* 143–148.

Leigh, J., & Fries, J. (1992). Health habits, health care use and costs in a sample of retirees. *Inquiry, 29,* 44–54.

Leigh, J., Richardson, N., Beck, R., Kerr, C., Harrington, H., Parcell, C. L., & Fries, J. F. (1992). Randomized controlled study of a retiree health promotion program: The Bank of America study. *Archives of Internal Medicine, 152,* 1201–1206.

Lorig, K., Mazonson., P., & Holman, H. (1993). Evidence suggesting that health education for self-management in patients with chronic arthritis has sustained health benefits while reducing health care costs. *Arthritis and Rheumatism, 36,* 439–446.

Lusk, S. L. (1990). Corporate expectations for OHN activities. *American Association of Occupational Health Nurses Journal, 38,* 368–374.

Lusk, S. L. (1992a, November). *Preventing injury and illness and promoting health in the workplace.* Paper presented at the National Center for Nursing Research Conference on Research Priorities for Nursing Practice, Bethesda, MD.

Lusk, S. L. (1992b). Selling health promotion programs: Recommendations for occupational health nurses. *American Association of Occupational Health Nurses Journal, 40,* 414–418.

Lusk, S. L. (1993, December). *Integrated services to prevent injury and illness and to promote health in the workplace.* Paper presented at the National Institute of Nursing Research Priority Expert Panel on Community-Based Models, Rockville, MD.

Lusk, S. L., Disch, J. M., & Barkauskas, V. H. (1988). Interest of major corporations in expanded practice of occupational health nurses. *Research in Nursing & Health, 11,* 141–151.

Lusk, S. L., & Kerr, M. J. (1994). Conducting worksite research: Methodological issues and suggested approaches. *American Association of Occupational Health Nurses Journal, 42,* 177–181.

Lynch, W. D., Gilfillan, L. A., Jennet, C., & McGloin, J. (1993). Health risks and health insurance claims costs. *Journal of Occupational Medicine, 35,* 28–33.

Lynch, W. D., Golaszewski, T. J., Clearie, A. F., Snow, D., & Vickery, D. M. (1990). Impact of a facility-based corporate fitness program on the number of absences from work due to illness. *Journal of Occupational Medicine, 32,* 9–12.

Mayer, J. A., Jones, J. A., Eckhardt, L. E., Haliday, J., Bartholomew, S., Slymen, D. J., & Hovell, M. F. (1993). Evaluation of a worksite mammography program. *American Journal of Preventive Medicine, 9,* 244–249.

O'Donnell, M. P. (1988). View point: Cost benefit analysis is not cost effective. *American Journal of Health Promotion, 3,* 74–75.

O'Hara, P., Gerace, T. A., & Elliott, L. L. (1993). Effectiveness of self-help smoking cessation guides for firefighters. *Journal of Occupational Medicine, 35,* 795–799.

Pelletier, K. A. (1991). A review and analysis of the health and cost-effective outcome studies of comprehensive health promotion and disease prevention programs. *American Journal of Health Promotion, 5,* 311–313.

Pelletier, K. R. (1993). A review and analysis of the health and cost-effective outcome studies of comprehensive health promotion and disease prevention programs at the worksite: 1991–1993 Update. *American Journal of Health Promotion, 8,* 50–62.

Prochaska, J. O., Norcross, J. C., Fowler, J. L., Follick, M. J., & Abrams, D. B. (1992). Attendance and outcome in a work site weight control program: Processes and stages of change as process and predictor variables. *Addictive Behaviors, 17,* 35–45.

Pruitt, R. H. (1992). Effectiveness and cost efficiency of interventions in health promotion. *Journal of Advanced Nursing, 17,* 926–932.

Pruitt, R. H., Bernheim, C., & Tomlinson, J. P. (1991). Stress management in a military health promotion program: Effectiveness and cost efficiency. *Military Medicine, 156,* 51–53.

Rosen, R. (1991). *The healthy company: Eight strategies to develop people, productivity, and profits.* Los Angeles: Tarcher.

Salina, D., Jason, L. A., Hedeker, D., Kaufman, J., Lesondak, L., McMahon, S. D., Taylor, S., & Kimball, P. (1994). A follow-up of a media-based, worksite smoking cessation program. *American Journal of Community Psychology, 22,* 257–271.

Sciacca, J., Seehafa, R., Reed, R., & Mulvaney, D. (1993). The impact of participation in health promotion on medical costs: A reconsideration of the Blue Cross and Blue Shield of Indiana Study. *American Journal of Health Promotion, 7,* 374–384.

Sheeshka, J. D., & Woolcott, D. M. (1994). An evaluation of a theory-based demonstration worksite nutrition promotion program. *American Journal of Health Promotion, 8,* 253, 263–264.

Shi, L. (1992). The impact of increasing intensity of health promotion intervention on risk reduction. *Evaluation and the Health Professions, 15*, 3–25.

Shi, L. (1993a). A cost-benefit analysis of a California county's back injury prevention program. *Public Health Reports, 108*, 204–211.

Shi, L. (1993b). Worksite health promotion and changes in medical care use and sick days. *Health Values: The Journal of Health Behavior Education and Promotion, 17*, 9–17.

Shi, L. (1993c). Health promotion, medical care use, and costs in a sample of worksite employees. *Evaluation Review, 17*, 475–487.

Shipley, R., Orleans, C., & Wilbur, C. (1988). Effects of the Johnson & Johnson Live for Life Program on employee smoking. *Preventive Medicine, 17*, 475–482.

Sorensen, G., Lando, H., & Pechacek, T. F. (1993). Promoting smoking cessation at the workplace. *Journal of Occupational Medicine, 35*, 121–126.

Sorensen, G., Morris, D., Hunt., M., Herbert, J. R., Harris, D. R., Stoddard, A., & Oekene, J. K. (1992). Work-site nutrition intervention and employees' dietary habits: The Treatwell Program. *American Journal of Public Health, 82*, 877–880.

Towers, A. M., Kishchuk, N., Sylvestre, M., Peters, C., & Sourgault. (1994). A qualitative investigation of organizational issues in an alcohol awareness program for blue-collar workers. *American Journal of Health Promotion, 1*, 56–63.

U.S. Department of Health, Education, and Welfare, Public Health Service. (1979). *Healthy People: The Surgeon General's report on health promotion and disease prevention* (DHEW Publication No. 79–55071). Washington, DC: U.S. Government Printing Office.

U.S. Department of Health and Human Services, Public Health Service. (1980). *Promoting health/Preventing disease: Objectives for the nation.* Washington, DC: U.S. Government Printing Office.

U.S. Department of Health and Human Services, Public Health Service. (1991). *Healthy People 2000: National health promotion and disease prevention objectives* (DHHS Publication No. PHS91–50212). Washington, DC: U.S. Government Printing Office.

U.S. Department of Health and Human Services, Public Health Service. (1993). 1992 National survey of worksite health promotion activities: Summary. *American Journal of Health Promotion, 7*, 452–464.

Warner, K. E., Wickizer, T. M., Wolfe, R. A., Schildroth, J. E., & Samuelson, M. H. (1988). Economic implications of workplace health promotion programs: Review of the literature. *Journal of Occupational Medicine, 30*, 106–112.

Wheat, J. R., Graney, M. J., Shachtman, R. H., Ginn, G. L., Patrick, D. L., & Hulka, B. S. (1992). Does workplace health promotion decrease medical claims? *American Journal of Preventive Medicine, 8*, 110–114.

Whitmer, R. (1992). The city of Birmingham's wellness partnership contains medical costs. *Business & Health, 10*(4), 60–66.

Wilbur, C. S. (1983). The Johnson & Johnson program. *Preventive Medicine, 12*, 672–681.

Wilson, M., Edmunson, J., & DeJoy, D. (1992). Cost-effectiveness of work-site cholesterol screening and intervention programs. *Journal of Occupational Medicine, 34,* 642–649.

Zwerling, C., & Ryan, J. (1992). Pre-employment drug screening: The epidemiological issues. *Journal of Occupational Medicine, 34,* 595–599.

APPENDIX A:

FOCI OF PROGRAMS

Alcohol Use: Fries, Fries, Parcell, & Harrington, 1992; Herbert et al., 1993; Holzbach et al., 1990; Kischuk et al., 1994; Leigh & Fries, 1992; Shi, 1992, 1993b.

Assertiveness Training/Self-Esteem Enhancement: Aldana et al., 1993a, 1993b.

Back Injury Prevention: Bertera, 1990b; Conrad, Riedel, & Gibbs, 1990; Harvey et al., 1993; Shi, 1993a; Wheat et al., 1992; Whitmer, 1992.

Blood Pressure Control: Aldana et al., 1993a; Aldana et al., 1993b; Aldana, Jacobson, Kelley, & Quirk, 1994; Bertera, 1990b; Bertera, 1993; Conrad et al., 1990; Ellis, Koblin, Irvine, Legare, & Logan, 1994; Erfurt et al., 1990; Erfurt, Foote, & Heirich, 1991a, 1991b; Fielding, Knight, Mason, Klesges, & Pelletier, 1994; Foote & Erfurt, 1991; Gomel, Oldenburg, Simpson, & Owen, 1993; Harrell, Cornetto, & Stutts, 1992; Harvey et al., 1993; Henritze, Brammell, & McGloin, 1992; Holzbach et al., 1990; Jones, Bly, & Richardson, 1990; Knight et al., 1994; Pruitt, 1992; Shi, 1992, 1993b; Wheat et al., 1992; Whitmer, 1992.

Cancer Screening, Awareness, and Risk Prevention: Bertera, 1990b, 1993; Conrad et al., 1990; Wheat et al., 1992.

Case Management: Shi, 1993b.

CPR Classes: Wheat et al., 1992.

Drug Screening: Zwerling & Ryan, 1992.

Employee Assistance Program: Burton & Conti, 1991.

Environmental/Policy Changes: Bertera, 1993; Brigham, Gross, Stitzer, & Felch, 1994; Erfurt et al., 1990; Gleason-Comstock, Lando, McGovern, Pirie, & Rooney, 1994b; Jeffery et al., 1994; Shi, 1992, 1993b.

Exercise/Fitness: Aldana et al., 1993a, 1993b, 1994; Bertera, 1990a, 1990b, 1993; Conrad et al., 1990; Fries et al., 1992; Golaszewski, Snow, Lynch, Yen, & Sdomita, 1992; Harvey et al., 1993; Heirich, Foote, Erfurt, & Konopka, 1993; Henritze et al., 1992; Holzbach et al., 1990; Jones et al., 1990; Knight et al., 1994; Lynch, Golaszewski, Clearie, Snow, & Vickery, 1990; Sciacca, Seehafa, Reed, & Mulvaney, 1993; Shi, 1992, 1993a, 1993b, 1993c; Wheat et al., 1992; Whitmer, 1992.

First Aid Classes: Wheat et al., 1992.

Health Education for Self-Care: Aldana et al., 1993a, 1993b; Conrad et al., 1990; Fries et al., 1992; Fries, Harrington, Edwards, Kent, & Richardson, 1994; Golaszewski et al., 1992; Harvey et al., 1993; Leigh & Fries, 1992; Shi, 1992; Wheat et al., 1992; Whitmer, 1992.

Health Risk Appraisals: Aldana et al., 1993a, 1993b, 1994; Bertera, 1990b, 1993; Conrad et al., 1990; Fries et al., 1994; Goetzel et al., 1994; Golaszewski et al., 1992; Gomel et al., 1993; Harvey et al., 1993; Henritze et al., 1992; Holzbach et al., 1990; Jones et al., 1990; Leigh et al., 1992; Leigh & Fries, 1992; Sciacca et al., 1993; Shi, 1992, 1993b; Wheat et al., 1992; Whitmer, 1992.

Lactation Program: Cohen & Mrtek, 1994.

210

Martial Arts: Conrad et al., 1990.

Nutrition Education/Cholesterol Reduction/ Lower Fat/High Fiber Diets: Aldana et al., 1993a, 1994; Baer, 1993; Bertera, 1990a, 1990b, 1993; Briley & Montgomery, 1992; Conrad et al., 1990; Fries et al., 1992; Goetzel et al., 1994; Gomel et al., 1993; Harrell, Cornetto, & Stutts, 1992; Hartman, McCarthy, & Himes, 1993; Harvey et al., 1993; Henritze et al., 1992; Herbert et al., 1993; Holzbach et al., 1990; Hunt et al., 1993; Jones et al., 1990; Knight et al., 1994; Larsen & Simons, 1993; Sciacca et al., 1993; Sheeshka & Woolcott, 1994; Shi, 1992, 1993b; Sorensen et al., 1992; Wheat et al., 1992; Whitmer, 1992; Wilson, Edmunson, & DeJoy, 1992.

Occupational Safety: Aldana et al., 1994.

Prenatal Education & Gynecologic Program: Burton, Erickson, & Briones, 1991.

Promotion of Breast Cancer Screening: Bertera, 1990; Falvo & Tippy, 1993; Kurtz, Kurtz, Given, & Given, 1994; Mayer et al., 1993.

Risk Factor Screening: Kingery, Ellsworth, Corbett, Bowden, & Brizzolara, 1994.

Seat Belt Use: Bertera, 1990b, 1993.

Sexual Awareness: Conrad et al., 1990.

Smoking Cessation: Aldana et al., 1993a, 1993b, 1994; Bertera, 1990a, 1990b; Bertera et al., 1990, 1990b, 1993; Conrad et al., 1990; Erfurt et al., 1991a, 1991b; Erfurt et al., 1990; Fisher et al., 1994; Fries et al., 1992; Gleason-Comstock et al., 1994; Goetzel et al., 1994; Golaszewski et al., 1992; Gomel et al., 1993; Harrell et al., 1992; Henritze et al., 1992; Holzbach et al., 1990; Jeffery et al., 1993a; Jeffery et al., 1993b; Jones et al., 1990; Knight et al., 1994; Leigh & Fries, 1992; O'Hara, Gerace, & Elliott, 1993; Salina et al., 1994; Sciacca et al., 1993; Shi, 1992, 1993a, 1993b; Sorensen, Lando, & Pechacek, 1993; Wheat et al., 1992.

Stress Abatement/Management: Aldana et al., 1993a, 1993b, 1994; Bertera, 1990b, 1993; Conrad et al., 1990; Fries et al., 1992; Golaszewski et al., 1992; Harvey et al., 1993; Holzbach et al., 1990; Jones et al., 1990; Knight et al., 1994; Pruitt, 1992; Pruitt, Bernheim, & Tomlinson, 1991; Shi, 1992, 1993a, 1993b; Wheat et al., 1992; Whitmer, 1992.

Vision/Glaucoma Screening: Wheat et al., 1992.

Weight Control/Body Fat: Aldana et al., 1993a, 1993b, 1994; Anderson, Mavis, Robison, & Stoffelmayr, 1993; Baer, 1993; Bertera, 1990a, 1990b, 1993; Briley & Montgomery, 1992; Conrad et al., 1990; Erfurt et al., 1990, 1991a, 1991b; Fries et al., 1992; Goetzel et al., 1994; Golaszewski et al., 1992; Gomel et al., 1993; Harvey et al., 1993; Holzbach et al., 1990; Hunt et al., 1993; Jeffery et al., 1993a, 1993b; Jones et al., 1990; Knight et al., 1994; Prochaska, Norcross, Fowler, Follick, & Abrams, 1992; Sciacca et al., 1993; Shi, 1992, 1993b; Wheat et al., 1992; Whitmer, 1992.

APPENDIX B:

OUTCOMES MEASURED

Absenteeism: Bertera, 1990a, 1990b; Bertera, 1993; Burton et al., 1991; Conrad et al., 1990; Golaszewski et al., 1992; Jeffery et al., 1993b; Jones et al., 1990; Knight et al., 1994; Lynch et al., 1990; Zwerling & Ryan, 1992.

Aerobic Capacity: Aldana et al., 1994; Breslow et al., 1990; Gomel et al., 1993; Larsen & Simons, 1993.

AIDS Knowledge/Attitudes: Barr & Warshaw, 1994.

Alcohol Awareness: Towers, Kishchuk, Sylvestre, Peters, & Bourgault, 1994.

Alcohol Intake: Bertera, 1993; Fries et al., 1992; Herbert et al., 1993; Shi, 1992.

Benefit-to-Cost Ratio: Aldana et al., 1993b; Bertera, 1990b; Ellis et al., 1994; Erfurt et al., 1991a; Erfurt et al., 1991b; Fries et al., 1993; Golaszewski et al., 1992; Pruitt, 1992; Pruitt et al., 1991; Wilson et al., 1992; Zwerling & Ryan, 1992.

Blood Pressure Control: Aldana et al., 1993, 1994; Baer, 1993; Bertera, 1993; Briley & Montgomery, 1992; Erfurt et al., 1990; Erfurt et al., 1991; Fielding et al., 1994; Fries et al., 1992; Gomel et al., 1993; Harrell et al., 1992; Harvey et al., 1993; Heirich et al., 1993; Henritze et al., 1992; Larsen & Simons, 1993; Pruitt, 1992; Pruitt et al., 1991; Shi, 1992.

Breast-feeding Duration and Rates: Cohen & Mrtek, 1994.

C-Section/Laparoscopy/D & C Rates: Burton et al., 1991.

Cholesterol Levels: Aldana et al., 1993a, 1993b, 1994; Baer, 1993; Bertera, 1993; Briley & Montgomery, 1992; Fries et al., 1992; Goetzel et al., 1994; Gomel et al., 1993; Harrell et al., 1992; Hartman, McCarthy, & Himes, 1993; Harvey et al., 1993; Henritze et al., 1992; Larsen & Simons, 1993; Shi, 1992; Sorensen et al., 1992; Wilson et al., 1992.

Clinical Breast Exam: Kurtz et al., 1994.

Cognitive Changes in Regard to Nutrition: Sheeshka & Woolcott, 1994.

Dietary Intake: Aldana et al., 1993; Baer, 1993; Bertera, 1993; Briley & Montgomery, 1992; Fries et al., 1992; Fries et al., 1994; Harrell et al., 1992; Hartman et al., 1993; Harvey et al., 1993; Henritze et al., 1992; Hunt et al., 1993; Larsen & Simons, 1993; Shi, 1992; Sorensen et al., 1992; Wilson et al., 1992.

Disability/Illness: Bertera, 1993; Bertera, 1990b; Conrad et al., 1990; Jones et al., 1990; Leigh & Fries, 1992; Lynch et al., 1990; Shi, 1993b, 1993c.

Exercise: Bertera, 1993; Breslow et al., 1990; Fries et al., 1992; Fries et al., 1994; Heirich et al., 1993; Henritze et al., 1992; Lynch et al., 1993.

Fitness Facility Membership: Lynch et al., 1990.

Frequency of Medical Care Visits: Aldana et al., 1993; Burton & Conti, 1991; Leigh et al., 1992; Leigh & Fries, 1992; Shi, 1993b, 1993c.

Health Risk Behavior Scores: Aldana et al., 1993; Bertera, 1993; Fries et al., 1993; Harvey et al., 1993; Henritze et al., 1992; Jasheway & Sirota, 1993; Larsen & Simons, 1993; Leigh et al., 1992; Lynch, Gilfillan, Jennet, & McGloin, 1993.

Hospitalizations: Shi, 1993b, 1993c.

Injuries: Aldana et al., 1993b; Shi, 1993b; Zwerling & Ryan, 1992.

Job Satisfaction: Holzbach et al., 1990; Shi, 1993a.

Mammography Intention Rates: Falvo & Tippy, 1993; Kurtz et al., 1994; Mayer et al., 1993.

Medical/Health Care Claims/Costs: Aldana et al., 1993b; Burton & Conti, 1991; Erfurt et al., 1991a, 1991b; Foote & Erfurt, 1991; Fries et al., 1993; Fries et al., 1994; Harvey et al., 1993; Kingery et al., 1994; Leigh & Fries, 1992; Leigh et al., 1992; Lynch et al., 1993; Sciacca et al., 1993; Shi, 1993c; Wheat et al., 1992.

Mortality/Morbidity Rates: Bertera, 1990b; Golaszewski et al., 1992.

Offering of Smoking Cessation Programs: Gleason-Comstock et al., 1994.

Participation Rates in Programs: Anderson et al., 1993; Erfurt et al., 1990b; Jasheway & Sirota, 1993; Jeffery et al., 1993a, 1993b; Knight et al., 1994; Mayer et al., 1993; Prochaska et al., 1992.

Productivity: Golaszewski et al., 1992.

Program Costs: Bertera, 1990b; Bertera, Oehl, & Telepchak, 1990; Fries et al., 1992; Henritze et al., 1992; Jeffery et al., 1993; Pruitt, 1992; Pruitt et al., 1991; Wilson et al., 1992.

Seat Belt Use: Bertera, 1993b; Breslow et al., 1990; Fries et al., 1994; Leigh & Fries, 1992.

Smoking Policies/Smoke-Free Environment: Gleason-Comstock et al., 1994.

Smoking Status: Anderson et al., 1993; Bertera, 1990, 1993; Bertera et al., 1990; Breslow et al., 1990; Brigham et al., 1994; Erfurt et al., 1991; Fisher et al., 1994; Fries et al., 1992; Fries et al., 1994; Goetzel et al., 1994; Gomel et al., 1993; Harrell et al., 1992; Harvey et al., 1993; Henritze et al., 1992; Jeffery et al., 1993a, 1993b; Jeffery et al., 1994; Jones et al., 1990; O'Hara et al., 1993; Prochaska et al., 1992; Salina et al., 1994; Shi, 1992; Sorensen et al., 1993.

Speeding: Shi, 1992.

Stress Levels/Symptoms/Psychological State: Aldana et al., 1993a; Fries et al., 1992; Pruitt, 1992; Pruitt et al., 1991.

Tardiness: Conrad et al., 1990.

Turnover: Zwerling & Ryan, 1992.

Weight/Body Fat: Aldana et al., 1993a, 1994; Baer, 1993; Briley & Montgomery, 1992; Erfurt et al., 1991a, 1991b; Fries et al., 1992; Fries et al., 1994; Goetzel et al., 1994; Jeffery et al., 1993a, 1993b.

Workers' Compensation Claims: Conrad et al., 1990.

PART III

Other Research

Chapter 9

Nursing at War: Catalyst for Change

QUINCEALEA BRUNK
SCHOOL OF NURSING
THE PENNSYLVANIA STATE UNIVERSITY

ABSTRACT

From the first development of nursing research agendas, scholars have called for historical inquiries into nursing's heritage and the influences that have affected the development of the profession. Because war leaves an indelible and distinct mark on the era in which it occurs, periods of significant development and change in nursing's heritage can be linked to involvement in war. This review explores the published scholarship about American nurses in wartime, from the War for Independence through the Persian Gulf War and notes the most significant changes that have come as a result of this involvement. Although particular wars and wartime nursing is a popular topic for historical inquiry, there are still eras that need to be further explored for contributions to the profession of nursing as it is today.

Keywords: Military Nursing, History of Nursing, Nursing and War

As the number of clinical nursing studies have exploded over the last two decades, so have studies that examine historical phenomena regarding the nursing profession. In previous writings, authors have called for historical inquiries into nursing's heritage and the influences that have affected the development of the profession (Austin, 1958; Newton, 1965; I. S. Palmer, 1986). The reciprocal relationship between nursing and war have left indelible marks on the status of women, the professional development of nursing, and the national environment of health care.

As early as the Crusades, nursing orders were established to care for the sick and wounded left in the path of war. Nightingale's contribution to the

217

development of modern nursing during the Crimean War (1854–1856) is legendary. Americans have participated in wartime nursing activities since the colonial era, consistently contributing to the development of the profession. The influence of American nurses' participation in wars serves as the basis for this review.

Historical analyses of nursing activities in the literature have proliferated over the last 2 decades. The diversity of nursing-related topics available for study has necessarily limited the depth of historical narratives in any one area of interest and expanded the breadth of topics in the literature. Because wars have left such indelible marks on nursing, published historical scholarship is more abundant on these topics than on clinical activities.

Budding recognition of the value of historical inquiry within the discipline of nursing has been paralleled by a honing of the skills needed to artistically synthesize and communicate the findings of historical inquiry. The published research reports included in this review mirror the evolution of historical inquiry within nursing. The efforts of the earliest authors reflected more narrative breadth, whereas more recent historical scholarship efforts added depth to the topics being explored. Although this is one explanation for the varying depth and breadth in the historical annals of nursing and wars, this development of technique cannot explain why there is relatively little published about the modern wars that have had such dramatic impact on the last several generations. One possible interpretation of this deficiency is that the wounds of memory are too fresh. Unpopular in American culture, the wartime activities of the last half of the 20th century are not far enough in the past to diminish the personal nature of the experience for either participants or scholars.

Selections for this review were generated from a MEDLINE search from 1966 through 1994; cumulative indexes of the professional literature over the same period; the ''invisible college'' of nurse historians; and the ancestral approach generated by the database search (Cooper, 1982). Keywords used were military nursing, history of nursing, nursing, and war. Review materials were limited to those found in nationally circulated journals, printed in English, focusing on American nurses' involvement in wars. Unpublished reports, book-length works, and narratives based entirely on secondary sources were excluded from this review. Clarity, scholarship, the use of primary sources, and documentation in the form of notes and bibliography were used as selection criteria for the review of materials.

THE COLONIAL PERIOD

American military nursing predates Florence Nightingale's wartime activities by approximately 75 years, to 1775 and the formation of the Continental Army during the War for Independence. In Colonial America, the health care system was rudimentary at best. Hospitals were few, physicians were usually trained as apprentices, and medical practices consisted primarily of bloodletting, purging, blistering, and poultices. Nursing care was provided in the home by female family members.

During the Revolution, nursing care for the army's sick and wounded was provided by fellow soldiers or "camp followers." Nursing care was:

> a combination of laundering, emptying slop pails, scrubbing floors, providing cooked meals, and washing dishes. "In fact, women were almost an essential ingredient of eighteenth century military life." . . . It was highly desirable to have female camp followers around to perform such tasks as mending, washing, cleaning, cooking, and nursing. (Selavan, 1975, p. 592)

Numerous records verified that women were sought out and paid as army nurses in the earliest stages of the new democracy. The Continental Congress authorized a hospital and the position of matron to supervise nursing care activities on 27 July 1775. Over the next 7 years, the Congress continued to authorize remuneration levels for nurses as they cared for the army. In spite of this authorization, Selavan (1975) noted that care for the sick and wounded was frequently provided by convalescent soldiers, depleting the military forces for battle:

> At various times in the course of the war Washington attempted to release soldiers who had been serving as orderlies and replace them with female nurses. In 1778 he suggested that women be enlisted for the same money paid to soldiers, "for he can no longer bear having an army on paper and not have them in the field." (p. 594)

Although historical accounts of nursing during the War for Independence are few, it is significant to note that nursing care for the military was first introduced in 1775 in what would become the United States. Furthermore, it is a credit to the men who served in the Continental Congress that the need for nursing care was recognized and remuneration offered for the services of this pioneering group (Sarnecky, 1989).

After the War for Independence, nurses disappeared from American military rolls until the mid-19th century. However, Gurney (1987) noted that ships' records document the presence of two nurses who served on board the warship *United States* during the War of 1812.

THE AMERICAN CIVIL WAR

At the midpoint of the 19th century, Victorian mores dominated sociocultural expectation in England and America. Care for the sick or injured was provided in the home by women as part of their domestic role. Hospitals in the United States were relatively few: primarily "pest-houses" for those with communicable diseases, "almshouses" for the indigent, or asylums for the mentally ill. Trained physicians made house calls for the sick, leaving orders for their care with the woman in charge of domestic management.

Between 1854 and 1856, Florence Nightingale brought international attention to the importance of women participating in military nursing. Designed to be read by the domestic nurse, Nightingale's (1860) *Notes on Nursing* highlighted the basic principles of sanitation, hygiene, and dietary considerations when caring for the sick. Thus, the American housewife gained a monopoly of knowledge in caring for the sick.

Women had not been maintained on military rolls nor participated as an authorized part of the standing army since the end of the Revolutionary War. With the outbreak of the War Between the States in April 1861, the standing army forces were unprepared for the numbers of sick and wounded that flowed into makeshift military hospitals after the initial battles. The army medical system initially provided care for the soldiers of the blue and the gray by detailing other recuperating or unfit soldiers as nurses (Brunk, 1992).

Multiple studies have reconstructed the sequence of events that led up to a loosely organized group of women nurses for the Union (Austin, 1975; Culpepper & Adams, 1988; P. A. Kalisch & B. J. Kalisch, 1976a; Wood, 1972). A few days after the fall of Fort Sumter, President Lincoln called for 75,000 volunteers to support the standing army of the United States. Dorothea Dix, the well-known crusader for reforms in the care of the mentally ill, volunteered her services as the Superintendent of Women Nurses of the Union Army. Shortly thereafter, the United States Sanitary Commission was formed to monitor sanitary conditions in the army camps and hospitals, provide relief supplies, and assign women nurses to the military hospitals (Matejski, 1986).

In one of the earliest projects detailing Civil War nursing, Wood (1972) analyzed the transition of nursing from the lay role at home to the professional endeavor in the military system. Focusing on several biographical citations to support the premise that there was generalized distaste for medical and bureaucratic "red tape," Wood stated:

> As Northerners, the nurses who followed the Union Army reckoned the Confederacy to be the enemy, but in daily practice their battles were more often with the ponderous war machine of their own menfolk and with the bureaucratic professionals—military and medical—who struggled to maintain it. (p. 199)

Although Wood related multiple examples of disregard for masculine authority, she did not clearly substantiate her thesis that women conjured up their more feminine attributes to expand woman's sphere in the 19th century.

Several thousand women eventually served as nurses during the War Between the States. P. A. Kalisch and B. J. Kalisch (1976a) identified several categories that could be applied to the appointments received by the women of the North. These included: (a) appointments by Miss Dix or another government official, (b) nuns of Holy Orders, (c) women employed to do menial hospital chores, (d) Black women employed under General Orders of the War Department, (e) women who served as uncompensated volunteers, (f) women camp followers, and (g) women employed by the various relief organizations. The women nurses of the South, in contrast, were a force consisting entirely of volunteers.

The women nurses of the Civil War acted during a period of political and cultural upheaval. Leaving the domain of their home, women risked social ostracism and instigated change in a resistant army medical system that desperately needed their services—even if these services were initially unsolicited. Armed only with good intentions, a patriotic spirit, and, perhaps, Nightingale's words of wisdom or government sanction, the women entered the hospital wards of the chaotic army medical system.

Although many diaries and collections of anecdotes were published in the late 19th century, the first published research reports focusing on Civil War nursing concentrated on the role of organizations and a few notorious women who performed nursing activities. A few celebrated women have been lauded repeatedly in both the popular literature for Civil War enthusiasts and in early scholarly works. Dorothea Dix, Clara Barton, Mary Ann Bickerdyke, Sally Tompkins, Kate Cumming, and the Woolsey sisters are names that most frequently appear on the rolls of the Civil War nursing "Hall of Fame." Historical studies encompassing the Civil War era are replete with descriptions of primitive conditions in the military camps and hospitals, the swift organization of women's relief societies, and the challenges faced by women as they entered the wards to render care to the sick and wounded soldiers (Austin, 1975; Culpepper & Adams, 1988; P. A. Kalisch & B. J. Kalisch, 1976a; Matejski, 1986; Wood, 1972).

Emphasizing the popularity of the Civil War in American culture, authors of recent scholarship have continued to analyze elements related to this 4-year period in American history. Going beyond the simple narrative of Civil War experiences, methodological and thematic issues of importance to modern nursing have been framed within an historical context and incorporated into the analyses. Exploring diaries and memoirs as valid sources for historical data, Parsons (1983) described the activities of Kate Cumming, Hannah Ropes, and Phoebe Yates Pember. Basing analytical comments on the women's diaries or memoirs, Parsons validated earlier scholarship and noted that the women nurses of the Civil War had no love lost for bureaucratic "red tape."

Focusing on thematic issues, Rogge (1987) described the interrelationship of political power and the activities of a select group of Civil War nurses. Particular attention is given to the power wielded by Clara Barton and Hannah Ropes, and supported in brief descriptions of the activities of Cordelia Harvey, Juliet Hopkins, and Sally Tompkins. Woodward (1991) questioned the traits possessed by 17 Civil War nurses that saw these women through to live until old age. Eliminating parentage/birth order, social/economic status, marital status/children, education/travel, service to nursing, other vocational work, health status/cause of death, religion, and authorship as viable interpretations, she concluded that the "pioneering spirit" that sustained the women nurses through the war also contributed to increased longevity.

With an emphasis on making the invisible women of history more visible, studies have been published that expose the hidden women who nursed during the Civil War. Gangwer (1988) detailed a neglected biography in her discussion of Emily Haines Harrison, a nurse working in Ohio hospitals, as an enlisted "spy" for the Union, and later a nurse on the Kansas prairie. Wall (1993) has highlighted the nursing activities of one order of Catholic sisters who provided services during the War Between the States. She concluded the exposé: "War holds a fascination throughout history, and war heroes are revered by their compatriots and readers of history. Yet war heroes are not limited to soldiers and their commanders; they include many others" (p. 83).

Nurse historians also suggest that the full story has not been told about Civil War nursing. Pokorny (1992) explained that as primitive and resistant as the Union army medical system was, the nurses who served as nurses for the Confederacy faced compounding challenges. The number of hospitals and trained surgeons was inadequate in the Confederacy; supplies, medicines, and daily necessities were scarce due to the Union blockade; and the South lacked the organizational structures that coordinated nursing efforts in the North. Although Pokorny used few primary sources, she exposed the need for further analyses that compare conditions and personalities of the warring factions.

Popular myth and scholarship have traditionally held that Dorothea Dix was the first woman to perform nursing services for the Union. New evidence suggests that this was not the case. While Dix was en route to Washington, DC, Adeline Blanchard Tyler offered the first nursing services to Union soldiers wounded in the Baltimore riots. Efforts have also been made to establish a similar honor for the first nurse of the Confederacy. Although the evidence is not as compelling, Sallie Chapman Gordon Law was credited as the first nurse for the Confederacy when she served as matron for a Memphis hospital that opened in April 1861 (Brunk, 1994).

Recently an historical analysis has been published that reconsiders the traditional and nontraditional relationships between men and women as they related to the United States Sanitary Commission. Through the experiences of Katharine Prescott Wormeley, Giesberg (1995) described the Sanitary Commission cohort as pivotal figures in the struggle between private and public, volunteer and professional, women and men. Giesberg poetically described the essence of these struggles:

> Katharine Prescott Wormeley and the women with whom she worked were active participants in this frontier struggle, sometimes accepting the limits defined by the men of the commission, sometimes rejecting them outright, and yet oftentimes reveling in the confusion that resulted from the commission's failure or inability to define its purpose. (p. 44)

The War Between the States was a pivotal period in the development of the national attitude and views about the roles of women in society. The Civil War would be the last war that American nurses would enter as "untrained but undaunted" (P. A. Kalisch & B. J. Kalisch, 1976a, p. 4). During the Reconstruction, philanthropic futurists continued to agitate for nurse training programs until the first was established in 1873. In describing nursing as a practical gift conferred on the women of the United States, P. A. Kalisch and B. J. Kalisch (1976a) paid tribute to the women nurses for the Blue and the Gray: "Although most were rank amateurs, their humble efforts and the positive effects of their femininity upon the sick men in the hospitals made it legitimate for respectable women to enter the field of nursing and helped create a new profession" (p. 30).

AMERICA AT WAR WITH SPAIN

Shortly before the turn of the century, America was embroiled in another war. Although short-lived, the Spanish–American War, which began in 1898, resulted in further changes for military nursing. P. A. Kalisch (1975) recounted that Congress had authorized the enlistment of men for a Hospital Corps in 1887. When Spanish warships sunk the U.S.S. *Maine* in February 1898, indignation among the American people mounted, and war was declared in April of that year. Firmly grounded in remnants of Victorian standards, the Army Medical Department initially refused an offer from the Daughters of the American Revolution (DAR) executive board to recruit and screen trained female nurses for military assignments.

Less than 2 months into the war, typhoid fever, yellow fever, dysentery, and other tropical diseases were taking their toll on the soldiers in Southern training camps and those stationed in Cuba. Woefully inadequate numbers of men in the Hospital Corps were supplemented by detailed squads of infantrymen for ward duty in camp hospitals: "These detail men, usually the dregs of their units, were worse than useless in caring for patients, and their neglect of elementary sanitary precautions helped spread diseases such as typhoid through the camps" (P. A. Kalisch, 1975, p. 413).

The high mortality rates from typhoid epidemics soon resulted in the wider employment of women in military hospitals. As the DAR screened applicants and coordinated contracts for qualified, trained nurses, the women were called on to use their energy, resources, and training to alleviate the wretchedness associated with tropical diseases. Once again, the women battled unsanitary conditions, worked long, exhausting hours, and attempted to avoid becoming ill themselves in order to return soldiers to active duty (P. A. Kalisch, 1975; Wall, 1995).

Spain signed the armistice on 12 August 1898, but the epidemics in camp continued to demand greater numbers of nurses than were already contracted to the Army. Nursing activities continued in the camps, hospitals, and on board the hospital ship *Relief*. By mid-September 1898, there were 1,158 nurses contracted to the army. After September, the typhoid epidemic began to subside. Many contracts for nursing services were annulled; however, 686 nurses were still enrolled at 27 different sites on 31 December 1898 (P. A. Kalisch, 1975).

Few historical analyses exist that recount the contributions of Catholic sisters to war efforts. Wall (1995) has added depth to the scholarly understanding of nursing activities during the Spanish–American War period with insight surrounding the activities of the Sisters of the Holy Cross.

Shortly after the end of the war, President William McKinley appointed the Dodge Commission to investigate the conduct of the War Department during the war with Spain. Testimonials were offered to the benefits and quality of care rendered by trained female nurses. A significant outcome of the Dodge Commission was the recommendation that a reserve corps of select trained nurses be associated with the Medical Department of the Army. Although acceptance of the nurse corps was tenuous through 1899, petitions to Congress during that year and through 1900 led to the establishment of the Army Nurse Corps as a permanent, female unit of the Medical Department on 2 February 1901. Within just a few years, the contributions of nurses who served aboard "floating hospitals" were acknowledged when the Navy Nurse Corps was officially established in 1908 (P. A. Kalisch, 1975).

Popular opinion supported these developments with a wide acceptance of the professional female nurse as the preferred caregiver in military hospitals, no matter what their location: "Woman was the natural nurse, and nowhere did she appear grander or nobler than when she was ministering to the sick and dying of any army in active warfare" (P. A. Kalisch, 1975, p. 418).

Although patriarchal opinions of the military medical system posed obstacles along the way, the "splendid little war" of 1898 firmly established the benefits of using trained female nurses during wartime. In establishing the Army Nurse Corps, and eventually the Navy Nurse Corps, the government at last recognized the need to have a standing complement of trained female nurses at the ready, to care for the sick and wounded soldiers during wartime activities.

NURSING IN THE FIRST WORLD WAR

When a shot fired in Sarajevo (Serbia) in 1915 ignited a war that engrossed most of Europe, the United States sought to remain neutral in regard to military involvement. However, political neutrality did not deter nurses from answering their own call to duty to serve the sick and injured. American nurses traveled to Europe and offered their services through the Red Cross as the war escalated. Entering the war as a belligerent in 1917, the United States called on the Army and Navy Nurse Corps to supply nurses for the ever-increasing demands placed on military medical services. In May 1917, the first nurses embarked for duty overseas. Within 6 months, there were 1,100 nurses stationed in overseas facilities and the Red Cross Nursing Service supplied nurses as the reserve corps (P. A. Kalisch & B. J. Kalisch, 1986).

Although the published historical reports related to nursing activities during World War I are not plentiful, the nature of the research is diverse. Baer (1987) offered insight into the depth of feeling of nurses stationed overseas for their training schools as she reconstructed events surrounding correspondence to Miss Katharine Sanborn, superintendent at the St. Vincent's Hospital in New York. Analysis of the correspondence portrays the problems of censorship during wartime, patriotic themes associated with wartime nursing, descriptions of the work, problems and privations endured by the military nurse, and, finally, the attachment the nurses felt for their training school and superintendent.

Beeber (1990) analyzed the aftershocks of the World War I nursing experience. She described the women nurses as being immersed in and confronted by the male homosocial structures that wanted to maintain women and nurses in a Victorian model. In analyzing reports of World War I (WWI) nursing activities, Beeber identified three major issues:

> First, the nurses were confronted with demands for autonomous practice unlike any they had ever known. Second, the disparity between their values as healers and the goals of the state at war became evident. Third, the nurses confronted sex-based inequality in the context of equal danger. (p. 37)

Each of these issues has been analyzed in other scholarly literature related to World War I nursing duties. P. A. Kalisch (1976) detailed the strife and struggles to acquire military rank for nurses. In October 1917, M. Adelaide Nutting, director of the Department of Nursing at Teachers College, Columbia University, began a crusade to gain commissioned officer rank for army nurses. Believing that the nurses were severely handicapped without rank, while bearing a great burden of responsibility, Nutting sought to elevate the status of the profession and give the Army nurse authority over complacent enlisted corpsmen. Gaining support from Annie W. Goodrich (future Dean of the Army Training School) and Lillian Wald (founder of the Henry Street Settlement), the "triumvirate" continued to press for officer rank for nurses even after the armistice of 11 November 1918 ended World War I. After much work, *relative rank* for nurses was finally made official on 4 June 1920. As implemented, relative rank gave the rights and privileges of all regular officers but did not provide an equivalent pay scale with male officers (P. A. Kalisch, 1976).

By the time the armistice was signed in 1918, there were approximately 20,000 Army, Navy, and Red Cross nurses stationed abroad. Yet this number of nurses was far exceeded by the demand. Not only was there an acute shortage of nurses in the military but domestic demands were escalating as well. In a timely analysis of a recurring problem in nursing, Malone (1994) examined the role of Jane A. Delano, head of the Red Cross nursing service, in the conflict over assigning minimally trained civilian aides to duty in Red Cross and military hospitals during World War I. Taking a stance against M. Adelaide Nutting and Annie W. Goodrich, Delano desired to use voluntary aide detachments to supplement nursing numbers in wartime hospitals. Nutting and Goodrich, however, argued that the professional status of nursing was yet too tentative to allow a "watering-down" method of delivering care.

Nutting and Goodrich instead supported proposals for the Vassar training program and the Army School of Nursing to rapidly supplement the number of trained nurses available for military assignments. After government acceptance of these two proposals, Nutting and Goodrich took a more tolerant approach to "the aide question." Although late in coming, the proposal for the training of hospital assistants was accepted in September 1918. Delano continued to work at a frenzied pace to supply the ever-increasing demand for trained nurses. Malone (1994) summarized the long-term effect of assistive personnel: "The aide question, however, as evidenced by the American Medical Association's late and little-lamented proposal for Registered Care Technicians to solve a nursing shortage, has never been put to rest" (p. 89). Although the war was over, the issues surrounding a nursing shortage would linger.

AMERICAN NURSES' INVOLVEMENT IN THE SPANISH CIVIL WAR

In a unique contribution to the literature addressing military nursing, Patai (1995) recounted some of the experiences of 46 nurses who participated in providing philanthropic care for those involved in the Spanish Civil War (1936–1939). Just on the eve of World War II, the Spanish Republic had called for international volunteers to help defend democracy and halt the progression of Fascism. Although enlightening with regard to a virtually unknown military involvement, Patai extended a "leap of faith" when she attributed a significant role in the halting of fascist activities to the 46 women who were overworked and underrecognized for their efforts in providing humanitarian nursing services to the sick and wounded in Spain.

THE IMPACT OF NURSING IN WORLD WAR II

Although Europe had been embroiled in conflict and war for several years, Americans were reluctant to admit that involvement in yet another war was inevitable. The bombing of Pearl Harbor on 7 December 1941 brought about a rapid response from civilians and military personnel alike. Grace Lally, later referred to as "Tugboat Annie," was present in Pearl Harbor during the bombing. Serving as a leader through the crisis of that day and others, Lally established a standard for others to emulate as a member of the Navy Nurse Corps (Hawkins & Matthews, 1991). Several changes in military nursing are revealed in the scholarly literature related to World War II: "In the midst of the war, relative rank was temporarily abandoned, the recruitment responsibilities were removed from the Red Cross, and nurses were brought more closely into the military services system" (Bullough, 1976, p. 120).

An acute shortage of nurses in the military and civilian sectors was again manifested, escalated by a greater demand for nurses due to increasing industrialization, availability of health insurance, societal health problems, and wartime job opportunities for women. Several scholars offered insight about contemplated solutions to the nursing shortage during World War II. The first of these was the Cadet Nurse Corps. Established under the Bolton Act in 1943, the government financed a vast campaign to supply 125,000 students who would enter an accelerated training program with all educational expenses, related necessities, and a stipend. All that was required of the cadet nurse, after training completion, was service as a nurse until war's end

(Brueggemann, 1992; B. J. Kalisch & P. A. Kalisch, 1976). Government funds also were made available for refresher courses in nursing and postgraduate training.

In an amazing media campaign, the Movietonews launched a positively oriented recruitment campaign for nursing services (Stevens, 1990). Working in collaboration with the government, Movietonews appealed to potential recruits with " 'the highest calling in the service of humanity [demanding] a sincerity of purpose and depth of understanding unmatched by any other profession' . . . who wanted to learn, join a profession, preserve health, and pursue a science-based discipline" (p. 47).

P. A. Kalisch and B. J. Kalisch (1973) analyzed another government solution to the nursing shortage that escalated during World War II: the Nurses' Selective Service Bill of 1945. Gravely concerned by the manpower shortage of civilian and military hospitals, President Franklin D. Roosevelt proposed a nurse's draft in his State of the Union message to Congress on 6 January 1945. Drawing support from various sectors, the bill went before subcommittees in both houses of Congress. Katherine Densford, then president of the American Nurses Association, even went on record in support of the "nurse's draft" if the Army was unable to get the necessary number of volunteers through any other methods. "She testified that 'the association would accept a draft of nurses as a first step, but, only as a first step, in a Selective Service Act for all women' " (P. A. Kalisch & B. J. Kalisch, 1973, p. 408). While the bill was still being debated in Congress, all the other drastic means of nurse recruitment became fruitful, and V-E (Victory in Europe) Day was near at hand. With this upswing in numbers, the nurse's draft bill was recalled from Congress.

One "first" to occur during World War II was the initiation of flight nursing with the U.S. Army Air Forces. In a series of historical analyses, Barger (1979, 1980, 1991a, 1991b) reconstructed the pioneer flight of air evacuation, detailed coping behaviors of Army flight nurses, and proposed lessons that can be learned from this particular group of nursing pioneers. Through this series, Barger brought challenges of the past into the present to make them relevant within a modern context.

Yet another dramatic but tragic "first" was discussed in the scholarly literature dedicated to World War II nursing activities. For the first time since the War for Independence, American military nurses were held as Japanese prisoners of war in the Philippines between 1942 and 1945 (P. A. Kalisch & B. J. Kalisch, 1976b; Norman & Eifried, 1993, 1995). These reports are graphic with details of the hospital bombings, the Bataan Death March, tunnel life at Corregidor, and privations of internment at Santo Tomas in Manila. Seventy-nine American nurses fell victim to the hardships and nightmarish realities of primitive administration of nursing services, starvation, bombings, loss of privacy, and isolation from the outside world during their imprisonment. Yet, they survived. Drawing support from the group and calling on their training as nurses to adapt and persevere, all of the women returned home after being freed in February 1945 (P. A. Kalisch & B. J. Kalisch, 1976b; Norman & Eifried, 1993, 1995).

Norman and Eifried (1993) paid tribute to the "Angels of Bataan" in stating:

> These nurses also add to our understanding of valor. Wartime heroism is neither gender nor occupation specific. . . . Through the bombings, the illnesses and the hunger they quietly persevered in the jungle. They also were scared. They wanted to live. They missed the men they knew and, sometimes loved, who were killed. They missed their homes and families. In short, we learn that true heroes are also very human. It might have been their very humanness that enabled them to perform so valiantly. (p. 125)

WARTIME NURSING DURING THE COLD WAR YEARS

In spite of the popularity of military nursing as a topic for scholarly inquiry, no studies exist that explicate the role of nursing during the Korean conflict (1950–1953). Although the Korean conflict was not a "popular" war effort for many Americans, the military buildup in the Far East that would follow but a decade later was even less popular. As the conflict in Vietnam escalated, more troops were sent to preserve democracy, and more medical units were established to care for the casualties.

As the silence over Vietnam has been broken in American culture during the last 10 years, so has the focus of scholarly inquiry. Unlike previous wars, assignment to duty in Vietnam was usually for 1 year, rotating through Southeast Asia as individuals rather than entire units of combat or medical personnel (Paul, 1985). The focus of nursing inquiry has been turned toward exploring commonalities between nurses and combat personnel and explicating the qualities that made military nursing different during this war.

Recognizing posttraumatic stress disorder (PTSD) in Vietnam veterans, the earliest published reports related to nursing activities in Vietnam also establish that nurses were susceptible to this particular problem. Analyzing data in a subset of a larger program, Stretch, Vail, and Maloney (1985) estimated that 3.3% of the sample of Vietnam veteran nurses still manifest PTSD symptomology. With this rate comparable to that found among nonnurse active duty Army Vietnam veterans, the investigators suggest that danger and exposure to violence contribute to stress reactions such as PTSD, even among noncombatants, and that social support acts as a moderating factor in attenuation of PTSD symptoms.

Paul (1985) also identified the presence of PTSD in Vietnam nurse veterans. Using a content-analysis approach, Paul classified eight stressors for the nurse veterans, including limited experience prior to assignment, exposure to severe casualties, survivor guilt, and threat to life. A list of 14 adverse aftereffects (common symptoms of PTSD) were also identified as being exhibited by some of the nurse veterans. Paul further suggested in the conclusion of this report that the different style of assigning personnel to duty in Vietnam may have limited the sense of peer support, thus increasing the potential for stress disorder problems.

Schwartz (1987) has contributed a more global perspective to the literature about nursing during the Vietnam War. Citing that approximately 11,000 women are estimated to have served in Vietnam in either a military or civilian capacity, Schwartz incorporated oral communications to detail the women's experiences with the casualties, the war, and the return home to the United States. Although the report was not entirely focused on nurses or nursing activities, this piece of literature added depth to the accumulating knowledge about the Vietnam nursing experience.

The most complete analysis of military nurses in Vietnam between 1965 and 1973 has been contributed by Norman (1986, 1988, 1989, 1990). Reporting the comprehensive findings in *Women at War*, Norman (1990) has also contributed individual elements by reporting in scholarly journals. Through interviews and surveys of 50 nurses from all branches of the military nurse corps, Norman (1986) concluded that there were personal and professional, good and bad, difficult and rewarding experiences associated with the time served in Vietnam. In a statistically analyzed subset report, Norman (1988) revealed that several nurses of the 50 participants suffered from PTSD in the past or even continue to do so at present. By exploring similarities and differences in the nurses' experiences, Norman (1989) synthesized the similarities as exposure to gruesome casualties, moral dilemmas, a special sense of camaraderie, and development of professional skills. Differences among the military branches were described as being the location of service and the year of service when rotated for duty in Vietnam.

Although the silence has now been broken about the Vietnam nursing experience, the full story has not yet been told. The experiences of nurses who served in Vietnam are just beginning to be explored by historians and others with an interest in military ordeals. The similarities and differences between combatants and noncombatants are just now beginning to take on meaning. Although changes undoubtedly occurred in nursing, the memories may still be too painful to warrant a full exploration of the impact of the Vietnam nursing experience.

NURSING IN THE PERSIAN GULF

As the United States has looked toward the next century, yet another military engagement has sent nurses to confront the casualties of war. Because this is the most recent military engagement, few studies have been published that analyze or synthesize the nursing experience during the Persian Gulf War of 1991. As participants in the nursing effort during Desert Storm, Dahl and O'Neal (1993) initiated the first exploration of stressors and coping behaviors that were used by a nursing unit in the desert war setting. Limited in scope, Dahl and O'Neal reported that stressors included environmental conditions, a lack of recognition, and a perceived lack of organization and leadership. Coping behaviors were identified as exercise and recreation, psychological coping skills, support, patient care activities, and spiritual activity. As in wars past, nurses adapted and coped with the military experience.

CONCLUSION AND DIRECTIONS FOR FUTURE RESEARCH

A theme of change is consistently interwoven in any exploration of military nursing and the catalyst facet of war. Within United States history, nursing activities have been noted during every military engagement. As early as the War for Independence, nursing care was recognized as a necessity in caring for the casualties of battle. Military nursing has consistently heralded change in the role of women in society, nursing education, and nursing practice. The Civil War left its mark in opening an acceptable avenue of work for women, allowing them to go beyond the suffering, swooning, and ornamental status of social expectations. The need for formal nursing education was recognized and programs were first established in 1873 as an outcome of nursing activities during the Civil War.

The Spanish–American War confirmed the need to establish military nursing corps and reaffirmed the value of nurses being attached to the military during engagements. After World War I, women gained the franchise and began to make political inroads, aided in part by a demonstration of competency and adaptability by women for nurses. World War II heralded the change of employment patterns for women in general (illustrated by ''Rosie the Riveter'') and for nurses in particular. The awarding of full military rank for nurses also enhanced the political base for the profession. A trend toward advanced education for nurses, particularly in the university setting, was also a result of World War II. Returning nurses from Vietnam further inflated the number of nurses holding advanced educational degrees in the United States.

Although Norman (1989) specifically attributed an underlying theme of role conflict to nursing during the Vietnam war, the comment can legitimately be linked to any wartime nursing experience:

> The nurses in a war zone were regarded as caregiver, but they were also looked on as surrogate mothers, sisters, wives—all the roles women provided back in the United States. The nurses gladly assumed these multiple roles, but assuming these roles added to the stress of wartime nursing. (p. 226)

Throughout history, there has existed a basic conflict between the carnage and devastation of war and the basic essence of healing and humanity attributed to nursing activities. Even limited research focusing on the experiences of nurses during any particular military engagement indicates that nurses have consistently been adapting, supportive of each other, and caring in the face of war's devastation and wholesale carnage.

P. N. Palmer (1991) has poetically summed up the impact of war, especially on the profession of nursing:

> War leaves permanent scars on everything it touches. For nursing, those scars have been mixed. Along with the loss of life, it raised public consciousness about the contributions of nurses, opened new fields of specialization, enhanced education, and accelerated nursing's growth as a profession. (p. 658)

Although the depth and breadth of knowledge about nursing during wartime is expanding, scholars have not yet exhausted the possibilities of sources, made all of the invisible heroes or heroines visible, nor learned all the lessons of the past. Continued research is needed to fully understand the role of nurses and nursing during war, the most powerful catalyst of social change.

Several periods of military nursing activities have been underrecognized in the development of the scholarly literature base. Interested scholars should be encouraged to further analyze the nursing activities associated with the War for Independence, the Spanish–American War, and World War I. A glaring void in the literature is any discussion of nursing activities during the Korean conflict. Enthusiasts of modern history should revel in the opportunity to make a significant contribution to enhancing the understanding of nursing's heritage through oral histories and other methods while first-hand participants in this military activity can still be located and utilized.

At present, historical research reports related to military nursing have focused primarily on the roles and activities of White women nurses. Expansion of the discipline's scholarly base would be well served to further explore the role of minorities and males in military nursing annals. A single attempt to rectify this marked neglect appeared in a brief piece in the *American Journal of Nursing* over a decade ago (Carnegie, 1984). Scholars have by no means exhausted the available possibilities for exploring the area of minority service to the military nursing effort.

Nurses' activities during periods of war are too complex to be fully explored in one brief volume. The organizational structure, activities, and individual leadership aspects of the nurse corps would each be worthy of study. At present, more comprehensive histories are in progress for the Army Nurse Corps and the Air Force Nurse Corps. However, the noble work of participants in the Navy Nurse Corps has yet to be fully explicated.

New scholars with an interest in nursing history and nursing activities during wars are consistently growing in number. Multiple masters' theses and doctoral dissertations already exist, and these scholarly endeavors continue to expand through the nurturing support of those who value and treasure nursing's heritage. Fortunately, some of these works have been published and are noteworthy for helping to get the true message of what nursing *is*, what nurses *do*, and *why* nurses continue to do "it" to the public. But the work is far from ended.

Sufficient markers of the territory covered by military nursing in the United States exist. However, depth in any number of areas can further contribute to a basic understanding of what defines nursing, where the essence of nursing commitment may lie, and the value of nursing within the sociocultural realm: "As nursing looks to the future and the technological promises that lay in store, it also needs to look to its past and remember the legions of nursing pioneers who remind us that nursing is, first and last, a human service" (Wall, 1993, p. 83).

REFERENCES

Austin, A. L. (1958). The historical method in nursing. *Nursing Research, 7*, 4–10.

Austin, A. L. (1975). Nurses in American history: Wartime volunteers 1861–1865. *American Journal of Nursing, 75*, 816–818.

Baer, E. D. (1987). Letters to Miss Sanborn: St. Vincent's Hospital nurses of World War I. *Journal of Nursing History, 2*(2), 17–32.

Barger, J. (1979). Origin of flight nursing in the United States Army Air Forces. *Aviation, Space, & Environmental Medicine, 50*, 1176–1178.

Barger, J. (1980). U. S. Army Air Forces flight nurses: Training and pioneer flight. *Aviation, Space, & Environmental Medicine, 51*, 414–416.

Barger, J. (1991a). Coping behaviors of U. S. Army flight nurses in World War II: An oral history. *Aviation, Space, & Environmental Medicine, 62*, 153–157.

Barger, J. (1991b). Preparing for war: Lessons learned from U. S. Army flight nurses of World War II. *Aviation, Space, & Environmental Medicine, 62,* 772–775.

Beeber, L. S. (1990). To be one of the boys: Aftershocks of the World War I nursing experience. *Advances in Nursing Science, 12*(4), 32–43.

Brueggemann, D. (1992). *The United States Cadet Nurse Corps 1943–1948: The Nebraska experience.* Unpublished master's thesis, University of Nebraska at Omaha.

Brunk, Q. (1992). *Forgotten by time: An historical analysis of the unsung lady nurses of the Civil War.* Unpublished doctoral dissertation, The University of Texas at Austin.

Brunk, Q. (1994). Caring without politics: Lessons from the first nurses of the North and South. *Nursing History Review, 2,* 119–136.

Bullough, B. (1976). Nurses in American history: The lasting impact of World War II on nursing. *American Journal of Nursing, 76,* 118–120.

Carnegie, M. E. (1984). Nurses and war: Black nurses at the front. *American Journal of Nursing, 84,* 1250–1252.

Cooper, H. M. (1982). Scientific guidelines for conducting integrative research reviews. *Review of Educational Research, 52,* 291–302.

Culpepper, M. M., & Adams, P. G. (1988). Nursing in the Civil War. *American Journal of Nursing, 88,* 981–984.

Dahl, J., & O'Neal, J. (1993). Stress and coping behavior of nurses in Desert Storm. *Journal of Psychosocial Nursing and Mental Health Services, 31*(10), 17–21.

Gangwer, C. W. (1988). A sketch of Emily Haines Harrison: Civil War nurse, spy, and nurse on the Kansas prairie. *Journal of Nursing History, 3*(2), 22–34.

Giesberg, J. A. (1995). In service to the fifth wheel: Katharine Prescott Wormeley and her experiences in the United States Sanitary Commission. *Nursing History Review, 3,* 43–53.

Gurney, C. (1987). Military nursing: 211 years of commitment to the American soldier. *Imprint, 34*(5), 36–41.

Hawkins, J. W., & Matthews, I. (1991). "Tugboat Annie": Nursing's hero of Pearl Harbor: Grace Lally (1897–1983). *IMAGE: Journal of Nursing Scholarship, 23,* 183–185.

Kalisch, B. J., & Kalisch, P. A. (1976). Nurses in American history: The Cadet Nurse Corps in World War II. *American Journal of Nursing, 76,* 240–242.

Kalisch, P. A. (1975). Heroines of '98: Female Army nurses in the Spanish-American War. *Nursing Research, 24,* 411–429.

Kalisch, P. A. (1976). How Army nurses became officers. *Nursing Research, 25,* 164–167.

Kalisch, P. A., & Kalisch, B. J. (1973). The women's draft. An analysis of the controversy over the nurses' Selective Service Bill of 1945. *Nursing Research, 22,* 402–413.

Kalisch, P. A., & Kalisch, B. J. (1976a). Untrained but undaunted: Women nurses of the Blue and the Gray. *Nursing Forum, 15*(1), 4–33.

Kalisch, P. A., & Kalisch, B. J. (1976b). Nurses under fire: The World War II experience of nurses on Bataan and Corregidor. *Nursing Research, 25,* 409–429.

Kalisch, P. A., & Kalisch, B. J. (1986). *The advance of American nursing* (2nd ed.). Boston: Little, Brown.

Malone, R. E. (1994). Jane A. Delano: Saint or sellout? *Nursing History Review*, 2, 67–97.

Matejski, M. P. (1986). Ladies' Aid Societies and the nurses of Lincoln's Army. *Journal of Nursing History*, *1*(2), 35–51.

Newton, M. E. (1965). The case for historical research. *Nursing Research*, *14*, 20–26.

Nightingale, F. (1860). *Notes on nursing: What it is, and what it is not*. New York: D. Appleton and Company.

Norman, E. M. (1986). A study of female military nurses in Vietnam during the war years 1965–1973. *Journal of Nursing History*, *2*(1), 43–60.

Norman, E. M. (1988). Post-traumatic stress disorder in military nurses who served in Vietnam during the war years 1965–1973. *Military Medicine*, *153*, 238–242.

Norman, E. M. (1989). The wartime experience of military nurses in Vietnam, 1965–1973. *Western Journal of Nursing Research*, *11*, 219–233.

Norman, E. M. (1990). *Women at war: The story of fifty military nurses who served in Vietnam*. Philadelphia: University of Pennsylvania Press.

Norman, E., & Eifried, S. (1993). The angels of Bataan. *IMAGE: Journal of Nursing Scholarship*, *25*, 121–126.

Norman, E. M., & Elfried, S. (1995). How did they all survive? An analysis of American nurses' experiences in Japanese prisoner-of-war camps. *Nursing History Review*, *3*, 105–127.

Palmer, I. S. (1986). Nursing's heritage. In H. H. Werley, J. J. Fitzpatrick, & R. L. Taunton (Eds.), *Annual review of nursing research* (Vol. 4, pp. 237–257). New York: Springer Publishing Co.

Palmer, P. N. (1991). Wars leave indelible marks on the nursing profession. *AORN Journal*, *53*, 657–658.

Parsons, M. E. (1983). Mothers and matrons. *Nursing Outlook*, *31*, 274–278.

Patai, F. (1995). Heroines of the good fight: Testimonies of U. S. volunteer nurses in the Spanish Civil War, 1936–1939. *Nursing History Review*, *3*, 79–104.

Paul, E. A. (1985). Wounded healers: A summary of the Vietnam Nurse Veteran Project. *Military Medicine*, *150*, 571–576.

Pokorny, M. E. (1992). An historical perspective of Confederate nursing during the Civil War, 1861–1865. *Nursing Research*, *41*, 28–32.

Rogge, M. M. (1987). Nursing and politics: A forgotten legacy. *Nursing Research*, *36*, 26–30.

Sarnecky, M. T. (1989). A history of volunteerism and patriotism in the Army Nurse Corps. *Military Medicine*, *154*, 358–364.

Schwartz, L. S. (1987). Women and the Vietnam experience. *IMAGE: Journal of Nursing Scholarship*, *19*, 168–173.

Selavan, J. C. (1975). Nurses in American history: The Revolution. *American Journal of Nursing*, *75*, 592–594.

Stevens, S. Y. (1990). Sale of the century: Images of nursing in the Movietonews during World War II. *Advances in Nursing Science*, *12* (4), 44–52.

Stretch, R. H., Vail, J. D., & Maloney, J. P. (1985). Posttraumatic stress disorder among Army Nurse Corps Vietnam veterans. *Journal of Consulting and Clinical Psychology, 53*, 704–708.

Wall, B. M. (1993). Grace under pressure: The nursing Sisters of the Holy Cross, 1861–1865. *Nursing History Review, 1*, 71–87.

Wall, B. M. (1995). Courage to care: The Sisters of the Holy Cross in the Spanish-American War. *Nursing History Review, 3*, 55–77.

Wood, A. D. (1972). The war within a war: Women nurses in the Union army. *Civil War History, 18*, 197–212.

Woodward, W. (1991). New surprises in very old places: Civil War nurse leaders and longevity. *Nursing Forum, 26*(1), 9–16.

Chapter 10

Long-Term Vascular Access Devices

Janet S. Fulton
College of Nursing and Health
Wright State University

ABSTRACT

Introduced in the 1970s, long-term vascular access devices are used in both adults and children, with about 500,000 devices placed annually. This integrative review of research on dressings to minimize infectious catheter-related complications showed that current practices were adapted from knowledge derived from short-term central venous and peripheral catheters without thorough investigation. Summary and critique of recent, as well as older significant studies, provide guidance for future research. Specifically, future research should demonstrate greater confidence in outcome measures with attention to reliability of laboratory methods, diagnostic criteria, and interrater reliability. Continuing research efforts are needed to capture unique design features of various devices, qualify device performance across prolonged time, examine nuances within patient subgroups, and address underrepresented patients and settings. Confounding and interacting variables require greater attention in study design and analysis.

Keywords: Vascular Access Device, Infection, Complications, Dressings, Interventions, Nursing Procedures

In the United States approximately 500,000 long-term venous access catheters are inserted into adults and children annually (Alexander, 1994). Designed to be left in place for years, they are used to administer fluids, nutrition, medication, blood, and blood products. They are also instrumental in the removal of blood for laboratory analysis.

The first long-term devices, introduced during the 1970s, were tunneled catheters; these were followed by implanted ports, and recently by a new generation of peripherally inserted central catheters (PICC). These long-term catheters vary in design, placement, materials, and clinical indications.

Health care professionals—nurses, surgeons, oncologists, infection-control practitioners, nutritionists, and pharmacists—have descriptively and experimentally studied access catheters during the past 25 years. Topical areas of research included: (a) indications for use, (b) insertion techniques, (c) mechanical complications, (d) infectious complications, (e) thrombolytic complications, and (f) routine–care procedures to prevent or to minimize complications.

The focus of this review is limited to research involving dressing procedures to either prevent or to minimize infectious complications associated with long-term venous access devices. Furthermore, it is especially directed to nurses, as dressing procedures are a major nursing responsibility.

An extensive MEDLINE search of both nursing and nonnursing sources from 1976 to 1995 identified research articles involving dressing techniques. No subheading *directly* identified *dressing procedures*; the subheadings adverse effects, nursing, and infectious complications were used. In addition, device manufacturers' and expert practitioners' opinions about landmark works and outstanding authors enhanced and supported the findings of the electronic search.

SIMILARITIES AND DIFFERENCES IN TYPES OF DEVICES

When considering dressings to prevent or to minimize infectious complications, similarities and differences between devices are important. Long-term central venous access devices represent three distinct designs: tunneled catheters, implanted ports, and peripherally inserted central catheters.

Tunneled catheters usually are either thick-walled silicone rubber (Silastic® [Dow Corning Corp., Midland, MI]) or polyurethane (Vialon® [Becton-Dickinson, Franklin, NY]), and of single, double, or triple lumen. Placed in the subclavian vein, the tip terminates in the superior vena cava. The nonvascular portion is tunneled under subcutaneous chest tissue. The port exits midsternum. The catheter is anchored by growth of fibrous tissue around a Dacron® (DuPont Inc., Wilmington, DE) cuff that circles the tunneled portion. The cuff and tunnel create a barrier against migration of microbes into the vasculature. Routine heparin flush maintains catheter patency.

Implanted venous ports are unique. All portions are surgically implanted beneath the skin. Although arterial, peritoneal, and epidural ports are available, this review includes only venous ports. Venous ports are placed using a percutaneous technique, locating the tip in the superior vena cava, and tunneling the catheter under the subcutaneous tissue. The access port, a chamber approximately 14 mm high by 34 mm in diameter with a silicone rubber septum, is placed subcutaneously and parallel to the skin. Percutaneous puncture of the chamber septum with a noncoring needle creates venous access. Ports are palpable under the subcutaneous tissue; access relies on placement location by palpation. Chamber design and material vary, including stainless steel, titanium, plastic, and silicone. Catheters are silicone. Double-lumen designs are available. Patency is maintained by routine heparin flush.

Peripherally inserted central catheters—as the name implies—are long-term catheters peripherally inserted into the basilic or cephalic venous networks near the antecubital fossa. These PICC lines should terminate in the superior vena (Ryder, 1993). Lines that terminate in the axillary vein at midclavicular region or at a point 6 to 8 inches from the antecubital area are called *peripherally inserted catheters* (PIC) or midline catheters (Markel & Reynen, 1990). Dressing care for both PICC and midline catheters is reviewed.

With no complications, PICC lines—available in silicone, polyurethane, and polyurethane–hydrogel mix (Aquavene® [Menlo Care, Menlo Park, CA])—are usable for extended periods of several months. Insertion techniques vary, but all catheters are inserted by percutaneous puncture of skin and threaded into the peripheral vasculature. Nylon sutures anchor catheters to the skin at the insertion site for the duration of catheter use.

INFECTIOUS COMPLICATIONS ASSOCIATED WITH LONG-TERM DEVICES

Infections related to long-term vascular access devices are serious and can be life-threatening. Infectious complications reportedly range from 0% to 60% (Alexander, 1994; Merritt et al., 1981; Mirro et al., 1989; Shapiro, Wald, Nelson, & Spiegelman, 1982; Winters, Peters, Coila, & Jones, 1990). The nature of catheter-related infections is an important consideration in understanding dressings as agents to prevent or to minimize infections.

Skin flora such as *Staphylococcus epidermidis*, *Staphylococcus aureus*, *Streptococcus* species, and *Candida* species are organisms most commonly isolated with peripheral intravenous catheters (Craven et al., 1985), percutaneous short-term central catheters (Conley, Grieves, & Peters, 1989; Maki & Band, 1981; Young, Alexeyeff, Russell, & Thomas, 1988), and in all types of long-term devices for both adult (Begala, Maher, & Cherry, 1981; Keung et al., 1994; Pegues et al., 1992) and pediatric populations (Becton, Kletzel, Golladay, Hathaway, & Berry, 1988; Dawson et al., 1991; Ingram, Weitzman,

Greenberg, Parkin, & Filler, 1991; Mirro et al., 1989). Implicating skin flora as a causative agent suggests that the etiology of infection may be related to these organisms' ability to overwhelm a susceptible host. Perhaps microbes enter through the catheter-induced break in skin integrity. To help prevent infectious complications, therefore, dressings are placed at exit sites—where skin integrity is interrupted.

Catheter-related infections include three types: exit site, tunnel or port pocket, and catheter-related sepsis (Alexander, 1994). Exit-site infections— that occur and remain wherever skin integrity is broken—manifest by erythema, swelling, warmth, and tenderness without systemic signs of infection. Tunnel or pocket infections—that represent a suppurative process in the subcutaneous tissue surrounding a portion of a catheter tunnel or port chamber— exhibit varying degrees of cellulitis, purulent drainage, and systemic signs of infection. Port pocket infections—that originate at the site of percutaneous needle puncture of port access—are believed to result from microbes migrating along the needle track into subcutaneous tissue surrounding the port chamber. Catheter-related sepsis—that becomes suspect when blood cultures show bacteremia—manifests clinical symptoms of infection, most often with fever and chills.

Although catheter colonization is one factor in the pathogenesis of catheter-related infection, the sources of catheter colonization remain controversial. It has been proposed, however, that both catheter site skin colonization and catheter hub contamination may be factors.

Colonization of the catheter may result from microbes migrating along the surface of the catheter from an exit site. Using an animal model, Cooper, Schiller, and Hopkins (1988) demonstrated that *Staphylococcus aureus* and *Streptococcus* species inoculated at the puncture site of subdermally placed polytetrafluroethylene (Teflon® [DuPont Inc., Wilmington, DE]) catheters can be identified at the tips of the catheters within 1 hour. Using an in vitro model of nutrient agar, polyethylene catheters, and *Pseudomonas aeruginosa*, Harris, Rosenquist, and Kealey (1992) demonstrated that capillary action occurs along catheters in an agar tunnel. In cases of catheter-related bacteremia involving percutaneously inserted central venous catheters, investigators demonstrated a strong association between isolates obtained from exit sites and catheter tip (Bjornson et al., 1982; Snydman et al., 1982). Although the above general distinctions may differentiate among types of catheter-related infections, no standard diagnostic criteria are available. Thus, determination of catheter-related infection remains subject to clinician discretion. Investigators rarely obtain independent determinations of infection or report interrater reliability scores.

Microbes can adhere to and multiply on the surface of catheters (Sheth, Rose, Franson, Buckmire, & Sohnle, 1983). All types of long-term catheter materials (silicone, polyurethane, and polyurethane–hydrogel mix) have been associated with microbial colonization (Becton et al., 1988; Keung et al., 1994; Rasor, 1991), although no research documented the degree of adherence by type of catheter material. Catheters with antimicrobial or bacteriostatic agents reduced incidence of intravascular, catheter-related infections for percutaneously placed central venous and arterial catheters (Kamal, Pfaller, Rempe, & Jebson, 1991; Maki, 1988).

Although catheter materials are considered thromboresistant and nonhemolytic, these properties vary by types of catheter material used. The insertion of any catheter introduces a foreign material into the body, and microbial adherence may begin almost immediately, following a sequence of events summarized by Ryder (1993). Initially, the catheter surface becomes coated—by plasma, tissue proteins, and fibrin—creating a sleeve of biofilm rich in substances highly adherent to selected microbes, including *Staphylococcus aureus* and *Staphylococcus epidermidis*. Microbial production of a glyacocalyx material, known as extracellular slime, enhances and promotes adherence of additional organisms. Extracellular slime also binds together microcolonies within fibrous exopolysaccharide matrix. Due to an expanding biofilm that coats the catheter, eradicating the microbes with systemic antibiotics becomes difficult (Kamal et al., 1991). Biofilm does not cause overt infections, but it can encourage infection if host resistance mechanisms do not overcome excessive microbial growth (Costerton et al., 1987). Thus, organisms that originate at external sites may migrate and reside in the biofilm adherent to long-term venous catheters as a source of catheter-related bacteremia.

Using an animal model and silicone catheters, Lloyd, Shanbhogue, Sutherland, Hart, and Williams (1993) compared microorganisms introduced before a biofilm sheath developed with microorganisms already protected by a fibrin sheath. Investigators suggested a possible protective role of biofilm. These results may indicate the need for very rigorous aseptic dressing techniques immediately following insertion of a catheter device.

On the other hand, not all infections related to long-term access devices are caused by resident skin flora. Evidence demonstrates that a variety of microorganisms may cause infectious complications, including bacteria, yeast, and fungi (Barber, Brown, Kiehn, Edwards, & Armstrong, 1993; Bottino, McCredie, Groschel, & Lawson, 1979; Prichard et al., 1988; Wade et al., 1981). Furthermore, not all catheter-related infections originate from direct invasion of microbes at the exit site. Microbes sometimes enter via catheter hub (Liñares, Sitges-Serra, Garau, Perez, & Martin, 1985; Salzman, Isenberg, Shapiro, Lipsitz, & Rubin, 1993), contaminated fluids (Maki, 1991), or hematogenous seeding from other infections such as wound infections within the body (Bjornson et al., 1982). Most catheter-related yeast infections are believed to be the result of hematogenous dissemination from another site (Hampton & Sherertz, 1988). In addition, other identified risk factors include: duration and use of the catheter, number of catheter manipulations, and number of catheter lumens, as well as individual experience in catheter insertion. Concurrent diagnoses and therapies that alter immunocompetence of the host pose additional risk factors (Hampton & Sherertz, 1988; Maki, 1991). The prevention of catheter-related infection does not solely depend upon dressing procedures. Consider other relevant variables—catheter materials, product designs, and host factors—when designing or evaluating research.

DRESSING TECHNIQUES TO MINIMIZE INFECTION

Initial Directions and Related Interests

Current interest in catheter dressings began with nurse investigators and others studying the relationship between dressing procedures and central venous catheter (CVC)-related infections. The use of percutaneously inserted CVC lines markedly increased during the 1960s. Serious and fatal septicemia was documented as a result of CVC line placement (Ryan et al., 1974). At the same time, the expanding use of intravenous (IV) therapy prompted a parallel interest in techniques for the care of peripheral IV sites. Dressing techniques for long-term venous access devices were adapted from knowledge and experience about CVC and peripheral IV catheter care. A complete discussion of CVC and IV catheter-care techniques is beyond the scope of this review. Selected findings from related work that support the research involving long-term devices are presented for discussion.

Initial interests in IV dressing techniques were demonstrated in studies that examined use of antibiotic ointment to prevent infectious complications related to peripheral IV devices (Norden, 1969; Zinner et al., 1969). Investigators determined that antibiotic ointment did not significantly reduce the rate of catheter-related infection. As a result of the study's emphasis on catheter care, however, Zinner et al. serendipitously noted that catheters receiving *inadequate* care had significantly and statistically greater positive tip cultures than those receiving *adequate* care.

In an early study of CVC, a team of physicians and nurses evaluated 200 subjects receiving total parenteral nutrition (TPN) via a polyethylene catheter inserted in the subclavian vein. They found a statistically significant lower sepsis rate among catheters carefully cared for according to protocol. Conclusion: Dressing care is an important variable. Their dressing care included rigorous skin preparation, antibiotic ointment, and an air-occlusive dressing (Ryan et al., 1974). Initial research efforts, therefore, gave evidence that routine, attentive dressing care is superior to random care.

Next, investigators explored the effectiveness of antibiotic ointments, skin preparation agents, frequency of dressing changes, and type of dressing material used with catheter-related, infectious complications. Jarrard and Freeman (1977) examined effects of antibiotic ointments applied under dressings. They noted that broad spectrum antibiotic ointments did suppress skin flora. Maki and Band (1981) further examined use of antimicrobial ointments on catheter insertion sites. They demonstrated that topical ointment confers some, but only marginal, protection against catheter-related infection.

To remove microbial contaminants and debris around the catheter insertion site, reported procedures often included use of antimicrobial agents such as: povidone iodine, alcohol, chlorhexidine, acetone, and ether. Jarrard and Freeman (1977) demonstrated reduction in skin flora using povidone iodine. Maki, Ringer, and Alvarado (1991) associated incidence of positive semiquantitative catheter tip cultures by type of skin preparation. Chlorhexidine, alcohol, and povidone iodine showed lowest incidence of positive tip cultures. Chlorhexidine was superior to povidone iodine as a skin preparation agent. Questioning the effects of removing normal fatty acid secretions from the skin's microbial ecosystem, Maki and McCormack (1987) evaluated the use of an organic solvent—acetone—to remove skin lipids and to disinfect CVC insertion sites. According to these researchers, acetone increased local skin inflammation, increased subject discomfort, did not improve microbial removal, and did not reduce incidence of catheter-related infection.

Jarrad, Olson, and Freeman (1980) examined the effects of daily dressing changes on skin flora under CVC dressings. Conclusion: Daily dressing changes eliminated all skin organisms from beneath dressings.

In the late 1970s, transparent adherent dressings (TAD) replaced many traditional types. Created as a wound dressing, the first TAD dressing, Op-Site® (Smith and Nephew Ltd, Largo, FL) gained popularity as a catheter dressing. Many nurses preferred its adhesive properties to tapes, and its transparency that enabled them to visualize the site. Prior to Op-Site® the only transparent dressing material was Saran Wrap® (vinylidene polymer plastic [Dow Brand, Indianapolis, IN]). Aly, Shirley, Cunico, and Maibach (1978) wrapped subjects' arms and demonstrated that several factors affecting bacterial survival on skin could be altered, such as hydration, pH, CO_2 emission rate, and skin surface lipids. Microbial flora changed. Some species increased; others decreased. TAD dressings were semipermeable (moisture vapor permeable) polyurethane and concluded to be safer than a dressing with totally occlusive properties.

Initial investigations supported the use of Op-Site® as a dressing material for CVC catheters (Palidar et al., 1982; Schwartz-Fulton, Colley, Valanis, &

Fischer, 1981; Thomas, 1977). These investigators all reported that infectious complications were low and suggested weekly dressing changes. Powell, Regan, Fabri, and Ruberg (1982) compared Op-Site® changed every 7 days to standard gauze and tape dressing changed Monday, Wednesday, and Friday. Conclusion: Op-Site® should be changed more frequently than every 7 days. On the other hand, Maki and Will (1984) drew different conclusions when they compared Tegaderm® (3–M Health Care, St. Paul, MN) TAD dressing changed every 2 days or every 7 days with gauze and tape dressings changed every 2 days. There was a statistically significant greater colonization of the skin under the Tegaderm® dressings changed every 7 days. The rate of catheter-related bacteremia, however, was similar in all three groups. Investigators concluded Tegaderm® could be safely used and changed every 7 days. To evaluate longevity and usefulness, Vazquez and Jarrard (1984) left Op-Site® dressings in place on CVC catheters for as long as 11 days, averaging a dressing life of 5.3 days for silicone catheters and 4.3 days for polyvinyl chloride catheters. They gave no explanation for the varying life of dressing by catheter material.

In addition to these studies involving CVC catheters, several investigators examined the use of TAD dressings for peripheral IV site care. Three separate investigators demonstrated a reduced incidence of phlebitis for subjects treated with Op-Site® when compared to gauze dressings (Gantz, Presswood, Goldberg, & Doern, 1984; Nicola & DeChairo, 1984; Peterson & Freeman, 1982). Kelsey and Gosling (1984) compared Op-Site® to gauze dressing using three different catheter brands representing two types of catheter materials. Conclusion: Catheter material, method of manufacture, and clinical use of the catheter were more important determinants of catheter-related complications than type of dressing.

Several investigators examined the effects of catheter-related dressing materials and antimicrobial agents on intact skin. Aly, Bayles, and Maibach (1988) demonstrated that 3 days following a povidone iodine and alcohol skin preparation, resident skin flora do not return to normal population densities. No significant quantitative differences between TAD and gauze dressings were noted. All dressings maintained flora at one-tenth the population of the uncovered site. Rhame, Feist, Muller, Steere, and Cameron (1983) concluded that TAD dressings, in combination with povidone iodine ointment, inhibited the growth of normal flora, and did not promote growth of nonresident microbes. Holmström and Svensson (1987) demonstrated significantly fewer microbial counts under TAD dressings when the skin was cleaned with chlorhexidine. Conclusion: Collective findings of these investigators suggested that the ability to maintain low bacterial skin counts under TAD dressings definitely was related to use of microbial agents.

In an isolated study that examined inert bactericidal activity of TAD dressings, Holland, Davis, Ingham, and Gowland (1984) used an in vitro model to determine the ability of Tegaderm® and Op-Site® to activate the complement system. In bacterial killing tests, Op-Site® was superior to Tegaderm®. Only Op-Site® activated C3 complement in human serum, which suggests that properties of the material could aid in killing microbes and facilitate opsonization and phagocytosis.

Maki and Ringer (1987) evaluated gauze, a TAD dressing, and an iodophor-treated, transparent dressing on peripheral IV sites. Stepwise, logistic multivariate analysis identified significant risk factors for catheter-related infection as cutaneous colonization of insertion site, contamination of catheter hub, moisture under the dressing, and prolonged catheterization. Investigators recommended that TAD dressing be more permeable to reduce accumulation of moisture beneath the dressing, and reduce risk of infection due to cutaneous colonization.

Early in the 1990s, moisture vapor permeability was modified by Smith and Nephew Ltd. of Largo, FL. With the new product, Op–Site IV 3000®, moisture vapor permeability became three to eight times greater than that of other TAD dressings. Evaluated as a dressing for pulmonary artery catheters, cutaneous colonization beneath the dressing was lowest with gauze, intermediate with the highly permeable Op–Site 3000®, and highest with a traditional TAD dressing (Maki, Stolz, Wheeler, & Mermel, 1994).

These studies highlight information gained through research on a variety of venous catheter dressings. Even so, comparisons among findings are difficult. Studies varied in the overall dressing procedure, as well as in skin preparation, antimicrobial ointment, type of dressing, and frequency of change. Catheters also differed in material, location, and use. Underreporting of variables was common. These difficulties are noted in a meta-analysis conducted to estimate the impact of TAD dressings on catheter-related infections (Hoffman, Weber, Samsa, & Rutala, 1992). Results of the meta-analysis demonstrated an increased risk of catheter-related infections; however, inconsistencies among and underreporting of study variables threatened the findings.

Tunneled Catheters

To secure a tunneled catheter after placement, a temporary skin suture is used at the exit site. It remains for 5 to 7 days—or longer for patients with impaired healing—as the cuff forms a fibrous attachment to the subcutaneous tissue. Because of the wound, exit sites routinely are dressed after catheter insertion; however, the practice of continuously dressing a healed site has been the subject of controversy (Lucas, 1994). The skin surface of a well-healed exit site may be likened to a healed, pierced ear that lacks any signs of inflammation or irritation. The cuff-and-tunnel technique were designed to prevent infection. Some clinicians, therefore, stated that there is no need to dress a healed exit site (Baranowski, 1993; Marcoux, Fischer, & Wong, 1990). On the other hand, some clinicians cite the possibility of infection and advocate dressings (Anderson, Aker, & Hickman, 1982; Johnstone, 1982). Exit-site and tunnel-track infections caused by skin flora also have been documented (Begala et al., 1981; Christensen et al., 1993).

Early reports of the successful use of tunneled catheters advocated rigorous dressing procedures (Bottino et al., 1979; Merritt et al., 1981; Shapiro et al., 1982; Wade et al., 1981). For example, Johnstone (1982) reviewed the incidence of tunneled catheter infections for 260 patients over a 2-year period and reported a low infection rate following use of daily gauze dressing changes, povidone iodine and hydrogen peroxide skin preparation, and povidone iodine ointment. Though dressing procedures were not systematically evaluated, the investigator suggested that they definitely relate to the successful use of the catheters.

According to Johnstone's (1982) report, initial dressing procedures for tunneled catheters were similar to CVC catheter-dressing procedures. After Carelli and Herink (1984) reviewed the literature and sampled hospital procedures, they determined that recommended dressing materials included gauze (87%), TAD (7%), and no dressing on healed sites (9%). Frequency of dressing change was daily (33%), every other day (45%), twice a week (14%), and weekly (7%). Commonly recommended skin preparation agents were alcohol, povidone iodine, and hydrogen peroxide. Frequently, povidone iodine ointment was also recommended.

Using a prospective nonrandomized two-group design, Jones (1987) examined two steps within dressing procedures—hand washing and masking—for adults with cancer and demonstrated that neither step was significantly associated with catheter-related infections. In this study, most of the subjects were immunosuppressed due to antineoplastic chemotherapy. A neutrophil count of under 22% increased the risk for infection. Erythema at the catheter site occurred in 70% of the subjects. Exit-site erythema of 1.1 to 3.0 cm was correlated with local catheter infection.

Petrosino, Becker, and Christian (1988) used a four-group experimental design to study dressing techniques for tunneled catheters in persons with cancer diagnoses. Dressing materials included Tegaderm®, Op-Site®, gauze, or no dressing. The rationale for no dressing: infections seldom develop in clean wounds when left exposed. To rate infection, investigators used a composite of indicators that included pain, erythema, skin cultures, oral temperature, and purulent drainage. These indicators were ranked, weighted, and given separate infection scores for each observation. Conclusion: Investigators demonstrated no statistically significant differences in infection rates among dressing groups, and the no-dressing group performed as well, presenting a simpler and less costly alternative for further investigation.

Shivnan et al. (1991) examined dressings on exit sites of persons with long-term catheters during bone marrow transplant. Investigators stratified 98 subjects by age, type of transplant, and location of catheter placement, then randomized them into two groups. One group received a TAD dressing changed every 4 days. The other received a daily change of gauze dressing. Both groups used a hydrogen peroxide and povidone iodine skin preparation, a skin protectant barrier, and a triple antibiotic ointment. All subjects received broad-spectrum antibiotic support. Only one case of catheter-related infection was reported. Investigators noted no significant differences between the two dressings in the incidence of local infection determined by skin cultures. Skin irritation appeared statistically greater for gauze dressings, and TAD dressings cost less.

Two studies specifically evaluated dressing procedures in pediatric populations. Freiberger, Bryant, and Marino (1992) compared the effects of two different antiseptics used to clean the skin (povidone iodine and chlorhexidine), and two different dressings (TAD and gauze) to cover the exit site of catheters in children with cancer. Dressings were changed on Mondays, Wednesdays, and Fridays. Skin cultures were taken at the time of dressing I and again during dressing V. No statistically significant differences occurred in the incidence of bacterial growth between types of dressings or between types of antiseptic skin preparation. Using a randomized, experimental, crossover study design, Hutchinson, Waskerwitz, Martin, Faubion, and Revesz (1990) compared sterile occlusive dressing to clean, nonocclusive dressing applied to the exit site of tunneled catheters in children with cancer. Conclusion: Investigators noted no significant difference in infectious complications between the two types of dressings.

In the above-mentioned studies, all dressing care procedures performed well in preventing catheter-related infection. All investigators used infectious complications as an outcome measure—each defining it slightly differently. These combined results support previous findings that a consistently applied care routine is effective in preventing infectious complications. What is less clear, however, is the rationale for choosing various procedural steps, dressing products, and antimicrobial agents in selected populations.

Several investigators identified cutaneous complications associated with rigorous dressing procedures. Schwartz-Fulton and Tischenko (1985) documented that persons with cancer experienced difficulty tolerating a procedure that included acetone, alcohol, povidone iodine skin preparation, povidone iodine ointment, tincture of benzoin, and an occlusive Elastoplast® tape (Beiersdorf Corp., Norwalk, CT). Of 24 subjects, 20 (83%) experienced skin irritation at their exit sites. These irritations related to products used in the dressing procedure. Povidone iodine ointment (62.5%) and Elastoplast® (58%) showed the highest frequencies of irritation.

Investigators questioned the degree to which the dressing procedure disrupted integrity of the skin. Conclusion: Investigators suggested that the rigorous dressing procedure left the skin more vulnerable to irritation, colonization, and infection. These results are consistent with the Maki and McCormack (1987) findings that acetone caused skin irritation and inflammation.

Bagnall-Reeb and Ruccione (1990) studied dressing-related cutaneous reactions experienced by 238 pediatric subjects on either tunneled catheters or on implanted ports. They observed 20 episodes of cutaneous reactions—defined as erythema, swelling, tenderness, discharge, or rashes—along with 13 episodes of local infection—defined as positive skin cultures in the presence of a cutaneous reaction. In each case, the dressing procedure included an alcohol and povidone iodine skin preparation, povidone iodine ointment, and a TAD dressing. Tunneled catheter dressings were changed every other day and accessed-port dressing but twice a week. From these data, investigators constructed an algorithm for managing cutaneous reactions to dressing procedures.

Implanted Ports

Port access is obtained by placing a needle through the skin and port septum, thereby creating a direct entry route for migrating microbes to enter the pocket. Ports may be accessed for varying lengths of time—short-term access and long-term access. Short-term access involves preparing the skin, inserting the needle, performing a limited procedure such as administering a drug or withdrawing a blood specimen, and removing the needle. Typically, dressings are not used for short-term access. Recommended skin preparation includes alcohol and povidone iodine (Bagnall & Ruccione, 1987; Gyves et al., 1984; Long & Ovaska, 1992; Schulmeister, 1987). Separate investigators examined port access procedures for short-term access. Schulmeister (1987) demonstrated no incidence with either the manufacturer's recommended rigorous, sterile procedures or with similar, less costly clean procedures. Long and Ovaska compared a sterile procedure, using a commercially available access kit, to a clean procedure. No port-related infections were reported for either group.

Long-term access involves leaving a needle in place for days or weeks. The implications of using a clean technique for prolonged access are not clear.

Microbial contamination introduced during a clean technique and covered by a dressing could create a potential source of infection. No studies examining infectious complications related to long-term port access dressings were located; however, recommendations for care included needle changes every 5 to 10 days, antibiotic ointment placed at the needle puncture site, and an occlusive dressing of either gauze-and-tape or TAD dressing (Baranowski, 1993; Ecoff, Barone, & Simons, 1983; Lokich, Bothe, Benotti, & Moore, 1985; Moore, Erikson, Yanes, Franklin, & Gonsalves, 1986). As with reports of tunneled catheters, investigators did not systematically evaluate the relationship between dressing procedures and catheter outcomes (Ecoff et al., 1983; Gyves et al., 1984; Lokich et al., 1985; Moore et al., 1986). Although some investigators reported no infectious complications (Ecoff et al., 1983; Gyves et al., 1984), others documented port-pocket and catheter-related infections (Bagnall & Riccone, 1987; Becton et at., 1988; Brothers et al., 1988; Lokich et al., 1985).

Several investigators compared infectious complications of tunneled catheters to implanted ports (Bagnall & Ruccione, 1987; Keung et al., 1994; May & Davis, 1988; Mirro et al., 1989; Pegues et al., 1992). Collective results demonstrated a trend toward fewer infectious complications in subjects with implanted ports.

PICC Catheters

For the duration of a PICC catheter placement, the catheter exit site is dressed. Placement of a PICC catheter creates a direct route for microbes to enter the vasculature. Infectious complications related to PICC lines have been reported (Abi-Nader, 1993; Myers & Kyle, 1993; Prichard et al., 1988).

Dressing care for PICC catheter exit sites appears to be derived from knowledge of CVC and peripheral IV catheter care. No investigations were located that specifically evaluated dressing procedures for PICC catheters. Investigators used descriptive designs to document the success of PICC catheters. They often discussed dressing care as a reason for minimal complications, but did not systematically evaluate dressing procedures (Abi-Nader, 1993; Andrews, 1991; Lawson, Bottino, & McCredie, 1979; Myers & Kyle, 1993; Rutherford, 1988).

Investigators recommended that dressing procedures include skin preparation using alcohol and povidone iodine, povidone iodine ointment, and occlusive dressing with gauze and TAD dressings. Furthermore, they recommended frequency of dressing change from 3 to 7 days (Andrews, 1991; Legha, Haq, Rabinowits, Lawson, & McCredie, 1985; Myers & Kyle, 1993; Prichard et al., 1988). Two investigators reported that subjects experienced localized skin reactions to povidone iodine (Harwood, Greene, Kozakowski-Koch, & Rasor, 1992; Prichard et al., 1988).

Several investigators described infection and phlebitis as complications related to the use of PICC catheters. Markel and Reynen (1990) followed 130 home care subjects in 16 states for a total of 2652 catheter years and reported low rates of both infection and phlebitis. Abi-Nader (1993) prospectively followed 97 consecutive PICC insertions in critical care subjects and reported low rates of catheter-related infection. Five subjects developed phlebitis upon insertion that resolved without catheter removal. Other investigators reported phlebitis as a PICC catheter complication (Andrews, 1991; Graham, Kelder-mans, Klemm, Semenza, & Shafer, 1991; Myers & Kyle, 1993). Andrews (1991) reported a lower rate of phlebitis associated with Aquavene® catheters compared to silicone catheters. Rutherford (1988) identified an association between days of catheter duration and localized skin inflammation. Phlebitis occurred more frequently in women during initial days following insertion of catheter (Abi-Nader, 1993; Hadaway, 1989; Rutherford, 1988). Phlebitis is thought to be caused by an irritating presence of a catheter. The development of mechanical phlebitis, however, can induce infection. Maki, Drinka, and Davis (1975) described incidences of catheter-related suppurative phlebitis. The relationship among dressings, local irritation, and phlebitis is not clear; however, phlebitis appears to be another variable of interest to include in dressing procedures for PICC lines. Investigators should differentiate between mechanical phlebitis and local irritation due to dressing products and antimicrobial agents.

RESEARCH ISSUES

Constructing a Scientific Rationale

The conceptual basis and scientific rationale for examining questions about dressing procedures emanate from the sciences of biology and physiology. Freiberger et al. (1992) offered Neuman's System Model as a conceptual framework. The model supports a general rationale for nurses' interests in preventing infectious complications. It is too abstract, however, to provide direction for study design or interpretation of results. In addition to Neuman's model, the investigators included microbiologic rationale for the study. Including Neuman's System Model seems superfluous and awkward.

Previous investigators made important contributions toward the construction of scientific rationale for clinical decision making regarding long-term catheter care. Unfortunately, their less-than-optimal research designs and data analysis inhibit interpretation of much of the research. When reviewing this literature, therefore, let future investigators be cautious regarding limitations of published findings.

Stating the Question

To state the question clearly and in advance provides focus for the study and encourages proper design and data analysis. Studies without a clearly delineated research question were little more than reports of personal experiences with patients in a given setting. Data from individual cases were summarized and discussed. Conclusions and directions for future research were not outlined (Becton et al., 1988; Brothers et al., 1988; Dawson et al., 1991; Graham et al., 1991; Harwood et al., 1992; Shapiro et al., 1982).

With no research question, data often were underanalyzed or overinterpreted. Underanalysis diminished the research effort. For example, when they reported observed catheter complications, Markel and Reynen (1990) could have explored the frequency of complications by a number of variables, such as age, type of device, and type of therapy, to maximize the effort of this multisite study. Brothers et al. (1988) reviewed the records of 300 persons with implanted ports and reported no relationship between complications and selected variables. It seems that investigators used individual correlation measures with arguably interactive variables, thus underanalyzing the data.

Using descriptive research designs to conclude interventions represents overinterpretation of data. For example, based on observations, Bagnall-Reeb and Ruccione (1990) recommended untested intervention algorithms for management of cutaneous reactions to various dressing materials and agents. As in this example, possible interventions suggested by initial findings need further controlled evaluation.

Measuring Outcome Variables

The most frequently cited outcome measure for catheter dressing studies is infection—local, tunnel, or port-pocket, or catheter-related sepsis. Multiple, inconsistent, and conflicting definitions prevail (Begala et al., 1981; Benezra et al., 1988; Press, Ramsey, Larson, Fefer, & Hickman, 1984).

Several influencing and interacting variables make it difficult to determine concise definitions of catheter-related infection. Five commonly used indicators, however, are fever, local inflammation, skin cultures, blood cultures, and catheter tip cultures. Not mutually exclusive, each indicator may occur in the presence or absence of another. Clinical suspicion of infection may result in treatment and prevent the complication from running its natural course. If so, expression of the indicator may not occur.

Use of these indicators is controversial for the following reasons:

1. Positive blood culture results do not necessarily indicate sepsis. Although catheter-related sepsis does not occur without bacteremia, bacteria in the blood does not always indicate sepsis. Blood taken from the catheter may yield a sample of resident organisms, known to reside in the slime formed on the catheter, and not reflect a true bacteremia. For comparison, investigators collect blood samples from both the catheter and peripheral blood. The usefulness of this practice may be questioned. Douard et al. (1991) used this paired-sampling method to evaluate febrile events in neutropenic children. From the catheter blood samples, 14% of the cultures demonstrated colony counts higher than from peripheral samples. Fourteen percent had identical counts from both specimens; 2% had positive results in only peripheral blood. Also, followup cultures are not always appropriate insomuch as the initiation of or change in antibiotic therapy can result in negative cultures.

2. The reliability of catheter-tip cultures can be questioned if the catheter is pulled through the insertion track. Using an in vitro model, Harris et al. (1992) confirmed that organisms can be dislodged from a catheter tip pulled through an agar tunnel. Possible results: A missed diagnosis, a missed causative organism, or a dislodged organism responsible for catheter sepsis replaced by a skin contaminant. Sensitivity of laboratory methods for determining catheter colonization varies (Raad, Sabbagh, Rand, & Sherertz, 1992). Nahass and Weinstein (1990) examined the predictive value of peripheral catheter cultures and concluded that many isolated organisms have no clinical relevance. Without the presence of other indicators, catheter-tip cultures provide insufficient evidence for diagnosis of catheter-related infection. Furthermore, infections related to long-term devices are curable without catheter removal, thereby eliminating an opportunity for catheter culture (Douard et al., 1991).

3. The strength of the relationship between positive skin cultures and subsequent development of catheter-related sepsis is questionable. Based on data primarily derived from peripheral catheters, Maki, Weise, and Sarafin (1977) and Maki and Ringer (1987) demonstrated an association between skin-and-catheter segment when semiquantitative culture counts were > 15 colony-forming-units (CFU). Where this association was established for central venous catheters, it was based on semiquantitative culture results of the tip and of proximal subcutaneous portions of the catheter (Bjornson et al., 1982; Snydman et al., 1982). Conley et al. (1989) found no significant association between > 15 CFU cultured from CVC catheter tips and any signs of local infection. Guidet et al. (1994), however, found skin cultures of > 15 CFU

useful for assessing catheter colonization. Skin cultures were always positive in cases of catheter colonization, and always negative in the absence of catheter colonization. Conclusion: The association between positive skin cultures and catheter-related infection for long-term access devices has only been theorized.

4.   Although recognized for its universal physiological response to infections, fever may be affected by several factors: medications, tumors, anesthesia, and surgical procedures (Cunha, 1985). Furthermore, persons with a hematologic malignancy may show little or no increase in body temperature, despite a life-threatening infection. Tumors can stimulate the hypothalamus to produce substances similar to endogenous pyrogens, and necrosis or infarction within a tumor can effect a low-grade fever. Too, the necrotic center of a solid tumor may become secondarily infected and cause fever (Cunha, 1985). Douard et al. (1991) demonstrated that over 50% of febrile episodes in children with cancer were microbiologically undocumented. Conclusion: The use of fever alone as an outcome indicator is questionable.

5.   A commonly used indicator of catheter-related infection is local inflammatory response—generally defined by pain, warmth, swelling, erythema, and purulent drainage. These indicators also are used to evaluate catheter-related phlebitis in peripheral venous catheters. The reliability and validity of these indicators, however, have not been demonstrated. Due to suppressed white cell function, immunocompromised persons may not form purulent drainage in the presence of infection. To judge erythema for persons with dark-skinned complexion may be difficult and underappreciated when compared to persons with lighter skin. To judge pain by either involuntary response or by direct questioning may be unreliable among subjects with diminished mental status or among those receiving systemic pain medication. Products used in dressing procedures such as skin preparation agents, ointments, and tapes, may induce an allergic reaction manifest as local inflammation, with either the active ingredient or the base compound as causative agent.

Investigators who rate or score local inflammatory response should address issues of interrater reliability. Determining catheter-related infection greatly depends upon clinician judgment. To demonstrate greater diagnostic reliability, therefore, obtain two or more independent judgments for each subject. Then, calculate an interrater reliability coefficient.

Controlling Extraneous Variables

Investigators' failure to address extraneous variables posed a common problem in both descriptive and experimental studies. Extraneous variables encompass properties or characteristics of persons, things, or situations that may prevent clear understanding of relational or causal dynamics within the study. Variables related to subject characteristics include age, gender, medical diagnoses, and concurrent medical therapies. Catheter-related variables include catheter use, duration of use, number of catheter lumens, type of catheter material, and number of catheter manipulations. As previously discussed, catheter-related variables are associated with outcome. At minimum, report extraneous variables. Investigators using experimental designs should control for extraneous variables, either by study design or method of analysis. In addition, studies are needed that use correlational and multivariate analyses to explicate relationships among these variables.

Sampling Issues

Persons who need long-term venous access devices differ greatly with respect to demographics, illness characteristics, and medical treatment. Population characteristics generally are not randomly distributed across a single setting. Many investigators recruited subjects from a single, tertiary-care setting. Single-site experimental studies threaten the generalizability of results. Recruiting subjects from multiple sites would have strengthened the credibility of findings.

Several investigators reported that members of their research team changed all dressing (Maki et al., 1994; Maki & Ringer, 1987; Schwartz-Fulton et al., 1981). Such close control compromises application of findings, as most care institutions have many nurses performing dressing care. In home care, patients and family members change the dressing.

Furthermore, the decision to use a long-term access device is based on clinician judgement. One prefers tunneled catheters; another recommends PICC lines for the same purpose. Investigators should consider the decision to use a device and selection of a device as bias reflected in the sample.

Experimental studies demonstrated a lack of attention to statistical power and sample size. Because investigators have repeatedly demonstrated that attentive care is superior to random care, statistical differences can be expected when comparing any consistently applied care technique to no consistent care. Given the evidence, it may seem unreasonable or unethical to create a *no-care* control group. The question becomes: Just how different are various dressing procedures? The effect size of one procedure over another is likely small to moderate, a situation that requires large sample sizes to detect a difference if one exists. In addition, with attentive care, incidence of infectious complications is low, further compounding a need for large sample sizes if infection becomes an outcome measure.

Few studies reported statistical power calculations. Using an effect size of 35%, a power of 80%, and a one-tailed alpha of 0.05, Shivnan et al. (1991) stated that 98 subjects were adequate for a two-group design. Freiberger et al. (1992) were unable to demonstrate differences among four groups and retrospectively calculated power. The effect size for the data was calculated to be 18%. The investigators determined that a sample size numbering 271 could provide sufficient power to detect true differences in the four dressing groups. They had 60 subjects.

SUMMARY AND FUTURE DIRECTIONS

As you already read, literature on dressing procedures for long-term venous access devices varies considerably according to type of dressing material, frequency of dressing change, and use of antimicrobial agents. Adapted from knowledge originally derived from short-term CVC and peripheral IV catheters, dressing procedures for long-term devices were applied without thorough investigation.

Increasing use of long-term venous access devices offers both opportunities and challenges for future investigators: (a) Design device-specific research that captures unique design features of each device; (b) Conduct longitudinal studies that follow devices in place for months or years. Although costly, longitudinal studies provide insight into variables that affect a device's success or failure; (c) Specify the population of interest. Pay attention to subgroups with samples; (d) Create multisite studies in underrepresented settings such as: home care, extended care, ambulatory care, and rural settings; (e) Increase confidence in outcome measures for determining infectious complications. Give greater attention to reliability of laboratory methods, diagnostic criteria, and interrater reliability; (f) Simplify comparison of results, and avoid duplication of effort—report all steps, materials, and agents used in dressing procedures; (g) Consider extraneous and interacting variables through research design and/or statistical analysis. Future research should focus on settings, unique conditions, and population variables that ultimately lead to successful use of long-term venous access devices.

ACKNOWLEDGMENTS

The author thanks Mary Christine Klekamp, BSN, RN, for her generous assistance with searching and locating the materials for this review.

REFERENCES

Abi-Nader, J. A. (1993). Peripherally inserted central venous catheters in critical care patients. *Heart & Lung, 22,* 428–434.

Alexander, H. R. (1994). Infectious complications associated with long-term venous access devices: Etiology, diagnosis, treatment, and prophylaxis. In H. R. Alexander (Ed.), *Vascular access and the cancer patient* (pp. 113–128). Philadelphia: Lippincott.

Aly, R., Bayles, C., & Maibach, H. (1988). Restriction of bacterial growth under commercial catheter dressings. *American Journal of Infection Control, 16,* 95–100.

Aly, R., Shirley, C., Cunico, B., & Maibach, H. I. (1978). Effect of prolonged occlusion on the microbial flora, pH, carbon dioxide and transepidermal water loss on human skin. *The Journal of Investigative Dermatology, 71,* 378–381.

Anderson, M. A., Aker, S. N., & Hickman, R. O. (1982). The double-lumen Hickman catheter. *American Journal of Nursing, 82,* 272–277.

Andrews, P. (1991). Increased dwell time with the Landmark® midline catheter: Clear indication of a technique-related learning curve. *Journal of Vascular Access Nursing, 1*(2), 14–19.

Bagnall, H., & Ruccione, K. (1987). Experience with a totally implanted venous access device in children with malignant disease. *Oncology Nursing Forum, 14*(4), 51–56.

Bagnall-Reeb, H. A., & Ruccione, K. (1990). Management of cutaneous reactions and mechanical complications of central venous access devices in pediatric patients with cancer: Algorithms for decision making. *Oncology Nursing Forum, 17,* 677–681.

Baranowski, L. (1993). Central venous access devices: Current technologies, uses, and management strategies. *Journal of Intravenous Nursing, 16,* 167–194.

Barber, G. R., Brown, A. E., Kihen, T. E., Edwards, F. F., & Armstrong, D. (1993). Catheter-related *Malassezia furfur* fungemia in immunocompromised patients. *The American Journal of Medicine, 95,* 365–370.

Becton, D. L., Kletzel, M., Golladay, E. S., Hathaway, G., & Berry, D. H. (1988). An experience with implanted port system in 66 children with cancer. *Cancer, 61,* 376–378.

Begala, J. E., Maher, K., & Cherry, J. D. (1981). Risk of infection associated with the use of Broviac and Hickman catheters. *American Journal of Infection Control, 10,* 17–23.

Benezra, D., Kiehn, T. E., Gold, J. W. M., Brown, A. E., Turnbull, A. D. M., & Armstrong, D. (1988). Prospective study of infections in indwelling central venous catheters using quantitative blood cultures. *The American Journal of Medicine, 85,* 495–498.

Bjornson, H. S., Colley, R., Bower, R. H., Duty, V. P., Schwartz-Fulton, J., & Fischer, J. E. (1982). Association between microorganism growth at the catheter insertion site and colonization of the catheter in patients receiving total parenteral nutrition. *Surgery, 92,* 720–726.

Bottino, J., McCredie, K. B., Groschel, D. H. M., & Lawson, M. (1979). Long-term intravenous therapy with peripherally inserted silicone elastomer central venous catheters in patients with malignant diseases. *Cancer, 43*, 1937–1943.

Brothers, T. E., VonMoll, L. K., Niederhuber, J. E., Roberts, J. A., Walker-Andrews, S., & Ensminger, W. D. (1988). Experience with subcutaneous infusion ports in three hundred patients. *Surgery, Gynecology and Obstetrics, 166*, 295–301.

Carelli, R. M., & Herink, E. (1984). Hickman/Broviac catheters: Results of survey and patient considerations. *NITA, 7*, 287–289.

Christensen, M. L., Hancock, M. L., Gattuso, J., Hurwitz, C. A., Smith, C., McCormick, J., & Mirro, J. (1993). Parenteral nutrition associated with increased infection rate in children with cancer. *Cancer, 72*, 2732–2737.

Conley, J. M., Grieves, K., & Peters, B. (1989). A prospective randomized study comparing transparent and dry gauze for central venous catheters. *The Journal of Infectious Disease, 159*, 310–319.

Cooper, G. L., Schiller, A. L., & Hopkins, C. C. (1988). Possible role of capillary action in pathogenesis of experimental catheter-associated dermal tunnel infections. *Journal of Clinical Microbiology, 26*, 8–12.

Costerton, J. W., Cheng, K. J., Geesey, G. G., Ladd, T. I., Nickel, J. C., Dasgupta, M., & Marrie, T. J. (1987). Bacterial biofilms in nature and disease. *Annual Review of Microbiology, 41*, 435–464.

Craven, D. E., Lichtenberg, D. A., Kunches, L. M., McDonough, A., Gonzales, M. I., Heeren, T. C., & McCabe, W. R. (1985). A randomized study comparing a transparent polyurethane dressing to dry gauze dressing for peripheral intravenous catheter sites. *Infection Control, 6*, 361–366.

Cunha, B. A. (1985). Significance of fever in the compromised host. *Nursing Clinics of North America, 20*, 163–168.

Dawson, S., Pai, M. K., Smith, S., Rothney, M., Ahmed, K., & Barr, R. D. (1991). Right atrial catheters in children with cancer: A decade of experience in the use of tunneled, exteriorized devices at a single institution. *The American Journal of Pediatric Hematology/Oncology, 13*, 126–129.

Douard, M. C., Arlet, G., Leverger, G., Paulien, R., Waintrop, C., Clementi, E., Eurin, B., & Schaison, G. (1991). Quantitative blood cultures for diagnosis and management of catheter-related sepsis in hematology and oncology patients. *Intensive Care Medicine, 17*, 30–35.

Ecoff, L., Barone, R. M., & Simons, R. M. (1983). Implantable infusion port (Port-a-Cath™). *NITA, 6*, 406–408.

Freiberger, D., Bryant, J., & Marino, B. (1992). The effects of different central venous line dressing changes on bacterial growth in pediatric oncology patients. *Journal of Pediatric Oncology Nursing, 9*, 3–7.

Gantz, N. M., Presswood, G. M., Goldberg, R., & Doern, G. (1984). Effects of dressing tape and change interval on intravenous therapy complication rates. *Diagnostic Microbiology & Infectious Disease, 2*, 325–332.

Graham, D. R., Keldermans, M. M., Klemm, L. W., Semenza, N. J., & Shafer, M. L. (1991). Infectious complications among patients receiving home intravenous therapy with peripheral, central, or peripherally placed central venous catheters. *American Journal of Medicine*, *91*(3B), 95S–100S.

Guidet, B., Nicola, I., Barakett, J., Gabillet, J. M., Snoey, E., Petit, J. C., & Offenstadt, G. (1994). Skin versus hub cultures to predict colonization and infection of central venous catheter in intensive care patients. *Infection*, *22*(1), 43–48.

Gyves, J. W., Ensminger, W. D., Niederhuber, J. E., Dent, T., Walker, S., Gilbertson, S., Cozzi, E., & Saran, P. (1984). A totally implanted injection port system for blood sampling and chemotherapy administration. *Journal of the American Medical Association*, *251*, 2538–2541.

Hadaway, L. (1989). Evaluation and use of advanced IV technology. Part I. Central venous access devices. *Journal of Intravenous Nursing*, *12*, 73–82.

Hampton, A. A., & Sherertz, R. J. (1988). Vascular-access infections in hospitalized patients. *Surgical Clinics of North America*, *68*(1), 57–71.

Harris, G. J., Rosenquist, M. D., & Kealey, G. P. (1992). An *in vitro* model for studying the effects of the subcutaneous tunnel and the skin exit site on the accuracy of central venous catheter tip cultures. *Journal of Burn Care and Rehabilitation*, *13*, 628–631.

Harwood, I. R., Greene, L. M., Kozakowski-Koch, J. A., & Rasor, J. S. (1992). New peripherally inserted midline catheter: A better alternative for intravenous antibiotic therapy in patients with cystic fibrosis. *Pediatric Pulmonology*, *12*, 233–239.

Hoffman, K. K., Weber, D. J., Samsa, G. P., & Rutala, W. A. (1992). Transparent polyurethane film as an intravenous catheter dressing: A meta-analysis of the infection risks. *Journal of the American Medical Association*, *267*, 2072–2076.

Holland, K. T., Davis, W., Ingham, E., & Gowland, G. (1984). A comparison of the in vitro antibacterial and complement activating effect of 'Op-Site' and 'Tegaderm' dressings. *Journal of Hospital Infection*, *5*, 323–328.

Holmström, B., & Svensson, C. (1987). Tegaderm dressings prevent recolonization of chlorhexidine-treated skin. *Journal of Hospital Infection*, *19*, 287–291.

Hutchinson, S. K., Waskerwitz, M., Martin, K., Faubion, W., & Revesz, S. (1990). Nonocclusive, clean permanent right atrial catheter dressing change procedures compared with occlusive, sterile permanent right atrial catheter dressing change procedures in children with cancer. *Journal of Pediatric Oncology Nursing*, *7*, 71.

Ingram, J., Weitzman, S., Greenberg, M. L., Parkin, P., & Filler, R. (1991). Complications of indwelling venous access lines in the pediatric hematology patient: A prospective comparison of external venous catheters and subcutaneous ports. *The American Journal of Pediatric Hematology/Oncology*, *13*, 30–136.

Jarrard, M. M., & Freeman, J. B. (1977). The effects of antibiotic ointments and antiseptics on the skin flora beneath subclavian catheter dressings during hyperalimentation. *Journal of Surgical Research*, *22*, 521–526.

Jarrard, M. M., Olson, C. M., & Freeman, J. B. (1980). Daily dressing change effects on skin flora beneath subclavian catheter dressings during total parenteral nutrition. *Journal of Parenteral and Enteral Nutrition*, *4*, 391–392.

Johnstone, J. D. (1982). Infrequent infections associated with Hickman catheters. *Cancer Nursing*, *5*, 125–129.

Jones, P. M. (1987). Indwelling central venous catheter-related infections and two different procedures of catheter care. *Cancer Nursing, 19,* 123–130.

Kamal, G. D., Pfaller, M. A., Rempe, L. E., & Jebson, P. J. R. (1991). Reduced intravascular catheter infection by antibiotic bonding: A prospective, randomized, controlled trial. *Journal of the American Medical Association, 265,* 2364–2368.

Kelsey, M. C., & Gosling, M. (1984). A comparison of the morbidity associated with occlusive and non-occlusive dressings applied to peripheral intravenous devices. *Journal of Hospital Infection, 5,* 313–321.

Keung, Y., Watkins, K., Chen, S., Groshen, S., Silberman, H., & Douer, D. (1994). Comparative study of infectious complications of different types of chronic central venous access devices. *Cancer, 73,* 2832–2837.

Lawson, M., Bottino, J. C., & McCredie, K. B. (1979). Long-term IV therapy: A new approach. *American Journal of Nursing, 70,* 1100–1103.

Legha, S. S., Haq, M., Rabinowits, M., Lawson, M., & McCredie, K. (1985). Evaluation of silicone elastomer catheters for long-term intravenous chemotherapy. *Archives of Internal Medicine, 145,* 1208–1211.

Liñares, J., Sitges-Serra, A., Garau, J., Perez, J. I., & Martin, R. (1985). Pathogenesis of catheter sepsis: A prospective study with quantitative and semi-quantitative cultures of catheter hub and segments. *Journal of Clinical Microbiology, 21,* 357–360.

Lloyd, D. A., Shanbhogue, L. K. R., Sutherland, D. D., Hart, C. A., & Williams, D. F. (1993). Does the fibrin coat around a central venous catheter influence catheter-related sepsis? *Journal of Pediatric Surgery, 28,* 345–349.

Lokich, J. J., Bothe, A., Benotti, P., & Moore, C. (1985). Complications and management of implanted venous access catheters. *Journal of Clinical Oncology, 3,* 710–717.

Long, C. M., & Ovaska, M. (1992). Comparative study of nursing protocols for venous access ports. *Cancer Nursing, 15,* 18–21.

Lucas, A. B. (1994). Routine maintenance and care of long-term vascular access devices. In H. R. Alexander (Ed.), *Vascular access and the cancer patient* (pp. 148–164). Philadelphia: Lippincott.

Maki, D. G. (1988). An attachable silver-impregnated cuff for prevention of infection with central venous catheters: A prospective randomized multicenter trial. *The American Journal of Medicine, 85,* 307–314.

Maki, D. G. (1991). Infection caused by intravascular devices: Pathogenesis, strategies for prevention [monograph]. *Royal Society of Medicine International Congress and Symposium* (Series No. 179).

Maki, D. G., & Band, J. D. (1981). A comparative study of polyantibiotic and iodophor ointments in prevention of vascular catheter-related infection. *The American Journal of Medicine, 70,* 739–744.

Maki, D. G., Drinka, P. J., & Davis, T. E. (1975). Suppurative phlebitis of an arm vein from a scalp vein needle. *New England Journal of Medicine, 292,* 1116–1117.

Maki, D. G., & McCormack, K. N. (1987). Defatting catheter insertion sites in total parenteral nutrition is of no value as an infection control measure. *The American Journal of Medicine, 83,* 833–840.

Maki, D. G., & Ringer, M. (1987). Evaluation of dressing regimes for prevention of infection with peripheral intravenous catheters: Gauze, a transparent polyurethane dressing, and an iodophor transparent dressing. *Journal of the American Medical Association, 258,* 2396–2403.

Maki, D. G., Ringer, M., & Alvarado, C. J. (1991). Prospective randomized trial of povidone iodine, alcohol, and chlorhexidine for prevention of infection associated with central venous catheters. *The Lancet, 338,* 339–343.

Maki, D. G., Stolz, M. S., Wheeler, S., & Mermel, L. A. (1994). A prospective, randomized trial of gauze and two polyurethane dressings for site care of pulmonary artery catheters: Implications for catheter management. *Critical Care Medicine, 22,* 1729–1737.

Maki, D. G., Weise, C. E., & Sarafin, H. W. (1977). A semi-quantitative method for identifying intravenous catheter-related infection. *New England Journal of Medicine, 296,* 1305–1309.

Maki, D. G., & Will, L. (1984, June). *Colonization and infection associated with transparent dressings for central venous catheters: A comparative trial.* Abstract presented at the Association for Practitioners in Infection Control, Washington, DC.

Marcoux, C., Fischer, S., & Wong, D. (1990). Central venous access devices in children. *Pediatric Nursing, 16,* 123–133.

Markel, S., & Reynen, K. (1990). Impact on patient care: 2652 PIC catheter days in the alternative setting. *Journal of Intravenous Nursing, 13,* 347–351.

May, G. S., & Davis, C. (1988). Percutaneous catheters and totally implantable access systems: A review of reported infection rates. *Journal of Intravenous Nursing, 11,* 97–103.

Merritt, R., Ennis, C. E., Andrassy, R. J., Hays, D. M., Sinatra, F. R., Thomas, D. W., & Siegel, S. E. (1981). Use of Hickman right atrial catheter in pediatric oncology patients. *Journal of Parenteral and Enteral Nutrition, 5,* 83–85.

Mirro, J., Rao, B. N., Stokes, D. C., Austin, B. A., Kumar, M., Dahl, G. V., Colten, M., Balas, L., Rafferty, M., Hancock, M., & Fairclough, D. (1989). A prospective study of Hickman/Broviac catheters and implantable ports in pediatric oncology patients. *Journal of Clinical Oncology, 7,* 214–222.

Moore, C. L., Erikson, K. A., Yanes, L. B., Franklin, M., & Gonsalves, L. (1986). Nursing care and management of venous access ports. *Oncology Nursing Forum, 13*(3), 35–39.

Myers, J. S., & Kyle, K. S. (1993). Intermediate term intravenous therapy: A pilot study. *Journal of Post Anesthesia Nursing, 8,* 21–25.

Nahass, R. G., & Weinstein, M. P. (1990). Qualitative intravascular catheter tip cultures do not predict catheter-related bacteremia. *Diagnostic Microbiology & Infectious Disease, 13,* 223–226.

Nicola, M., & DeChairo, D. (1984). A transparent polyurethane membrane used as an IV dressing. *NITA, 7,* 139–142.

Norden, C. W. (1969). Application of antibiotic ointment to the site of venous catheterization: A controlled trial. *Journal of Infectious Diseases, 120,* 611–615.

Palidar, P. J., Simonowitz, D. S., Oreskovich, M. R., Dellinger, E. P., Edwards, W. A., Adams, S., & Karkeck, J. (1982). Use of Op-Site as an occlusive dressing for total parenteral nutrition catheters. *Journal of Parenteral and Enteral Nutrition, 6,* 150–151.

Pegues, D., Alexrod, P., McClarren, C., Eisenberg, B. L., Hoffman, J. P., Ottery, F. D., Keidan, R. D., Boraas, M., & Weese, J. (1992). Comparison of infections in Hickman and implanted port catheters in adult solid tumor patients. *Journal of Surgical Oncology, 49,* 156–162.

Peterson, P. J., & Freeman, P. T. (1982). Use of transparent polyurethane dressing for peripheral intravenous catheter care. *NITA, 5,* 387–390.

Petrosino, B., Becker, H., & Christian, B. (1988). Infection rates in central venous catheter dressings. *Oncology Nursing Forum, 15,* 709–717.

Powell, C., Regan, C., Fabri, P. J., & Ruberg, R. L. (1982). Evaluation of Opsite catheter dressings for parenteral nutrition: A prospective, randomized study. *Journal of Parenteral and Enteral Nutrition, 6,* 43–46.

Press, O. W., Ramsey, P. G., Larson, E. B., Fefer, A., & Hickman, R. O. (1984). Hickman catheter infections in patients with malignancies. *Medicine, 63,* 189–200.

Prichard, J. G., Nelson, M. J., Burns, L., Kaplowitz, H. J., Caillouet, B. L., & Sanchez, M. A. (1988). Infections caused by central venous catheters in patients with Acquired Immunodeficiency Syndrome. *Southern Medical Journal, 81,* 1496–1498.

Raad, I. I., Sabbagh, M. F., Rand, K. H., & Sherertz, R. J. (1992). Quantitative tip culture methods and the diagnosis of central venous catheter-related infection. *Diagnostic Microbiology & Infectious Disease, 15,* 13–20.

Rasor, J. S. (1991). Review of catheter-related infection rates: Comparison of conventional catheter materials with Aquavene®. *Journal of Vascular Access Nursing, 3*(3), 3–16.

Rhame, F. S., Feist, J. F., Muller, C. L., Steere, K. J., & Cameron, S. (1983, May). *Transparent adherent dressings (TADs) do not promote abnormal skin flora.* Paper presented at the meeting of the Association for Practitioners in Infection Control, San Diego, CA.

Rutherford, C. (1988). A study of single lumen peripherally inserted central line catheter dwelling time and complications. *Journal of Intravenous Nursing, 11,* 169–173.

Ryan, J. A., Abel, R. M., Abbott, W. M., Hopkins, C. C., Chesney, T. M., Colley, R., Phillips, K., & Fischer, J. E. (1974). Catheter complications in total parenteral nutrition: A prospective study of 200 consecutive patients. *The New England Journal of Medicine, 290,* 757–761.

Ryder, M. A. (1993). Peripherally inserted central venous catheters. *Nursing Clinics of North America, 28,* 937–971.

Salzman, M. B., Isenberg, H. D., Shapiro, J. F., Lipsitz, P. J., & Rubin, L. G. (1993). A prospective study of the catheter hub as the portal of entry for microorganisms causing catheter-related sepsis in neonates. *The Journal of Infectious Diseases, 167,* 487–490.

Schulmeister, L. (1987). A comparison of skin preparation procedures for accessing implanted ports. *NITA, 10,* 45–47.

Schwartz-Fulton, J., Colley, R., Valanis, B., & Fischer, J. E. (1981). Hyperalimentation dressings and skin flora. *NITA, 4,* 354–357.

Schwartz-Fulton, J., & Tischenko, M. M. (1985). Hickman catheter exit site skin sensitivities in an oncology patient population. *NITA, 8,* 63–68.

Shapiro, E. D., Wald, E. R., Nelson, K. A., & Spiegelman, K. N. (1982). Broviac catheter-related bacteremia in oncology patients. *American Journal of Diseases in Children, 136,* 679–681.

Sheth, P. K., Rose, H. D., Franson, T. R., Buckmire, F. L. A., & Sohnle, P. G. (1983). *In vitro* quantitative adherence of bacteria to intravascular catheters. *Journal of Surgical Research, 34,* 213–218.

Shivnan, J. C., McGuire, D., Freedman, S., Sharkazy, E., Gosserman, G., Larson, E., & Grouleff, P. (1991). A comparison of transparent adherent and dry sterile gauze dressings for long-term central catheters in patients undergoing bone marrow transplant. *Oncology Nursing Forum, 18,* 1349–1356.

Snydman, D. R., Gorbea, H. F., Pober, B. R., Majka, J. A., Murray, S. A., & Perry, L. K. (1982). Predictive value of surveillance skin cultures in total parenteral nutrition related infection. *Lancet, 2,* 1385–1388.

Thomas, M. A. (1977). Op-Site wound dressing for subclavian line care. *Journal of Parenteral and Enteral Nutrition, 1,* 41.

Vazquez, R. M., & Jarrard, M. M. (1984). Care of the central venous catheterization site: The use of a transparent polyurethane film. *Journal of Parenteral and Enteral Nutrition, 8,* 181–186.

Wade, J. C., Newman, K. A., Schimpff, S. C., VanEcho, D. A., Gelber, R. A., Reed, W. P., & Wiernick, P. H. (1981). Two methods for improved venous access in acute leukemia patients. *Journal of the American Medical Association, 246,* 140–144.

Winters, V., Peters, B., Coila, S., & Jones, L. (1990). A trial with a new peripheral implanted vascular access device. *Oncology Nursing Forum, 17,* 891–896.

Young, G. P., Alexeyeff, M., Russell, D. M., & Thomas, R. J. S. (1988). Catheter sepsis during parenteral nutrition: The safety of long-term Op-Site dressings. *Journal of Parenteral and Enteral Nutrition, 12,* 365–370.

Zinner, S. H., Denny-Brown, B. C., Braun, P., Burke, J. P., Toala, P., & Kass, E. H. (1969). Risk of infection with intravenous indwelling catheters: Effect of application of antibiotic ointment. *Journal of Infectious Diseases, 120,* 616–615.

Chapter 11

Nursing Research in Taiwan

Shyang-Yun Pamela Koong Shiao
Frances Payne Bolton School of Nursing
Case Western Reserve University

Yu-mei Yu Chao
Bureau of National Health Insurance
Department of Health and School of Nursing
National Taiwan University

ABSTRACT

Nursing research in Taiwan has evolved over the past 30 years. This review focused on refereed publications, research published in English, and specifically the 27 studies produced by doctorally prepared first authors. Most investigators used surveys and interviews. Designs were at the levels of description, association, and evaluation, not at the level of experiment. Problems are identified for this body of research. Further evolution of nursing science in Taiwan needs to incorporate the scientific and technologic resources of the world to develop nursing knowledge.

Keywords: Nursing Research, Taiwan

Nursing research in Taiwan has developed a great deal over the past 30 years. The major areas of research in Taiwan are maternal–child nursing, medical-surgical nursing, psychiatric nursing, and community nursing. This review summarizes the current state of clinical nursing research in Taiwan and provides some direction for future studies. The review follows Cooper's (1982) guidelines for conducting integrative research reviews, in which the review is conceptualized as a research process and validity and reliability issues are emphasized.

A total of 740 studies were located from the past 30 years. After excluding 389 studies that were nonrefereed or that focused on nonclinical topics (administrative or educational research), 351 studies met the criteria for the review. Of those, 76 papers published in the past 3 years were examined in depth. Then, from the 280 nursing studies published since 1981 when the first doctorate in nursing was graduated from the United States in Taiwan, 27 refereed studies produced by doctorally prepared first authors were reviewed in detail.

LOCATING THE STUDIES

Studies conducted in Taiwan were identified from: (a) Volumes I and II of Abstracts of Nursing Research in Taiwan from 1966 to 1992 (Nursing Research Committee, Nurses' Association of the Republic of China, 1987, 1992); (b) two nursing research journals, *Nursing Research (Taiwan)* and *Journal of Nursing (Taiwan)* from 1992 to the summer of 1995; and (c) information solicited from nurse researchers in Taiwan by the second author of the review during the summer of 1995. Thus, a total of 740 studies published from 1966 to the summer of 1995 were located. Inter-rater reliability on the identification of nursing studies from existing sources was 98.92%.

CODING THE STUDIES

Studies were entered into the computer for coding using Paradox for Windows software (Borland, Scotts Valley, CA) and an investigator-developed codebook. Items coded included the year of publication, number and name(s) of authors, source of publication, title, area, design, sampling, number of subjects, unit of analysis, study method, and analyses. The review evaluated the appropriateness of the title; the methods section; and the overall presentations of sampling, method and design, results, and discussion.

DESCRIPTION OF STUDIES INCLUDED IN THE REVIEW

Nonrefereed studies included theses, dissertations, studies published in institutional newsletters, institutional papers and publications, summary reports, and chapters; as noted above, these were excluded from the review. Research on nursing administration and nursing education also was excluded because the review focused on the assessment of clinical nursing knowledge. Developments in educational and administrative research are reviewed in an excellent article by Y. Y. Lee, Wang, and Liu (1995) entitled ''Trend analysis of nursing research published in the *Journal of Nursing*: 1982–1992.'' A total of 351 refereed nursing research reports from Taiwan remained. The number of refereed research reports has increased substantially over the years: from 6 published in the years from 1966 to 1970, 26 from 1971 to 1975, 42 from 1976 to 1980, 102 from 1981 to 1985, 74 from 1986 to 1990, and 103 from 1991 to the first half of 1995. The major areas of published refereed research over the past 30 years, in rank order, are maternal-child nursing (129 papers); medical and surgical nursing (118); community nursing (78); and psychiatric nursing (26).

The 351 studies published over the past 30 years were primarily descriptive studies (67.3%), with about one-fifth of those descriptive studies being case studies (12.7%). A smaller proportion were correlational studies (22.1%), and a few were quasiexperimental (8.8%) or experimental studies (1.7%). The most commonly used methods (some studies used more than one design) were surveys (61.2%), interviews (29.6%), observations (23.3%), chart reviews (4%), and counts (1.4%). A few studies used equipment (5.9%), such as thermometers, sphygmomanometers, and rulers. A limited number of nursing studies done in Taiwan have been published in international or American journals, such as *Maternal-Child Nursing Journal* (four papers); *Cancer Nursing* (two papers); and *Journal of Advanced Nursing, Classification of Nursing Diagnoses, Rehabilitation Nursing, Intensive Care Nursing*, and *Oncology Nursing Forum* (one each).

THE STUDIES FROM THE PAST 3 YEARS

The journal *Nursing Research (Taiwan)*, which began publication in 1993, includes studies written in Chinese with English abstracts and, occasionally, English papers with Chinese abstracts, which is a unique style of research reporting. The journal is published quarterly, with eight papers in each issue. Papers in the journal *Nursing Research (Taiwan)* and papers from the past 3 years were assessed in depth and compared with the work over the past 30 years. In the past 3 years, areas with the most published research were maternal-child nursing (29 papers); medical-surgical nursing (24); psychiatric nursing (15); and community nursing (8).

When the 76 papers published in the past 3 years were examined for methodological types, the predominant design was descriptive (36.8%); 2.6% were case studies (however, this design was used significantly less often than over the past 30 years); and 44.7% were correlational (the use of this design was double that for the past 30 years). Quasiexperimental (7.7%) and experimental (1.3%) designs continued to be rarely used; and some of these studies were evaluation studies (6.6%), or pre- and postdesigns (2.6%). A few were instrument development studies (2.6%). The most commonly used methods were still surveys (50.6%), interviews (31.6%), and observations (23.7%); there were a few chart reviews (1.3%) and counts (5.2%).

Maternal–Child Nursing

There were 29 papers in maternal–child nursing published over the past 3 years: 19 related to pregnancy, and 10 in pediatrics. Among the 19 pregnancy-related papers, there were 10 descriptive, 5 correlational, and 4 quasiexperimental studies. The descriptive studies included seven studies during labor and delivery: two studies focused on fathers' experiences and needs (F. H. Chou, Chao, & Yee, 1994; Tzeng, Wang, & Shih, 1993), four on mothers' concerns and experiences (Tzeng & Chao, 1994; F. Y. Wu, Teng, & Shieh, 1994; Y. L. Yang & Chao, 1993; Y. O. Yang & Chao, 1994), and one on family function (S. C. Kuo, 1994). There also was one study of a breast-feeding program (Y. C. Su, Chen, Chang, Wu, & Chen, 1994), one on the subjective experience of infertility (T. J. Su, 1993), and another on the reproduction therapy experience (T. J. Su, Teng, & Yang, 1995). Five correlational studies focused on maternal-fetal attachment (T. Y. Lee, 1994); factors in breast-feeding at 1 month (Teng, Ho, & Kuo, 1994); postpartum depression (C-H. Chen, Tseng, Wang, & Lee, 1994); knowledge, affect, and behavior toward sexual behaviors during pregnancy (M. C. Chen, 1992); and hepatitis control (H. C. Chung, Chen, & Yen, 1992). Four quasiexperimental studies included mother–baby dyad care and mothers' satisfaction (Feng, 1993); the effects of rooming-in on breast-feeding at 1 month (Teng, Su, Yang, & Chang, 1995); the effects of a nursing intervention on psychosocial response and the stress of infertility (B. C. Kuo & Lee, 1992); and the effects of home visits and telephone contacts on breast-feeding (C-H. Chen, 1993). The studies of breast-feeding have special clinical significance and potential. In these studies, however, breast-feeding was the outcome variable, not an independent variable affecting outcomes for infants. Future research needs to focus on the effects of breast-feeding on infant health and development and mother–infant interactions.

The 10 pediatric papers included four descriptive studies on stress and coping of mothers (T. Y. Cheng, & Chen, 1993), appraisal of allergy-reduction injections in children with asthma (N. T. Chang & Huang, 1994), the families of Down syndrome children (L. H. Huang, 1994), and behaviors of preschool-ers after cardiac surgery (Y. J. Chang, Chen, Yu, & Mao, 1992). Four correlational studies included three studies of mother–infant feeding interactions (Feng, 1994; Shiau, Chang, Hung, & Yu, 1994; Teng, Kuo, & Ho, 1993) and one on pain perception in children (Chiang & Mao, 1994). Two evaluation studies included the effects of an alcohol sponge on the size of BCG immunization reactions (C. I. Chang & Chiang, 1992) and the effects of a brochure and phone education for G6-phosphorate-deficiency children (M. C. Huang, Chang, Kuo, & Lin, 1994). One of the most studied areas was mother–infant feeding interactions related to breast-feeding and bottle-feeding. Future studies need to explore the clinical implications of different feeding methods.

Medical–Surgical Nursing

There were 24 medical and surgical nursing papers: 9 in oncology, 7 in cardiovascular nursing, and 8 in general medical and surgical nursing. Among the nine oncology nursing papers, four descriptive studies examined the needs of oncology patients in regard to eating (H. Y. Lin & Chen, 1993), coping (Lu, Chin, & Huang, 1993), sexual behavior (Ma & Lo, 1993), and support of caregivers (Y. L. Lee, Chen, & Lin, 1993). Five correlational studies included two on the needs of breast cancer patients (S. Y. Cheng, 1995; H. P. Lee & Ku, 1992), two on caregivers (M. S. Su & Wang, 1993; L. B. Wu & Ku, 1994), and one on the health care needs of children with cancer (Y-C. Chen, Martinson, Chao, Lai, & Gau, 1992). Among the seven cardiovascular papers, five correlational papers examined the stress of cardiac surgery (Hwang, Lin, Liao, Hwang, & Chang, 1994), adjustment after myocardial infarction (B. C. Lin, 1992), family care for stroke patients (M. N. Lin & Chiou, 1995), physio-psychosocial support (Yu & Kao, 1992), and psychosocial self-care (B. J. Lin & Huang, 1993). Two quasiexperimental studies focused on teaching myocardial infarction patients (M. C. Lin & Ku, 1993) and cardiac rehabilitation (Kao-Lo, 1992). In the area of general medical and surgical nursing, there was one descriptive study on assessment in diabetes (Shiau, Chiang, Hong, & Chen, 1993). Additionally, there were seven correlational studies: two on psychological adjustment (Shiau, Chen, Tsai, Lin, & Tai, 1994) and stress and coping in diabetes (Y. L. Su, Chang, & Chen, 1994), three on the lives of those with chronic illnesses (H. C. Chang, Liu, & Huang, 1995; Hwu, 1994; C. S. Lin, Liu, & Liao, 1993), one on osteoporosis (S. Lin, 1994), and one on pressure sores (C. L. Huang, 1993). Commonalities among these studies included the use of the psychosocial concepts of stress and coping and emphasis on caregivers. Future studies need to examine findings on these common concepts.

Psychiatric Nursing

The 15 psychiatric papers included 6 descriptive studies. Three focused on couple therapy (M. F. Lin & Shiau, 1994; Shiau, Lin, & Chang, 1995; Shiau, Wu, Chang, & Song, 1994), one on the life space of offspring of schizophrenic patients (Shiau & Chang, 1993), one on the Quality of Life Index (QLI) (Ferran & Powers, 1985) in Chinese (Liu, 1993), and one on risk assessment of assault (S. C. Chen, 1993); four correlational studies focused on music therapy (S. Lee, Yeh, & Lie, 1993), the life satisfaction of psychiatric patients (Cheng-Younger & Yu, 1993), adjustment in schizophrenia (P. J. Chung & Shiau, 1995), and restraint use (M. S. Yang & Chung, 1993); and five evaluation studies were on relaxation therapy (Shiau, Teng, & Yang, 1993), social skills (S. Lee, Yeh, & Hung, 1994), family therapy (S. Lee & Yeh, 1992), and home care for schizophrenia (C. F. Chou, Hsung, & Huang, 1992a, 1992b). There were more evaluation studies in the psychiatric area than in other areas. Future studies need to investigate efficient and effective ways of delivering psychiatric nursing care.

Community Nursing

There were eight papers in community nursing, and they were the best written, with the fewest problems of internal and external validity. There were three descriptive studies of long-term care (Shyu, Hsiung, Dai, Chen, & Huang, 1993), home care (J. C. Chen, Lo, & Hu, 1994) and caregiver burden (Tang, Mao, Chou, Chen, & Liou, 1992); and five correlational studies on health behaviors (Hau, 1993), health promotion (M. Y. Chen, Chang-Liao, Liao, & Chou, 1994), caregiver burden (Hsu, Chang, Yang, & Huang, 1992), osteoporosis (Hsia & Yu, 1994), and pressure sores in home care (J. C. Chen & Lo, 1993). A common area seemed to be long-term care and health promotion in home settings. The community is currently being emphasized in nursing care as an alternative site for care delivery in Taiwan. Future studies in this area must further explore findings on chronicity, long-term care, and health promotion that are significant for home care as an alternative approach to care delivery.

RESEARCH REPORTED BY
DOCTORALLY PREPARED AUTHORS

To further assess the state of development of nursing science in Taiwan, studies done after the first nurse graduated with a doctorate degree in 1981 were examined in depth. Since 1981, 280 nursing studies have been published in refereed journals in Taiwan. This review examined the 27 refereed studies produced by doctorally prepared first authors.

These studies were produced by 11 different first authors. Six studies were published from 1982 to 1989, and 21 studies were published from 1990 to 1995. More than half (15) of these studies had multiple authors, ranging from two to five (C-H. Chen et al., 1994; Y-C. Chen & Lin, 1991; Y-C. Chen et al., 1992; S. L. Hwang et al., 1994; S. Lee & Chen, 1991; S. Lee & Yeh, 1992; S. Lee et al., 1994; S. Lee et al., 1993; Shiau & Chang, 1993; Shiau, Chang, et al., 1994; Shiau, Chen, et al., 1994; Shiau, Chiang, et al., 1993; Shiau, Lin, & Chang, 1995; Shiau, Teng, & Yang, 1993; Shiau, Wu, et al., 1994); and 12 studies had single authorship (Chao, 1983, 1984, 1987; C-H. Chen, 1990; L. H. Huang, 1994; Kao-Lo, 1986a, 1986b, 1992; T. Y. Lee, 1994; Liu, 1993; Mao, 1989; Shiau, 1991). Four studies were by multidisciplinary authors, including three physicians and one medical technologist; and one included an international author. These articles were published in the *Journal of Nursing (Taiwan)* (6), *Nursing Research (Taiwan)* (13), other Chinese journals in Taiwan (2 in the *Journal of Chinese Oncology*, and 1 in *Chinese Psychiatric Health*), and in international journals and books: *Journal of Advanced Nursing, Classification of Nursing Diagnoses, Cancer Nursing Conference Proceedings, Intensive Care Nursing*, and *Cancer Nursing* (5).

Eight studies were related to the topics of maternal child nursing, 11 were in adult acute and chronic care, and 8 in psychiatric nursing. There were 8 descriptive studies (including 1 case study), 12 correlational studies (including 3 pre–postevaluation studies), 4 studies aiming at the development/modification of instruments, and 3 quasiexperimental studies. Four studies used interviews as the research method, five used observation, nine used surveys, and three used psychometric instruments; three used both interview and observation, two used both observation and survey; and one used three methods, interview, observation, and survey.

Descriptive Studies

Eight descriptive studies were conducted by four first authors from one institution, the National Taiwan University (Chao, 1984, 1987; Y-C. Chen, 1990; Y-C. Chen & Lin, 1991; L. H. Huang, 1994; Shiau & Chang, 1993; Shiau et al., 1995; Shiau, Wu, et al., 1994). Since 1981, when she finished her nursing doctorate in the United States, Chao, the first nursing doctorate in Taiwan and a nursing faculty member of the National Taiwan University, has influenced the development of nursing research in Taiwan. Thus, it is not surprising that her efforts in descriptive design have been followed by others from the same institution. The following paragraph briefly summarizes the findings of these descriptive studies.

Two studies (Chao, 1984, 1987) described folk curing and caring strategies of cancer patients receiving radiation therapy. One study (Y-C. Chen & Lin, 1991) described the side effects of chemotherapy, which were multifaceted and invasive of body functions and body appearance; hematologic counts reached their lowest levels during the second and the third weeks of treatment and 50% of the high-risk group developed infections. A qualitative single case study (Y-C. Chen, 1990) described psychosocial support in intensive care and nurses' caring efforts to reduce the patient's and family's fear of the future and to increase their communication of needs and feelings. One study (L. H. Huang, 1994) explored parents' and siblings' needs and responses to children with Down syndrome. Parents' responses included sorrow, shock, an inability to accept the fact, fear, hopelessness, and disappointment; they needed to know more about Down syndrome and needed guides to raise these children. Another study (Shiau & Chang, 1993) was on the descriptions of the life space of offspring of schizophrenic patients reported by the patients and their spouses; while most patients believed that their disease did not interfere with their parenting and the growth of their children, most spouses felt the opposite. Two studies (Shiau et al., 1995; Shiau, Wu, et al., 1994) described the behaviors of functional adaptation and information transmission as well as ego transformation processing and affect bonding in couples undergoing group psychotherapy for schizophrenic patients.

The descriptive designs used in these studies, particularly participant-observed clinical field studies, have the advantage of providing insight into human behaviors in their unique cultural context, minimizing the imposition of the Western frame of reference held by the nursing graduates of Western nations and thus enabling more effective and therapeutic nursing care in Taiwan (Chao, 1995). The process of clinical field nursing research was used to promote the nurse-patient relationship, thus maximizing the effects of nursing education and nursing research in clinical nursing practice. However, if the reliability or quality of the measures used in research is not addressed, even in a descriptive design, then the data cannot serve as the building blocks of nursing science (Knapp, 1985; Lynn, 1985).

Among these descriptive studies, the attempts to explore cultural influences on the caring and curing actions of Chinese were inspiring for new directions in health care (Chao, 1984, 1987). All subjects in Chao's first study and 92% in the second study used at least one of the culturally known methods of the Chinese to deal with complications of cultural origin, for example, complaints of "hotness" and "loss of vital energy" when receiving radiation therapy. The radiation therapy was believed to cause "hotness" and thereby to weaken the body and cause a "loss of vital energy." A belief in the need for balance of the universal properties of "Yin and Yang" (cold and hot, weak and strong, flexible and rigid, etc.) to maintain healthy body function served as the basis for dealing with these complications. The complications were dealt with by using one or more of the following strategies to reach a balance in body function: Chinese or herbal medicine, food and dieting, religion and ritual, and Chinese exercise and breathing. To build upon these descriptive findings, the reliability and validity of the measures used must be addressed. Additionally, research using the next levels of design, correlation or association and experiment, must be planned to build the knowledge base for nursing in Taiwan. For example, a correlational study might be planned to explore the relationship between the use of one or more of the strategies listed above and the occurrence of culturally interpreted complications; or an experimental study might be designed to examine the effects of one or more of these strategies on the course of such complications.

Correlational Studies

Twelve correlational studies were conducted by eight researchers from four institutions in the field of maternal–child nursing (five studies) (Chao, 1983; C-H. Chen et al., 1994; Y-C. Chen et al., 1992; T. Y. Lee, 1994; Shiau, Chang, et al., 1994); adult critical and chronic care (four studies) (Hwang et al., 1994; Mao, 1989; Shiau, Chen, et al., 1994; Shiau, Wang, et al., 1993), and psychiatric nursing (three studies) (S. Lee & Chen, 1991; S. Lee et al., 1993; Shiau, Teng, & Yang, 1993). There were few commonalities among these studies. Future collaborative efforts and program development are needed to facilitate the development of nursing science.

One study (Chao, 1983) explored mothers' behaviors towards their newborn babies during feedings; 2300 records of mothers' behaviors were classified into the categories of orienting, evaluating infants' aspects of appearance, physical state, body function, and social characteristics. These mothers used more evaluating behaviors in regard to infants' appearance; Chinese mothers used less evaluating behaviors than American mothers.

Shiau, Chang, et al. (1994) explored factors influencing breast-feeding and infant development in 66 mother–infant dyads. Fewer employed than unemployed mothers were breast-feeding at 2 to 3 months postpartum; the breast-feeding group had better maternal behavior than the bottle-feeding group; and the infants of the breast-feeding group exhibited better socialized behavior than the bottle-feeding group.

Y-C. Chen et al. (1992) examined health care changes for 121 children with cancer from 1981 to 1991. The results indicated improved medical care, better pain control, and better acceptance of nurses and doctors by parents.

T. Y. Lee (1994) compared 40 mothers with a normal pregnancy to 37 mothers with a history of infertility and found different maternal–fetal attachment patterns from the first to second trimester. C-H. Chen et al. (1994) examined the prevalence of and factors in postpartum depression among 129 Taiwanese women at 6 weeks postpartum and found that 40.3% of the women were mildly to severely depressed. Predictors of postpartum depression included self-esteem, social support, perceived stress, and whether the pregnancy was planned or unplanned. Efforts in the maternal-child area may start with the perinatal care of mothers and infants.

Mao (1989) explored stress and related factors in 112 acutely burned adults and found that the severity of the burn affected stress perceptions. Hwang et al. (1994) explored the stressors of heart surgery for 30 patients as reported by the patients and by 22 nurses. The most important stressors for patients were physical discomfort, increasing burden to others, complications, surgery, and the threat of death. Nurses overestimated the stressors of their patients.

Shiau (Shiau, Chen, et al., 1994; Shiau, Wang, et al., 1993) conducted two related studies on insulin-dependent-diabetic patients. In the first study, Shiau, Wang, et al. (1993) assessed the needs of these patients through self-reports of 100 patients and reports of 25 nurses. In the second study, Shiau, Chen, et al. (1994) explored the psychological adjustment and family attitudes of 130 patients and parents; the results indicated that better psychological adjustment was related to better home care management. Physiological measurements need to be added to such studies to further establish the science of adult nursing in Taiwan.

Shiau, Teng, et al. (1993) evaluated the effects of a 12-session relaxation group (30 minutes each, three times a week for 4 weeks) on sleep difficulties of psychiatric patients, using a one-group pre–posttest design. The attendance rate for patients on the psychiatric unit was 20.85%; 48 subjects constituted the sample. Results indicated that subjects improved in their sleep.

S. Lee and Chen (1991) used a single-case repeated measures design to evaluate the effects of training on the social and communication skills of a 13-year-old schizophrenic patient, as observed by the subject, family, and health care personnel. The results indicated improved social skills; however, there were different responses from the three participants. S. Lee et al. (1993) evaluated the effects of 10 hours of music group therapy (three times a week for 2 weeks) on psychiatric symptoms and personal interactions of 40 psychotic patients using a one-group pre–post test design. Subjects improved in their personal interactions and showed fewer withdrawn and anxious behaviors, and nurses' satisfaction was improved.

These studies indicate the effects of interventions for psychiatric patients. However, a common basis for interventions for Chinese in Taiwan is lacking.

Future studies must incorporate the findings from these studies to build a cohesive body of nursing literature in Taiwan.

Quasiexperimental Studies

Three quasiexperimental studies have been conducted by two researchers from different institutions at the time of publication; two of the studies were focused on psychiatric patients (S. Lee & Yeh, 1992; S. Lee et al., 1994) and one on cardiac rehabilitation patients (Kao-Lo, 1992). Kao-Lo examined the effects of early cardiac rehabilitation on the progress of activity tolerance in 40 experimental subjects and 40 control subjects following acute myocardial infarction. More subjects in the experimental early rehabilitation group had recovered their activity tolerance at 2 weeks after the surgery and at the time of discharge; they performed more activities at discharge; had increased activity tolerance at 1, 3, and 6 months after discharge; and returned to work faster than subjects in the control group.

S. Lee et al. (1994) found that a social skills training program (30 minutes each, six times a week, for 5 to 8 weeks) improved expression and communication in psychotic patients. The content of the classes included social relations, self-expression, communication, and coping skills in specific situations. Twenty-eight subjects were randomly assigned to the experimental and control groups, and 24 subjects completed the study. S. Lee and Yeh (1992) evaluated the effects of a 6-week, 30-minutes per week family conference on the cognitive and coping skills of 165 family members of manic-depressive patients using a survey design. The self-selected experimental group demonstrated increased understanding of the disease course and improved cognitive and coping skills.

These quasiexperimental studies all present problems of internal and external validity. They clearly point the direction for nursing research in Taiwan. Future studies must pay increased attention to the credibility of measures, data collection procedures, and sampling procedures.

Studies of Instrumentation

Four instrumentation studies were conducted by three researchers from two different institutions; two were on sleep disturbances (Kao-Lo, 1986a, 1986b), one on the Quality of Life Index in Chinese (Liu, 1993), and another on the development of the Child Coping Behavior Scale (Shiau, 1991). Continuing her dissertation work, Kao-Lo validated the nursing diagnosis of sleep pattern disturbances using methodological triangulation in two separate studies (1986a, 1986b). Nurses in four hospitals (Kao-Lo, 1986a) and 31 faculty members and graduate students in medical-surgical nursing (Kao-Lo, 1986b) were surveyed for the defining characteristics and etiologies of sleep disturbances; and 25 cardiac patients were observed, examined, and interviewed about the problem. The study findings indicated a Cronbach's alpha of 0.821 for the total score, and 12 essential defining characteristics for this nursing diagnosis, but the author did not report the findings with these different methods.

Liu (1993) explored the psychometric properties of the Quality of Life Index with Chinese caregivers. The Quality of Life Index (Ferrans & Powers, 1985) was translated into Chinese and validated with 437 family caregivers using Cronbach's alpha, criterion validity, and factor analysis. Five factors were identified: psychosocial, health, environmental, intimacy, and family. Chinese caregivers reported most satisfaction with the intimacy factor and least satisfaction with the environmental factor.

Shiau (1991) developed the Child Coping Behavior Scale (CCBS) to assess the 30-month-old child's behavior in the context of a moderate-stress situation. The sample was socially disadvantaged. The 5-item scale was validated by reliability tests, factor analysis, convergent and discriminant validity (construct validity), and predictive power (criterion validity).

DISCUSSION

Nursing research has developed a great deal over the past 30 years in Taiwan. However, the development of nursing science is still in an early state. Much of the research continues to use the medical frame of reference of disease and nursing care of diseases, rather than focusing on systems and concepts important to nursing, such as the fundamental laws governing health. These laws encompass important dependent or outcome variables for nursing care, and nursing interventions that improve outcomes are important topics for inquiry.

Findings from the studies to date are in many different domains; programs of research still need to be developed. Further, physiological instrumentation and the measurement of physiologic variables was rarely observed in these studies. Most used surveys and interviews, and designs were at the levels of description, association, and evaluation, not at the level of experiment. Design issues include low reliability and validity and failure to acknowledge reliability and validity issues, procedural biases and errors, and sampling biases. In addition, the lack of outcomes-related experimental research hinders the development of knowledge for nursing.

Advanced nursing research generates knowledge and provokes in-depth thinking for the further evolution of research; current knowledge is incorporated into the research process, using the scientific and technologic resources of the world to further develop nursing knowledge. Over the past 15 years, great efforts have been made to advance nursing education in Taiwan. Currently, there are about 60 doctorally prepared nursing faculty in Taiwan; in 3 years, there will be at least 100 doctorally prepared nursing faculty, all graduates of schools of nursing in the United States of America. This critical mass of nursing faculty will be an important human resource for the continued development and advancement of nursing science in Taiwan.

From 1981 through 1992, 20,986 scientific papers (about 1,900 scientific papers per year) from Taiwan were published in international journals and cited in the Science Citation Index (Garfield, 1993). None of these papers, however, were produced by nursing scholars in Taiwan. Further development of nursing science must be fast-forwarded in Taiwan. Along with efforts to develop a nursing PhD program in the country, major efforts must be made to produce advanced nursing science and scholarship. Nursing research in Taiwan has made great advances over the past two decades, but there is still more to be done. Researchers who are willing to tolerate criticism to make their best work even better and a community of scholars who value continuous learning and growth (Downs, 1991; Gennaro & Vessey, 1994) are essential to the progress of nursing science and scholarship in Taiwan.

Nursing research in Taiwan has come a very long way in the last 30 years, and developments have been especially rapid in the last 3 years. This rapid development reflects both the development of nursing as a recognized scientific discipline and the improving context for nursing in Taiwan. Though primarily female occupations such as nursing once held little respect, today the world is open to women in nursing, as in other fields, in Taiwan. They are making great strides.

ACKNOWLEDGMENT

The authors acknowledge assistance in locating the literature by Ying-Ju Chang, Chi-Chun Chin, Jen-Juan Liao, and Li-Hua Lo, and the data coding by Ying-Ju Chang, Miao-Ju Chwo, Hua-Li Lin, and Li-Hua Lo. The authors also acknowledge the editorial assistance of Elizabeth Tornquist.

REFERENCES

Chang, C. I., & Chiang, C. M. (1992). Skin disinfection effect of alcohol on BCG vaccination in newborn and infants. *Journal of Nursing (Taiwan), 39*(1), 87–94.

Chang, H. C., Liu, H. E., & Huang, C. C. (1995). An exploration of the factors influencing the needs for the CAPD patients. *Nursing Research (Taiwan), 3,* 106–116.

Chang, N. T., & Huang, M. C. (1994). Appraisal of hyposensitization injection of school-age children with asthma. *Nursing Research (Taiwan), 2,* 191–202.

Chang, Y. J., Chen, Y. C., Yu, Y. M., & Mao, H. C. (1992). The communicative behaviors of the preschooler with congenital heart disease during the postoperative period. *Journal of Nursing (Taiwan), 39*(1), 77–86.

Chao (Yu), Y. M. (1983). Conceptual behavior of Chinese mothers in relation to their newborn infants. *Journal of Advanced Nursing, 8,* 303–310.

Chao (Yu), Y. M. (1984). Folk curing and caring activities practiced concomitantly by hospitalized gynecological patients receiving radio therapy. *Proceedings of 3rd International Conference on Cancer Nursing* (pp. 143–149). Melbourne, Australia.

Chao (Yu), Y. M. (1987). Folk curing and caring activities concurrently practiced by Chinese patients receiving radio therapy. *Cancer Nursing, 10 (Suppl. 1),* 146–152.

Chao (Yu), Y-M. (1995, July). *Unique care concept in Taiwan.* Paper presented at the Nursing from a Multicultural Perspective Conference, Zhuhai, China.

Chen, C-H. (1993). Effects of home visits and telephone contacts on breastfeeding compliance in Taiwan. *Maternal-Child Nursing Journal, 21*(3), 82–90.

Chen, C-H., Tseng, Y. F., Wang, S. Y., & Lee, J. N. (1994). The prevalence and predictors of postpartum depression. *Nursing Research, (Taiwan), 2,* 263–274.

Chen, J. C., & Lo, L. H. (1993). A study of home-care patients with pressure sores. *Nursing Research (Taiwan), 1,* 257–268.

Chen, J. C., Lo, L. H., & Hu, S. C. (1993). Using nursing process to deal with common nursing problems in hospital-based home nursing program: A study. *Nursing Research (Taiwan), 2,* 6–16.

Chen, M. C. (1992). A survey of pregnant women's knowledge, attitude, and behavior toward sexual activity during pregnancy. *Journal of Nursing (Taiwan), 39*(3), 77–88.

Chen, M. Y., Chang-Liao, J., Liao, J. H., & Chou, C. C. (1994). The preliminary study of health-promotion life-styles of public health nurses. *Nursing Research (Taiwan), 2,* 41–54.

Chen, S. C. (1993). Nurses' risk assessment of assault and caring competence in usual nursing problems with psychotic patients. *Nursing Research (Taiwan), 1,* 359–368.

Chen, Y-C. (1990). Psychological and social support system in intensive care medicine. *Intensive Care Nursing, 6,* 59–66.

Chen, Y-C., & Lin, K-H. (1991). Leukemia children: Chemotherapy-related side effects and caring needs. *Journal of Chinese Oncology Society, 7*(2), 11–25.

Chen, Y-C., Martinson, I. M., Chao, Y-M. Y., Lai, Y-M., & Gau, B-S. (1992). A comparative study of health care for children with cancer in 1981 and 1991 in Taiwan. *Journal of Chinese Oncology Society, 8*(3), 11–21.

Cheng, S. Y. (1995). A study of breast self examination for patients after mastectomy. *Nursing Research (Taiwan), 3,* 67–78.

Cheng, T. Y., & Chen, Y. C. (1993). Perceived stressors and coping behavior of mothers who have children with congenital imperforate anus or megacolon. *Nursing Research (Taiwan), 1*, 22–34.

Cheng-Younger, H. L., & Yu, W. Y. (1993). Life satisfaction of psychiatric in-patients. *Nursing Research (Taiwan), 1*, 269–278.

Chiang, L. C., & Mao, H. C. (1994). Assessing pain perception and pain responses of post-operative children. *Nursing Research (Taiwan), 2*, 239–253.

Chou, C. F., Hsung, B. C., & Huang, R. (1992a). The influence of home care on perceived stress of family with schizophrenic patient. *Journal of Nursing (Taiwan), 39*(1), 55–64.

Chou, C. F., Hsung, B. C., & Huang, R. Y. (1992b). The influence of home care on daily living of schizophrenic patients. *Journal of Nursing (Taiwan), 39*(3), 119–129.

Chou, F. H., Chao, Y-M. Y., & Yee, D. H. (1994). The lived experience of expectant fathers accompanying wives throughout labor and birth. *Nursing Research (Taiwan), 2*, 359–370.

Chung, H. C., Chen, C. M., & Yen, C. C. (1992). Knowledge-attitude-practice of hepatitis B control in pregnant women in Kaohsiung city. *Journal of Nursing (Taiwan), 39*(3), 53–62.

Chung, P. J., & Shiau, S. J. (1995). The attitude of young schizophrenic adults and their mothers toward life adaptation. *Chinese Journal, 14*, 256–267.

Cooper, H. M. (1982). Scientific guidelines for conducting integrative research reviews. *Review of Educational Research, 32*, 291–302.

Downs, F. (1991). Values. *Nursing Research, 40*, 132.

Feng, R. C. (1993). The nursing effectiveness of implementing the mother-baby dyad care. *Nursing Research (Taiwan), 1*, 71–82.

Feng, R. C. (1994). The neonatal perception and feeding interaction in Chinese mothers. *Nursing Research (Taiwan), 2*, 116–129.

Ferrans, C. E., & Powers, M. J. (1985). Quality of Life Index: Development and psychometric properties. *Advances in Nursing Science, 1*(1), 15–24.

Garfield, E. (April 25, 1993). Current comments: A citationist perspective on science in Taiwan: Most cited papers, institutions, and authors, 1981–1992. *Current Contents, 17*, 1718–1734.

Gennaro, S., & Vessey, J. A. (1994). Wanted: A few good jumblies. *Nursing Research, 42*, 269.

Hau, Y. J. (1993). The preliminary study of health consciousness and health behavior of adult people in small communities. *Nursing Research (Taiwan), 1*, 309–315.

Hsia, P. H., & Yu, S. (1994). Knowledge of osteoporosis among women and its influencing factors in community. *Nursing Research (Taiwan), 2*, 275–287.

Hsu, Y. Y., Chang, M., Yang, Y. M., & Huang, C. M. (1992). Family caregiver's burden and related factors of dependent elderly persons in urban and rural communities. *Journal of Nursing (Taiwan), 39*(3), 99–108.

Huang, C. L. (1993). Factors related to pressure sore occurrence of in-patients at a teaching hospital. *Journal of Nursing (Taiwan), 40*(4), 47–56.

Huang, L. H. (1994). The impact of raising a child with Down syndrome on the family. *Nursing Research (Taiwan), 2*, 253–262.

Huang, M. C., Chang, M. H., Kuo, C. H., & Lin, S. J. (1994). Effects of brochure and telephone counseling on cognitive change of parents having G-6-PD deficiency infants. *Nursing Research (Taiwan), 2,* 306–314.

Hwang, S. L., Lin, B. J., Liao, W. C., Hwang, S. F., & Chang, Y. (1994). Stressors associated with heart surgery: A follow-up and comparison study of patients' and nurses' perceptions of pre- and post-heart surgery stressor. *Nursing Research (Taiwan), 2,* 17–28.

Hwu, Y. J. (1994). Impact on and coping behaviors of patients with chronic illness. *Nursing Research (Taiwan), 2,* 140–152.

Kao-Lo, C. H. (1986a). Defining characteristics and etiologies of sleep pattern disturbances. *Journal of Nursing (Taiwan), 33*(1), 17–29.

Kao-Lo, C. H. (1986b). Construct validity of sleep pattern disturbances: A methodological approach. In M. E. Hurley (Ed.), *Classification of nursing diagnosis: Proceedings of the 6th Conference* (pp. 197–260). St. Louis: Mosby.

Kao-Lo, C. H. (1992). The effectiveness of the cardiac rehabilitation on the progress of activity tolerance. *Journal of Nursing (Taiwan), 39*(3), 63–76.

Knapp, T. R. (1985). Validity, reliability, and neither. *Nursing Research, 34,* 189–192.

Kuo, B. C., & Lee, M. S. (1992). Effects of nursing intervention on the psychosocial response and stress perceptions among infertile women receiving the treatment course of assisted reproductive technology. *Journal of Nursing (Taiwan), 39*(1), 95–104.

Kuo, S. C. (1994). Change in family functioning during perinatal period in high-risk pregnancy with preterm labor pattern. *Nursing Research (Taiwan), 2,* 106–115.

Lee, H. P., & Ku, N. P. (1992). Informational needs for breast cancer patients receiving chemotherapy. *Journal of Nursing (Taiwan), 39*(2), 55–66.

Lee, S., & Chen, B. C. (1991). Effects of social skill training on social functions of a schizophrenic patient in day care center: A controlled case study. *Journal of Nursing (Taiwan), 38*(4), 43–52.

Lee, S., & Yeh, M. Y. (1992). Effects of family therapy on improving levels of cognition and coping skills of families with MDP patients. *Journal of Nursing (Taiwan), 39*(3), 41–52.

Lee, S., Yeh, M. Y., & Hung, T. M. (1994). Effects of social skill training on improving expression and communication of hospitalized psychotic patients. *Nursing Research (Taiwan), 2,* 166–179.

Lee, S., Yeh, M. Y., & Lie, T. Z. (1993). Effect of music therapy on improving psychotic symptoms and personal interactions of psychotic patients. *Nursing Research (Taiwan), 1,* 145–157.

Lee, T. Y. (1994). Maternal-fetal attachment in normal and previously infertile Chinese women. *Nursing Research (Taiwan), 2,* 67–77.

Lee, Y. L., Chen, Y. C., & Lin, K. S. (1993). The supportive system perceived by primary caregivers of children with cancer. *Journal of Nursing (Taiwan), 40*(3), 59–69.

Lee, Y. Y., Wang, C. J., & Liu, S. Y. (1995). Trend analysis of nursing research published in the *Journal of Nursing*: 1982–1992. *Nursing Research (Taiwan), 3,* 161–170.

Lin, B. C. (1992). A preliminary study of life adjustment in survivors after acute myocardial infarction. *Journal of Nursing (Taiwan)*, *39*(1), 65–76.

Lin, B. J., & Huang, S. Y. (1993). A study of psychosomatic reactions, self-care, and related factors of post-op mechanical valve replacement patients one month later. *Journal of Nursing (Taiwan)*, *40*(4), 37–46.

Lin, C. S., Liu, H. E., & Liao, J. (1993). An exploration of the influencing factors of the quality of life of renal transplanted patients. *Nursing Research (Taiwan)*, *1*, 369–379.

Lin, H. Y., & Chen, Y. C. (1993). Eating problems and strategies used by nasopharyngeal cancer patients receiving radiotherapy in Taiwan. *Nursing Research (Taiwan)*, *1*, 158–165.

Lin, M. C., & Ku, N. P. (1993). Effects of group teaching programs on improving knowledge and lessening stress of myocardial infarction patients. *Nursing Research (Taiwan)*, *1*, 341–350.

Lin, M. F., & Shiau, S. J. (1994). The intervention skills of nurse therapist applied to the process of couple therapy. *Nursing Research (Taiwan)*, *2*, 288–298.

Lin, M. N., & Chiou, C. J. (1995). The quality of family care for the elderly homebound stroke victim. *Nursing Research (Taiwan)*, *3*, 138–148.

Lin, S. (1994). The impact of osteoarthritis and its related factors on the quality of life. *Nursing Research (Taiwan)*, *2*, 371–378.

Liu, H. E. (1993). An exploration of the psychometrics of the Quality of Life Index of Chinese family. *Nursing Research (Taiwan)*, *1*, 127–136.

Lu, K. Y., Chin, C. C., & Huang, H. P. (1993). Coping behaviors of women with breast cancer. *Nursing Research (Taiwan)*, *1*, 247–256.

Lynn, M. (1985). Reliability estimates: Use and disuse. *Nursing Research, 34*, 254–256.

Ma, H. J., & Lo, L. H. (1993). A preliminary study of bladder cancer patients' sexual concerns. *Nursing Research (Taiwan)*, *1*, 176–186.

Mao, C. L. (1989). Stress perception and its related factors in acutely burned adults. *Journal of Nursing (Taiwan)*, *36*(1), 71–84.

Nursing Research Committee, Nurses' Association of the Republic of China. (1987). *Abstracts of Nursing Research (Vol. I)*. Taipei, Taiwan: Author.

Nursing Research Committee, Nurses' Association of the Republic of China. (1992). *Abstracts of Nursing Research (Vol. II)*. Taipei, Taiwan: Author.

Shiau, S. J. (1991). The development of "Child Coping Behavior Scale." *Chinese Psychological Health (Taiwan)*, *5*(2), 45–51.

Shiau, S. J., & Chang, S. R. (1993). The life space of offsprings with schizophrenic parents: The primary study of patients' and spouses' perceptions. *Nursing Research (Taiwan)*, *1*, 218–230.

Shiau, S. J., Chang, G. L., Hung, W. C., & Yu, Y. M. (1994). The influence of feeding methods on feeding behaviors and infant development. *Nursing Research (Taiwan)*, *2*, 90–98.

Shiau, S. J., Chen, Y. C., Tsai, S. T., Lin, B. J., & Tai, T. Y. (1994). The association between psychological adjustment, family attitude and knowledge, and health outcome of persons with IDDM. *Nursing Research (Taiwan)*, *2*, 130–139.

Shiau, S. J., Chiang, Y. J., Hong, L. J., & Chen, Y. C. (1993). Screening assessment for self-management for IDDM patients. *Journal of Nursing (Taiwan), 40*(3), 49–57.

Shiau, S. J., Lin, H. Y., & Chang, S. R. (1995). The primary exploration of interactive phenomenon at the couple level in a couples group psychotherapy. *Nursing Research (Taiwan), 3,* 90–98.

Shiau, S. J., Teng, L. H., & Yang, L. M. (1993). Application and evaluation of relaxation group therapy in an acute psychiatric ward. *Nursing Research (Taiwan), 1,* 16–21.

Shiau, S. J., Wang, I. C., Hung, L. C., & Chen, Y. C. (1993). Screening assessment of self-management for IDDM patients. *Journal of Nursing (Taiwan), 40*(3), 49–57.

Shiau, S. J., Wu, H. Y., Chang, S. Z., & Song, W. T. (1994). A couple group psychotherapy for schizophrenic patients: Analysis of self-phenotype at the personal level. *Nursing Research (Taiwan), 2,* 349–358.

Shyu, Y. I., Hsiung, P. C., Dai, Y. T., Chen, Y. C., & Huang, J. M. (1993). Characteristics of residents in long-term care facilities. *Nursing Research (Taiwan), 1,* 7–15.

Su, M. S., & Wang, C. J. (1993). A study of clinical stress in caring for cancer patients. *Nursing Research (Taiwan), 1,* 351–358.

Su, T. J. (1993). The subjective experiences and nursing needs of infertile women when they decided to accept the treatment of assisted reproduction. *Nursing Research (Taiwan), 1,* 50–59.

Su, T. J., Teng, S. W., & Yang, Y. L. (1995). Types and experiences of medical treatment and folk curing of the receiving reproductive-treatment women who searched conception. *Nursing Research (Taiwan), 3,* 127–137.

Su, Y. C., Chen, W. T., Chang, S. C., Wu, T. H., & Chen, M. C. (1994). The promotion of breast feeding: An evaluation of a program in nursery. *Nursing Research (Taiwan), 2,* 217–226.

Su, Y. L., Chang, M., & Chen, Y. C. (1994). Stress perception and coping methods of non-insulin-dependent diabetic patients at the out-patient department of a medical center. *Nursing Research (Taiwan), 2,* 29–40.

Tang, L. Y., Mao, C. L., Chou, C. F., Chen, R. C., & Liou, H. C. (1992). Caregiver burden of demented elderly and related factors: An exploratory study. *Journal of Nursing (Taiwan), 39*(3), 89–98.

Teng, S. W., Ho, S. H., & Kuo, M. C. (1994). Factors influencing the breast-feeding mother's feeding method one month after delivery. *Nursing Research (Taiwan), 2,* 153–165.

Teng, S. W., Kuo, M. C., & Ho, S. H. (1993). Factors influencing the mother's selection of feeding method. *Nursing Research (Taiwan), 1,* 329–340.

Teng, S. W., Su, T. J., Yang, Y. L., & Chang, G. L. (1995). The impact of rooming-in care on the breast-feeding mother's emotional disturbance and feeding method one month after delivery. *Nursing Research (Taiwan), 3,* 181–193.

Tzeng, Y. L., & Chao, Y-M. Y. (1994). Subjective experience of the primipara mothers during the course of labor and delivery. *Nursing Research (Taiwan), 2,* 327–338.

Tzeng, Y. L., Wang, L. L., & Shih, Y. L. (1993). Preliminary study of the behavioral response and nursing care needs in labor and delivery process of the expectant fathers. *Nursing Research (Taiwan), 1,* 279–289.

Wu, L. B., & Ku, N. P. (1994). The needs of family members of hepatoma patients. *Nursing Research (Taiwan), 2,* 180–190.

Wu, F. Y., Teng, S. W., & Shieh, L. H. (1994). A study of the maternal concerns about themselves and their babies and their perception of nursing care during early postpartum period. *Nursing Research (Taiwan), 2,* 78–89.

Yang, M. S., & Chung, H. H. (1993). The attitudes and perception of patients and nurses toward restraint and seclusion: A comparative study. *Nursing Research (Taiwan), 1,* 193–204.

Yang, Y. L., & Chao, Y-M. Y. (1993). Concerning behaviors of multipara women with Cesarean sections in relation to both themselves and their infants during early postpartum period. *Nursing Research (Taiwan), 1,* 316–328.

Yang, Y. O., & Chao, Y-M. Y. (1995). Operational meaning of time for multipara during the early postpartum at home. *Nursing Research (Taiwan), 3,* 149–160.

Yu, B. R., & Kao, C. H. (1992). Changes in physical and psychological responses, social support and self-care ability of stroke patients during hospitalization. *Journal of Nursing (Taiwan), 39*(2), 67–76.

Index

Contents of Previous Volumes

ORDER FORM

Save 10% on Volume 16 with this coupon.

_____Check here to order the ANNUAL REVIEW OF NURSING RESEARCH, Volume 16, 1998 at a 10% discount. You will receive an invoice requesting prepayment.

Save 10% on all future volumes with a continuation order.

_____Check here to place your continuation order for the ANNUAL REVIEW OF NURSING RESEARCH. You will receive a prepayment invoice with a 10% discount upon publication of each new volume, beginning with Volume 16, 1998. You may pay for prompt shipment or cancel with no obligation.

Name _____

Institution _____

Address _____

City/State/Zip _____

Examination copies for possible adoption are available to instructors ''on approval'' only. Write on institutional letterhead, noting course, level, present text, and expected enrollment (include $3.50 for postage and handling). Prices slightly higher overseas. Prices subject to change.

_____

Mail this coupon to:
SPRINGER PUBLISHING COMPANY
536 Broadway, New York, N.Y. 10012

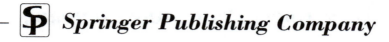

Springer Publishing Company

Advancing Nursing Education Worldwide

Doris Modly, RN, PhD, **Renzo Zanotti**, IP, AFD, Dott., PhD (C), **Piera Poletti**, & **Joyce J. Fitzpatrick**, RN, PhD, FAAN, Editors

The contributors of this comprehensive book describe global trends in nursing education, share innovative approaches to it, report and develop cross-cultural and collaborative research, and provide a model for future international collaborations in nursing. The book concludes with a blueprint for action that nurses can apply to improve the status of nursing education.

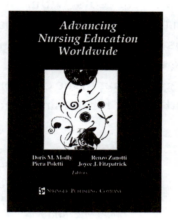

Partial Contents:

Part I: Nursing Education Requirements Worldwide. Global Trends in Nursing Education: A World Health Organization Perspective, *J. Salvage* • Broadening Nursing Boundaries Through Nursing Education and Nursing Education Research, *R. Zanotti*

Part II: Teaching Practices Worldwide. Designing Curriculum to Advance Nursing Science and Professional Practice, *D.M. Modly*

Part III: Issues Important to Nurse Educators Worldwide. Management Education for Nurses in the United States, *S.A. Ryan & C. Conway-Welch* • Computers in Nursing Education, *M. Tallberg* • Re-entry of Students, *D. McGivern*

Part IV: Advancing Research in Nursing Education. Pathways to Implementing Nursing Education Research Globally, *J.J. Fitzpatrick* • A Blueprint for Advancing Nursing Education Research Globally, *Scientific Committee Members*

1995   200pp   0-8261-8650-5   *hardcover*

536 Broadway, New York, NY 10012 • (212) 431-4370 • Fax (212) 941-7842

Springer Publishing Company

Clarifying Concepts in Nursing Research
Audrey G. Gift, PhD, RN, FAAN

This volume aims to improve the process nurses use to develop, identify, analyze, and define concepts within a nursing context. Chapters demonstrating many of these methods are presented. It is a guide to the evolving and dynamic nature of concept development leading to the creation of solid research and theory for nursing practice.

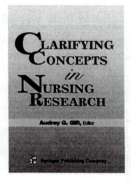

Contents:

I. Traditional Methods.

- Concept Analysis in Nursing: A Critique of Wilsonian Methods, *J.E. Hupcey, J.M. Morse, E.R. Lenz, and M.C. Tason*

- The Pediatric Physiological Stress Response: A Concept Analysis, *C.H. Rosenthal-Dichter*

- Exploring the Concept of Undocumentedness: The Meaning of a Person's Immigration Status to Nursing Care, *D.K.H. Messias*

II. Other Approaches, Future Directions.

- Choosing a Strategy for Concept Analysis in Nursing Research: Moving Beyond Wilson, *J.M. Morse, J.E. Hupcey, C. Mitcham, E.R. Lenz*

- Postpartum Fatigue: Clarifying a Concept, *R. Milligan, E.R. Lenz, P.L. Parks, L.C. Pugh, and H. Kitzman*

- Development of a Conceptual Model of Quality of Life, *C.E. Ferrans*

1997 144pp 0-8261-9980-1 hardcover

536 Broadway, New York, NY 10012-3955 • (212) 431-4370 • Fax (212) 941-7842

SP *Springer Publishing Company*

Home Care Nursing Services
International Lessons

Doris Modly, RN, MA, PhD, **Renzo Zanotti,** IP, AFD, PhD, **Piera Poletti,** and **Joyce J. Fitzpatrick,** RN, PhD, FAAN

With home healthcare becoming a fast growing industry in the U.S., readers of this volume can pick up valuable lessons for their own institutions about how home health nursing is managed and structured in other countries around the world. Home health nursing experiences in ten countries are profiled, from Zimbabwe to Australia, along with overviews of important aspects of home health nursing world wide (such as education and research). Contributors include Ida Martinson, Violet Barkauskas, and Tina Marelli.

Contents:

1997   272pp   0-8261-9600-4   hardcover

536 Broadway, New York, NY 10012-3955 • (212) 431-4370 • Fax (212) 941-7842